AF892833

The Human Impact of the COVID-19 Pandemic

Robert B. Burns

The Human Impact of the COVID-19 Pandemic

A Review of International Research

Springer

Robert B. Burns
Bli Bli, QLD, Australia

ISBN 978-981-99-1709-9 ISBN 978-981-99-1710-5 (eBook)
https://doi.org/10.1007/978-981-99-1710-5

© The Editor(s) (if applicable) and The Author(s), under exclusive license to Springer Nature Singapore Pte Ltd. 2023

This work is subject to copyright. All rights are solely and exclusively licensed by the Publisher, whether the whole or part of the material is concerned, specifically the rights of translation, reprinting, reuse of illustrations, recitation, broadcasting, reproduction on microfilms or in any other physical way, and transmission or information storage and retrieval, electronic adaptation, computer software, or by similar or dissimilar methodology now known or hereafter developed.
The use of general descriptive names, registered names, trademarks, service marks, etc. in this publication does not imply, even in the absence of a specific statement, that such names are exempt from the relevant protective laws and regulations and therefore free for general use.
The publisher, the authors, and the editors are safe to assume that the advice and information in this book are believed to be true and accurate at the date of publication. Neither the publisher nor the authors or the editors give a warranty, expressed or implied, with respect to the material contained herein or for any errors or omissions that may have been made. The publisher remains neutral with regard to jurisdictional claims in published maps and institutional affiliations.

This Springer imprint is published by the registered company Springer Nature Singapore Pte Ltd.
The registered company address is: 152 Beach Road, #21-01/04 Gateway East, Singapore 189721, Singapore

Contents

About the Author

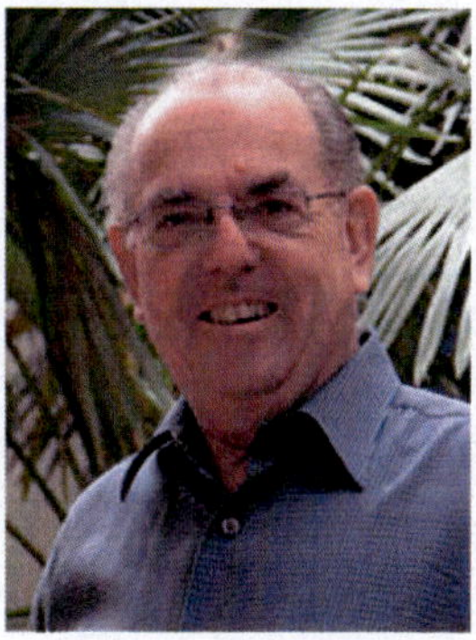

Dr. Robert B. Burns is a former professor, now retired in Australia. He spent 45 years in teaching, researching and senior management in universities in the UK, South Africa, Australia and Brunei. His field of academic expertise lies in psychology, and statistics and research methods as they applied to students in education, management, psychology and health fields. Dr. Burns is an experienced author with over 23 texts published by major publishing houses including Longmans, Sage, Allen and Unwin, Kluwer and Addison-Wesley. In this book, he was able to explore his interests in human behaviour in its response to a diverse set of entwined social, psychological and economic disruptive impacts on societies, groups and individuals from the flow on effects of not only the disease itself but also the indirect impacts stemming from mandated restrictions imposed by national governments.

CHAPTER 1

Definitions and Background Issues

Abstract This opening chapter provides a quick guide to the origins and spread of the pandemic, clarifies the terms pandemic, epidemic, endemic and explains the use of the R0 and Rt indices for measuring transmission rates. Social distancing, RAT tests and the use of masks are evaluated.

Keywords Pandemic · Epidemic · Endemic · Transmission rates · RAT tests · Social distancing · Masks

Introduction

At the outset be quite clear that this is not a medical text nor one for aspiring epidemiologists or virologists. It is an analysis of the indirect impacts of Covid-19 on individuals, communities and society from a social science perspective. Currently, the world is dealing with an intersecting rage of a real virus and socio-psychological and economic impacts creating pandemonium and disruption of normal life. It's no coincidence that the words '*viral*', '*virus*' and '*contagion*' have gained new metaphorical meaning in the digital age as ideas, thoughts, beliefs and behaviours spread the same way from person to person, just as rapidly and sometimes as dangerously as was intended in their original meaning. This discombobulating set of events, involving a revolving door of rising, falling then another rise in contagion levels matched by national roundabouts of alternating mandated restrictions then freeing up of policy settings, is increasingly stressful as populations become anxious or sometimes aggressive having very limited certainty of what the next move and its implications might be.

© The Author(s), under exclusive license to Springer Nature Singapore Pte Ltd. 2023

R. B. Burns, *The Human Impact of the COVID-19 Pandemic*,
https://doi.org/10.1007/978-981-99-1710-5_1

Involved in the pandemonium are:

SARS-CoV-2 (Covid-19). The initial virus that spawned globally. From this emerged:

1. A contagion of misinformation and conspiracy theories that accompanied the spread of the virus round the world,
2. A creeping authoritarianism worldwide as governments attempted to master, suppress and in some cases bunker down to eliminate the Covid virus,
3. A global spread of human suffering and distress in coping with death, disease and stringent restrictions on everyday routines of life,
4. A rapid escalation of research in many nations into all aspects of the above impacts led to low levels of peer review and methodological issues 'infecting' the quality of research with later withdrawal of many papers.

Each of these impacts metaphorically was akin to 'viruses' impacting globally, generating a degree of pandemonium everywhere. Consider some of the daily terminology expressing an overwhelming negativity that is in use throughout the world to describe our situation over the last three years, e.g. 'disaster', 'global health crisis', 'national emergency', 'case to death rates' 'lockdown', 'quarantine', 'stay-at-home order', 'mandated vaccination', 'mental stress' and 'draconian over-reach measures'. There is little question that internationally, steps to halt the spread of Covid have exacted a heavy toll on personal and community wellbeing in many nations. So much so that the security assessment of several Western governments was that China would try to seize the initiative as these global 'pandemic' impacts turned each nation's focus inwards on its own survival policy and simultaneously allow Beijing to continue imposing a slowly increasing grip on its strategic objectives particularly in its expansion of influence and in trade/economic pressures.

As can be seen from the chapter titles, the book essentially focusses on and discusses the effect of the impacts of the current Covid pandemic from a socio-psychological perspective on human responses in a variety of important areas of life and experience, involving

(a) beliefs and attitudes towards spread and control of the disease,
(b) impacts on education, employment, personal wellbeing, and bereavement offering coping mechanisms for present and future, helping people to manage their everyday life, now and in the future
(c) ethical and moral issues underlying government and public health decision-making in the Covid context.

This book may help lay persons realise that epidemics and pandemics are not something novel, but are more frequent that they might think, having littered human history for several millennia. Our predecessors had to deal with epidemics and pandemics without the public health procedures and medical advances we have now to see us through. Their experiences are likely to have been far more distressing than ours, resulting in many early Empires collapsing. It is essential that the way we manage Covid-19 does not impact similarly and deleteriously on our ability to maintain Western Democracy in face of other current worldwide political challenges. The Chinese initially praised the superiority of their authoritarian system in controlling their outbreak compared to the riotous situations in dithering democracies as cries for freedom sowed the seeds of discord in their handling of the contagion, fearful of electoral backlash. Now ironically through 2021/22, China reaped what it sowed originally in Wuhan, with a massive surge of contagion and millions of hapless citizen prisoners now revolting against the severity of numerous excessive total lockdown periods.

The current global pandemic has created a multifaceted set of experiences: a cacophony of conflicting voices, of personal and community dislocation and distress caused by restrictive mandates, of dis-established routines for work, school and play, of panic about catching a contagious disease and its ramifications for self and family. The book will be discussing and exploring some of the major components of this current social, economic and political bedlam with the assistance of what we know so far about solutions and management of them from a socio-psychological perspective. The research and knowledge referred to involves both pre-Covid studies of well-known socio-psychological information that help illuminate current conditions as well as studies undertaken in the last two years.

The Covid Virus. A Brief Travelogue

Towards the conclusion of 2019, a new coronavirus (*SARS-CoV-2*), originating in Wuhan, China sparked an epidemic of an acute respiratory syndrome (*COVID-19*) in humans (why can't we call it the Chinese virus? No-one objects to Japanese encephalitis, German measles or even Spanish flu even though that flu did not originate there!) By March 2020, the virus had spread to more than 118,000 cases and caused 4291 deaths in 114 countries, leading the World Health Organization to declare a global pandemic. New Year's Eve 2021 marked the first anniversary of China alerting the WHO to 27 cases of viral pneumonia of unknown origin in the city of Wuhan. Through the first half of 2022, the world was still in the middle of a massive health crisis, with a peak surge reached in mid-2022. China at the start of 2022 had to lock down millions of people in major cities to dampen infection there just prior to the Olympic Winter Games. Later in both April and August-November 2022, China has again physically locked down increasing millions of people in numerous cities as the infected numbers exceed anything yet experienced in China in a failing policy of trying to wipe out the pandemic. They relented in late November 2022 easing restrictions.

It is difficult to track *accurate* data of aspects like cases per period (e.g. day, week, month) or total cases to date or how many died over a particular period due to registration problems, inability to maintain accurate records often due to failure by relatives to report positive cases or cause of death. Therefore, only a small sample of statistics will be included in this text with the sole aim of depicting trends with the caveat that there could be a large element of unreliability in the data. There have so far been around 635 million confirmed cases infected globally and an estimated 6.59 million (approx. 1% or 1 in 100) have died, according to the daily updated WHO tally. These ratios do not significantly differ between developed nations. In three regions where there was inadequate reporting in some countries, only the African regional report as a whole revealed a greater death-to-case ratio, and many undeveloped African states did not report regularly so the ratio is probably much higher. The numbers are immense, and total cases and deaths may be well approaching double the reported figures due to an increasing number of individuals refusing to test and report in most countries (Table 1.1).

There has been massive global public health campaign responses launched to slow down the spread of the virus over the last two years by imposing mandated requirements including *inter alia* quarantine, lockdowns, closing down education, blocking national borders to travellers, increasing hand washing, reducing face touching, wearing masks in public and physical distancing. These were working well initially in controlling spread, but public discontent has led to weakening of such measures with laxity by individuals

Table 1.1 Gives some examples of case numbers and deaths in some major countries and world regions by 30 October 2022

	Global cases—635 million	*Global deaths—6.59 million*	*Approximate case to fatality ratio*
Location	*Total cases to date (M)*	*Total deaths to date*	*Percentage*
USA	96.0	1.06 M	0.011%
India	44.6	529 K	0.012%
Brazil	34.8	688 K	0.02%
UK	24.0	185 K	0.007%
France	35.7	153 K	0.004%
Australia	10.4	14.7 K	0.0015%
W. Pacific region	95	278 K	1. Low as mainly islands as border easily closed
S.E.Asian region	60	800 K	0.013%
African region	10	14.7 K	1.93% High due to less adequate health provisions

Selected data from WHO https://covid19.who.int/

Table 1.2 Basic reproduction number (*R0*) of some diseases

Disease	*R0. Basic reproduction number assuming no immunity in population*
Middle East respiratory syndrome (MERS coronavirus)	0.8
Influenza	1.5
Ebola	2.0
Severe acute respiratory syndrome (SARS coronavirus)	3.5
Mumps	4.5
Covid	5.7[a]
Rubella virus (German Measles)	6.0
Smallpox	6.0
Measles	16.0

[a]This number depends on the variant
Data collated by author from numerous documents

when mandates are removed, which inevitably has led to the sizeable increase in cases and deaths in mid- and late 2022 due to Omicron and its mutations.

Changes in case and fatality numbers have followed changes by jurisdictions in their policy settings. As countries relaxed so did the numbers of cases and deaths increase. For example, Australia had a rapid increase in Omicron variant cases in March and April 2022 consequent to the removal of most restrictions, a policy greeted with enthusiasm by many but with concern from medical authorities. A third major wave, with a massive impact on cases on hospitals already short on staff, then created a catastrophe in Australia in June/July 2022, exacerbated by a surge in influenza cases. By late August 2022, a steady decline in cases and deaths commenced. On 1 Nov 2022, only 3373 cases were registered in Australia with 6 deaths; the UK had 10,129 cases with 187 deaths and the USA 266,104 cases with 2,480 deaths reported in updated WHO data (https://covid19.who.int/). But a fourth surge has started as numerous variants of Omicron continue to proliferate in the form of *BA.1* through to *BA.5* and in late 2022 with a Christmas present of *XBB* (first reported in Singapore) and *BQ.1* (first detected in India) on the horizon, forming what has been termed ***a viral soup of infections,*** a not so welcome entrée to Xmas turkey dinner.

This melange of Omicron variants was driving up case numbers across the world late 2022, all with the ability to escape immunity. This fourth Covid wave is quite steep, and the world is in a different state of preparedness than Christmas 2021, with more variants, and lower population immunity from vaccinations six months past. It's likely that those who previously had Covid could be reinfected if they come into contact with one or more of the new strains. The newest variants while less severe in debilitating effects are extremely contagious, and governments re-invoked strong recommendations (but not mandates) around mask wearing, social distancing and vaccinations to counter the developed lackadaisical attitudes to these by their citizens.

Examples of the global mid-November 2022 surge is illustrated by the daily cases in the USA rising over 600% from 3679 to 21,017 new cases in the week ending 8 Nov 2022 (USA Covid Cases Today website). Similarly, the total of cases in Australia jumped 47.3% over the week November 1 to 8 according to Australian Government health alerts web site. To exacerbate matters in Australia, a cruise ship Majestic Princess docked in Sydney 11.11.22 disgorging 800 Covid infected passengers onto the mainland and dispersing who knows where!

Because the pandemic crisis requires large-scale behaviour change and places significant psychological burdens on individuals and organisations, valuable insights from the social and behavioural sciences can be used to understand human behaviour responses and help epidemiologists and public health experts provide policies and advice that will blend with these understandings to maximise adherence to requirements, otherwise human negative psychological reactance (and sometimes downright refusal) can jeopardise disease control and suppression.

So in the chapters that follow discussion focusses on topics that impact the current pandemic to help policy-makers, medical leaders and the public better understand how to manage health threats, depower fake news and misinformation, navigate different social and cultural contexts, gain greater compliance and persuasion through improved communication skills, align individual and collective interests, understand the social and economic distress caused inter alia to children unable to go to school, workers who have lost jobs or must work from home, and frontline health staff cope with the stress and mental illness, all of whom are in novel territory with the sudden disrupting of established routines. Most importantly, behavioural science can offer some direction on how to ensure greater adherence to public health advice and to the various measures advocated and mandated by democratic governments which are caught between a '*rock*' and a '*hard place*', the clash of personal freedom versus compliance with legally imposed restrictions for the public good, a conflict that offers difficult ethical and moral decision-making dilemmas.

Currently, we are finding in many nations across the world that rights and freedoms we have taken for granted appear to have been trampled on and managed in a previously unknown form of society by medical/ruling elites in the name of public health that promised so much in the initial panic, but often delivered a poorly planned and only partial suppression of Covid, while simultaneously imposing restrictive mandates for vaccinations, lockdowns, mask wearing, social distance, loss of travel freedoms, apps that trace where you have been, for all of which no cost/benefit arguments were offered and made inroads into the democratic tenets of equality, fairness, proportionality and personal responsibility, and in some peoples' views, taking over their lives (Chaps. 3 and 10).

Note that the issues discussed in the text currently identify as potentially relevant to pandemic responses for national populations, but are not exhaustive, with future data, new research findings and government regulations all changing rapidly as the pandemic twists and turns. Research on these topics is obviously still ongoing and, therefore, what we currently know and their implications for policy and practice should be interpreted cautiously given that published social science research on the Covid pandemic only covers two years. Thus, much of the research and information discussed often derives from earlier and different contexts than the current pandemic, for example, studies on compliance and persuasion that employed hypothetical scenarios, or on the known effects of job loss and isolation/loneliness, or on the management of stress and Post Traumatic Stress Disorder (*PTSD*).

Some Definitions: Pandemic, Epidemic and Endemic and Other Related Words

These terms cannot be avoided today as they crop up repeatedly on radio and TV, in newspapers, and in conversation whenever friends, neighbours, work colleagues and family get together. They are up there with the usual football and cricket scores, holidays, petrol prices and Royal dramas as common topics of everyday chat over a drink. As the current pandemic still continues to flow through all countries having mutated into *Delta, Omicron* and likely other future variants (really worry when we get to *Omega*), impacting and at times overwhelming testing procedures, health services, economies and social life, the terms are encountered more and more frequently, but sometimes inaccurately.

Many people use '*pandemic*' and '*epidemic*' interchangeably or incorrectly, but this is very understandable because both end with '*demic*' (which in my Lancashire slang meant a wreck), and are both used when there are serious disease outbreaks, but they have different implications. The key difference is geographical scale or spread. The *-demic* part of pandemic, epidemic and their little cousin endemic comes from the Greek *dêmos* meaning 'people of a district'. This root is also the basis for the English word '*democracy*'. While conversational use of these words might not require precise definitions, knowing the difference is important to better understand public health debate and appropriate public health responses.

What Is a Pandemic?

A pandemic is a disease that has spread across continents or the entire world with international boundaries no barrier, consequently affecting many millions of people. The word 'pandemic' derives from the Greek '*pándēmos*', meaning '*common, public.*' The World Health Organization (WHO) more specifically defines a pandemic as *a worldwide spread of a new disease* and was therefore clearly able to officially declare the COVID-19 outbreak a pandemic due to the global spread and severity of the disease on March 11, 2020. This was not the first pandemic, with the global spread of the 1918 Spanish flu pandemic estimated to have affected one-third of people across the entire globe with over 50 million deaths. 'Pandemic' is also used alone as a noun, implying 'a pandemic disease'. The classical definition implies nothing about other important accompanying factors such as *degree of contagiousness or disease severity.* As an adjective, pandemic can also mean '*general*' and '*universal*', with a negative connotation, e.g. '*a pandemic of drug addiction is current throughout the world*'. However, pandemic appears to be most commonly used in the context of epidemiology, which is concerned with infectious diseases.

What Is an Epidemic?

An epidemic disease is one that spreads from person to person infecting large numbers at the same time *in a more restricted locality* like a large conurbation or region of a State where the disease is not usual or permanently prevalent. WHO similarly specifies '*epidemic*' as occurring at the level of a region or community. Epidemics can occur quite regularly, as with the annual or almost annual epidemic outbreaks of influenza. Typical global death tolls for epidemic cases of influenza lie at around 21,000 lives. A recent epidemic was the 2003 Severe Acute Respiratory Syndrome (SARS) epidemic in the Middle East, which claimed the lives of nearly 800 people. In Greek '*Epi*' means '*in*'. Used all on its own as a noun '*epidemic*' commonly means '*a temporary prevalence of a disease.*' For example: '*The capital city was able to stop the flu epidemic before it spread across the state*' and '*The city had to close pre-schools to contain a measles epidemic*'. In another sense, 'epidemic' metaphorically is any fast moving spread or increase in the occurrence of something, often implying a negative or humorous connotation. For example: '*An epidemic of gentrification was preventing low-income persons from buying houses in the area*' or '*rugby league players are creating an epidemic of mullet hairstyles*'.

How Do Epidemics Differ from Pandemics?

The main way epidemics differ from pandemics is through the breadth of their reach. The latter cover most of the globe and affect far more people than an epidemic causing many more deaths than epidemics. But both create significant social disruption, economic loss, and hardship in general. One of the determining factors in what turns an outbreak into a pandemic is how infectious it is. Pandemics are usually caused by new viruses or new strains of viruses, which are foreign to humans who have no inbuilt immunity. This differs from epidemics, which often occur annually, with annual vaccination and built up immune systems defeating the epidemic infection limiting its range and impact in most cases as happens with influenza. From the perspective of relevant authorities, controlling a pandemic is extremely hard compared to controlling an epidemic. As has been seen during the current Covid pandemic, there is a need for more detailed calculations via statistical modelling on patient numbers requiring hospitalisation, how many hospital beds will be needed, and other equipment-related calculations plus drastic response measures in the community such as case and contact finding, quarantine/lockdowns, and measures to prevent infection in health facilities, nursing homes, and long-term care facilities.

However, many places in the world can also be massively at risk even from rapid spreading epidemics where public health measures, such as clean water, toilet facilities, handwashing etiquette are not possible and overcrowded ghettos exist. Similarly, these places are far more at risk during pandemic preparations because there may not be facilities to adequately test for diseases, or provide hospitalisation.

What Is Implied by Endemic?

Endemic as an adjective is perhaps most commonly used to describe a disease that is prevalent in, native to, or confined to a particular location, region or population. For example, yellow fever is said to be endemic in the Amazon Basin. It is also applied generally to a wide range of non-disease related characteristics of a people, place or situation, as in '*gender discrimination was endemic in that organization when I worked there*'.

The first records of endemic in English come from the mid-1600s. It comes from the Greek *éndēm(os)* in which the prefix *en-* means '*in or within*'. So the basic meaning of endemic is '*within a certain people*' or '*within a certain area*'.

Relationships Between the Three Terms

It's unsurprisingly easy to confuse these three words. For one, they all feature -demic, which can make it difficult to suss out which word should be used in which situation. Here's a handy rule of thumb repeating from the above material the meaning of the prefixes: pan-, epi- and en-. The Greek prefix '*pan*'- means '*all*'; '*epi*'- means '*on*' *upon, near, at*; while '*en*' means '*in*'.

The appropriate use of these prefixes enables health authorities, as the situation changes and the spread of the disease moves out from endemic to epidemic and perhaps eventually to pandemic, to label the event correctly which brings into force appropriate health measures. Sometimes as a disease progresses a regular endemic outbreak in a small area, can rapidly spread out to a region becoming an epidemic. As the epidemic spreads to infect a huge range of populations, across continents with a worldwide reach it becomes a pandemic. A pandemic can revert back to become an enduring endemic within small regions when eradication has occurred elsewhere, e.g. the current Covid situation may become endemic in parts of certain poorer countries in Africa, whereas other countries will have effectively controlled the virus through the use of vaccines annually like the flu. Currently, the policy of some governments in 2022 is to abandon any idea of eliminating Covid but to treat it like flu and to run with it so that it can be treated as an endemic disease in which eventual small flare ups can be contained in a '*hot spot*'.

Epicentre and Outbreak

An *'epicentre'* is a focal often start point of activity as in an earthquake. If a country or region is called the epicentre of a pandemic disease, that means more or an accelerating number of cases are being confirmed there than anywhere else in the world. Wuhan was initially the Covid epicentre from where the virus spread out, like a tsunami from the epicentre of the earthquake. This turned into an epidemic then with worldwide spread producing a pandemic.

The term *'outbreak'* is also used at the onset of the awareness of a disease present in the public. An outbreak is specifically a sudden rise in cases, especially when it is only as yet affecting a relatively localised area which is then often designated a *hot spot*. A particular site, such as a nursing home can be an epicentre or hotspot, where there is a sudden spate of new cases from where an outbreak can spread if not managed adroitly. An outbreak must be treated no less aggressively than a pandemic if it has the potential to expand beyond its borders, such as occurred with the Ebola virus.

Seasonal epidemics, despite crossing international boundaries and between hemispheres affecting a large number of people, are not considered pandemics. A true influenza pandemic occurs when almost simultaneous transmission takes place worldwide. In the case of pandemic influenza *A(H1N1)*, widespread transmission was documented in both hemispheres between April and September 2009. Transmission occurred early in the influenza season in the temperate southern hemisphere but out of season in the northern hemisphere. This out-of-season transmission is what characterises it as an influenza pandemic.

Many historically early disease outbreaks were not really epidemics or pandemics as the population and area through which they spread were localised, and the term *'plague'* which refers specifically to a contagious bacterial disease characterised by fever and delirium, such as bubonic plague, was usually applied to these historic outbreaks.

Disease Severity and Transmissibility

The pandemic–epidemic distinction is actually not the most important distinction. There are other variables that need considerable attention. These are *disease severity* and *transmissibility or level of contagion. Omicron* and its variants are very contagious (i.e. easy to catch) but less severe in outcome than the previous *Delta* variant. This lower severity of outcome has led to an evolution and reset of national responses globally, with lockdowns, close contact tracing and travel restrictions gradually loosened to limit effects on national economies, and placing the focus more on personal responsibility, emphasising self-testing and self-isolation.

Severity

Severity is estimated by the *Case to Fatality Ratio* (*CFR*), that is how many infected persons actually died. The number of lives lost in a pandemic depends on factors such as:

- How many people are infected.
- How severe an illness does the virus causes (its virulence).
- How vulnerable are certain groups of people like aged care, pregnant ladies and unvaccinated persons.
- What prevention efforts used, how effective they are and what level of compliance has been achieved.

The overall *CFR* for Australia for the initial Covid hit at 30 June 2020 was 1.31% (13 per 1000), and a year later 30 June 2021 was 2.97% (29.7 per 1000), but this was for *Delta*. Australia's overall *CFR* on 4 November 2021 dropped to 1.02% (10.2 per 1000) showing the improvement due to vaccination and other measures. The *CFR* can differ by key demographics, particularly age cohort, so that while the *CFR* in late 2021 for those aged under 60 years was 1 per 1000, the *CFR* among cases in the 70–79 age group was 69.7 per 1000. In the 80–89 group, it was 198.6 per 1000. In the 90-plus group, it was 323.1 per 1000 brought down from June's figure six months earlier of 500 per 1000 due to vaccination and better control measures in aged care facilities. The increasing dominance of *Omicron* and variants *BA.2* and *BA.5*. has also resulted in the overall *CFR* index figure in Australia to slump dramatically to just 0.15% per 100 (1.5 per 1000) early February 2022 although case numbers and deaths both rose in the first half of 2022 (Data above abstracted from tables in Mathieu et al. Our World in Data (2022)). A major study from South Africa found people who catch *Omicron* are 80% less likely to be hospitalised than those who get Delta. The real-world analysis of more than 160,000 people by South Africa's National Institute for Communicable Diseases revealed *Omicron* sufferers were also 70% less likely to end up in intensive care units (*ICUs*) or put on a ventilator (Madhi et al., 2022).

The trend in major countries with *Omicron* dominant appeared to be that younger people in the 19–29 age group were the most infected but often unvaccinated cohort; however, it is within the oldest members of society that failure to survive has amplified, often with known co-morbidities. Worldwide trends suggest infection numbers rose rapidly in early 2022 but death numbers fell considerably, except among the aged care groups where a huge spike occurred. By mid- to late 2022 case numbers globally generally fell due to increased booster vaccinations. Currently (late October 2022), there are around 3373 infected cases daily in Australia mainly people below 40 years of age and over 65 and around 6 deaths per day, while just over 10,000 now become infected each day in the UK, with 187 deaths and around 266,000 daily cases with around 2500 deaths in the USA. Remember it is hard to pin down these figures as perfectly accurate as there is sometimes a delay in identifying and reporting cases/deaths, but these figures do provide an impression of the magnitude and trends of the infection (Data above abstracted from tables in Mathieu et al. (2022) Our World in Data).

Transmissibility or Contagiousness: The R, R0 and Rt Indices–Tracking Infectiousness

Transmissibility tells us how many susceptible people, on average, each sick person will in turn infect. Scientists use a basic measure called the *reproduction number*, known as *R*, to track and rate the infectiousness of a disease or ability to spread. Rising global connections and interactions as a driving force humanity's reliance on one another has sparked opportunities for pandemic disease to spread. The move from small hunting and gathering communities to the metropolis and urbanisation in the developing world is bringing more and more people into denser neighbourhoods. At the same time, passenger air traffic doubled in the past decade while cruise ships carry and breed diseases around the world with both international transport systems like flying and floating Petri dishes. Australia has witnessed, with the Ruby Princess Covid outbreak, when disembarked passengers scattered widely within Australia and around the world taking infection with them when the cruise ended in Sydney in March 2020. These international travel trends had a profound impact on the spread of Covid in early 2020.

The Origins of the Concept of R

Employed almost a century ago in demography, *R* originally was designed to measure the reproduction of people, that is whether a population was growing or not. Transferred into epidemiology, the same principle applies, but it measures the reproduction or spread of infection in a population. *R* defines the average number of secondary cases generated by one primary case. If *R* is two, one infected person will on average infect two people who will, on average, go on to infect two more each, i.e. four others, who will infect eight others, and who will infect 16 others and so on. This does not seem too bad except that *R* can be much higher than 2. Different infections produce different *R* values. *R* is also rejigged as *R0* (*Rnought*) as it really represents the reproduction value at the onset of the disease *where no one has immunity*. That is *R0* is the base measure of the number of secondary cases initiated before any health actions are instituted.

Measles tops the list in Table 1.2 being the most contagious with a *R0* of around 16. This means a single person can infect, on average, 14–18 people *in an unvaccinated population*. While measles may be the most virulent, vaccination efforts and herd immunity can curb its spread. The more people become immune to a disease, the less likely it is to proliferate, making vaccinations critical to prevent the resurgence of known and treatable diseases. Let us look at a couple of examples of how this works.

With rubella *R0* is 6 and measles 16. Depicted below is the 'theoretical' rapid spread over a period of time with these larger figures developing on the assumption of no medical interventions. Luckily most people accept medical intervention and public health restrictions to prevent such devastating and rapid spread that would overwhelm medical and hospital services.

$$\text{Rubella } R0: \text{One person} \rightarrow 6 \rightarrow 36 \rightarrow 196 \rightarrow 1176$$
$$\text{Measles} R0: \text{One person} \rightarrow 16 \rightarrow 256 \rightarrow 16{,}896 \rightarrow 285{,}474{,}816$$

But there is no indication of the speed at which the infection grows and the above figures would likely stretch over a few months for the end calculated figures to be reached. There are also people who may already be immune, and others are less disposed to show symptoms (asymptomatic persons) so the real transmission figures will be less than the theoretical calculation above.

Mathematical modellers at Imperial College London (van Elsland and O'Hare. 17 March 2020) attempted to track how the *R0* number of Covid changed as isolation, social distancing and the full lockdown were introduced in the UK in spring of 2020. Before any measures came in, the global *R0* value of the original Covid virus was theoretically estimated to be about 5.7 or 5.8. This means conditions were ripe for a large outbreak as one Covid-infected person could on an average pass the disease on to five to six people, and these would pass it on to 25–30 others and so on if the virus was allowed to spread without any form of public health intervention. This base reproduction rate assumes that all individuals in the population are equally susceptible to catching the disease. That usually isn't true, although it might be not far off the mark at the time a new virus emerges with no-one immune. Vaccination of virtually the whole population is seen as the easiest and quickest way to block further infection as the virus cannot find a suitable host.

The initial *R0* of the *Omicron* variant was much higher, estimated at 15 in an unvaccinated, unprotected population, and it rapidly made its way around the world infiltrating 89 countries within three weeks of first being identified in late November 2019. This generated a huge surge in infected people recorded in most nations particularly through the early months of 2022, as many restrictions were beginning to be removed on cross border travel and contact tracing, with quarantine periods shortened, close contact redefined, and opening up of mass events over the 2921/2022 festive season. But as many nations had provided some vaccination protection in those countries the *R0* was less, overall about 9.5. *Omicron* variants ranging from *BA.1* through to *BA.5* of which *BA.2* and *BA.5* are the most prevalent now. New mutations give the virus an advantage if they can increase transmissibility as shown in the sequence below (all figures close estimates):

- The original Wuhan strain has an *R0* of 5.7.
- Delta has an *R0* of 5.1.
- Omicron *BA.1* has an *R0* of 9.5.

- *BA.2*, is 1.4 times more transmissible than *BA.1*, and so has an *R0* of about 13.3.
- *BA.4/5* is now dominant and research from South Africa suggests *BA.4/5* has a growth advantage over *BA.2* similar to the growth advantage of *BA.2* over *BA.1* (Wolter et al., 2022). The Royal Australian College of General Practitioners (*RACGP*) recently provided a false evaluation claiming *BA.5* with an *R0* of over 18.6. This would have placed the variant as more transmittable than the current most transmittable disease measles that has an *R0* value of 18. Fortunately, this horrendous *R0* was inaccurate as shown by a Reuters Factcheck Report (2022) with the verdict that the *R0* of the *BA.5 Omicron* variant was miscalculated and not greater than that of measles. It is now believed to be similar to that for *BA.2,* i.e. around 13, but the actual value remains uncertain.

An *R0* number above 1.0 is unwelcome news since it implies an increase in the number of cases. With an *R0* below 1.0, the disease will eventually stop spreading, because not enough new people are being infected to sustain the outbreak. This is why governments in the early stages were focussing on forcing the *R0* number down to below 1.0 by quarantine and vaccination and were keen to publicise such decreases to allay public fears. In general, a person testing positive for coronavirus would naturally infect others, but if placed in quarantine isolation then no transmission is likely to occur. This explains why mandated quarantine was perceived as the first line of defence in many countries alongside social distancing and gaining high vaccination rates, all of which protects others and keeps *R0* low.

Problems with R0

R0 therefore became regarded as a totemic figure in the Covid pandemic because it appeared to offer a clear undisguised, if rather simplistic picture of how things are going, quickly embraced by politicians seeking prestige and an aura of success, and the general public seeking an understandable form of reassurance. In many countries, in the first few months of Covid during 2021 the *R0* statistic was publicly reported almost on a daily basis, and with politicians and health officials nightly pointing to a TV '*R*' barometer, it was almost like looking in at the weather reports with temperature and rainfall figures, so important was it made to seem. Australia and the UK were prominent in featuring it on TV news and in newspapers to reassure the population that health measures taken were having positive effects in reducing contagion. Politicians have embraced it with enthusiasm because it is a simple visual demonstration of their effectiveness in '*saving the people*' that has been shown to boost their electability at the hustings.

Epidemiologists are quite keen on downplaying *R0* and believe fascination with it had turned into unhealthy political and media fixation. *R0* is an imprecise estimate as it is always a figure that relates to some days past and cannot capture the current status of an epidemic. It may also only reflect some mythical national average which hides local variations or special demographics like aged care homes, and dispersed agricultural communities. Too much attention to it could obscure the importance of other vital measures, such as trends in numbers of deaths to cases, hospital admissions, and ICU requirements.

It's also impossible to calculate a global *R0* and forecast the true global impact of the current pandemic, because as the outbreak is still ongoing, and as it is worldwide it is proliferating in countries that vary from possessing first rate medical and health service provision to places where treatment for even common complaints is rudimentary and limited geographically. In the former *R0* could be quite low, whereas for the latter it is likely to be high where there are no or few controls on rampant transmission.

Rt (Reff)

Another complexity arises when politicians and scientists talk about *R0*, they usually mean, without explaining it, another variant called *'Rt'* (sometimes called '*Reff*', or 'effective *R*'). *'Rt'* is the reproduction number at a particular time *'t'* since the start of the epidemic and captures the number of secondary infections generated from a population consisting of '***protected***' vaccinated persons and exposed ***non-protected*** (unvaccinated) as well as immune individuals It is calculated over time as an outbreak progresses and reflects a more realistic situation where some people might have gained immunity, perhaps because they have survived infection or been vaccinated, or mandated behaviours like social distancing and mask wearing are proving highly effective. The *Rt* or *Reff* effective reproduction number is a more realistic measure of how many other people on average each case infects when sound vigorous public health measures are in place.

Like *R0,* an *Rt* of less than 1.0 means the infection is not spreading and that the number of people being infected on average will get fewer over time and if this situation persists, the disease will eventually die out. An *Rt* value above 1.0 means the virus is spreading fast. So Rt is an estimate that will change in value over time, usually decreasing, and will always be less than the initial R0 measured when the virus first invades a country because of the effect of people following mandated health directions.

Rt can't be measured directly since you can't capture the moment people are infected, so it is usually estimated retrospectively: disease modellers look at current and previous numbers of cases and deaths, admittances to hospital or positive tests for the virus over time to estimate how easily the virus is spreading, make some assumptions that could explain the trend and then derive *Rt* from these. Trying to model future infection rates on the basis of very recent and current trends in Covid cases is tricky enough, but mortality data typically come with a longer lag, because of the extra time someone has the disease before they succumb to it and because of the paperwork involved in registering deaths, which can take weeks or months to file.

Such a time lag it's not going to be that useful as a real-time decision-making tool. You need to know if public health measures are working now, which are and which aren't. So researchers are concerned that the various *R* indices are looming too large, and being used for purposes for which they were never intended, nor do they clarify what health actions there are imposed or are not being taken. Other data on the pandemic's progress can feed into estimates of *Rt* by serving as proxies for infections and social behaviour, such as hospital and intensive care admissions, the trend in the number of new cases, ratio of infections to deaths (CFR) and ratio of discharged individuals in comparison with the number of new admissions. Another is results from random testing of a population to see how many people currently have Covid, or have had it. Researchers also conduct contact surveys, which ask people who they mix with, and can be used to infer changes in *Rt* on the basis of estimates of how many others an infected person could meet, although these are time-consuming and could cover only small groups of people. These difficulties in modelling help to explain why some modelling estimates are far from accurate when compared later with what actually eventuates.

An important aspect of *Rt* is that it represents only an estimated average across a nation. This average can miss regional clusters of infection. Conversely, high incidences of infection among a spatially distinct smaller subsection of a population can sway a larger region's *Rt* value. For instance, Germany's national *Rt* value jumped from just over 1 to 2.88 in one month (later revised down to 2.17) largely because of an outbreak in a meat-processing plant at Gütersloh in North Rhine-Westphalia. The Robert Koch Institute noted that national infections overall were still low, which is why the local outbreak had such an effect on the country's *Rt*, which had dropped below 1 again by the end of the following month. This made it impossible that the obtained *Rt* could be used validly to steer local lockdown policy at that time in Germany (Xinhua News Agency, 2020).

Most experts claim that the *Rt* for both the United Kingdom and Australia is artificially high due to the very large numbers of infections and deaths in care homes for older people, and does not reliably represent the risk to the general population. Another subtlety not captured by *Rt* is that many people never infect others, but a few '*superspreaders*' pass on the disease many more times than average, perhaps because they are very social persons who mingle in crowded, indoor events like choir practices, nightclubs, basketball matches, parties, weddings and funerals while church services stand out as notorious superspreading events within some sects despite attendees attempts to ward off disease by appeals to '*higher authority*'. As few as 10–20% of infected people seem to cause 80% of new Covid cases, that means bans on certain crowded indoor activities can have more benefit than blanket lockdown restrictions that have been too commonly introduced whenever the *Rt* value hits above 1.

Groups of epidemiologists each have their own approach to combining and using these disparate sources of data to work out *Rt*, relying on their own statistical models to look at trends in presumed infections. To calculate the official *Rt* of the UK, about ten groups present the results of their models to a dedicated government committee, which reaches consensus on a possible range. The figures are presented in that range, showing how uncertain the estimates are, but the individual model details are not released.

All these issues tend to demote the usefulness of *R* and *Rt* in deciding policy. Most countries have abandoned publicising the index now. It's far more important to identify clusters of cases, trace and test their contacts, isolate those infected, and vaccinate as many as possible than to watch a beaming politician point to the needle swinging lower on a colourful dial. Health-care management, and deeper understanding of the factors that incubate pandemics have been powerful tools in mitigating their impact than statistical 'guesstimates'.

To summarise these variations of *R*:

- *R0* or *R-naught* is the initial reproduction number of the virus at the beginning of the pandemic before health actions are taken.
- *Rt* refers to the reproduction number at a particular point in time when known effective health actions are in place.

Provide Sensible Reassuring Statistics

Every day people globally listen to politicians, read newspapers, watch TV news where daily figures are presented on the Covid saga with numbers of cases, admissions to hospitals, ICU admissions and death rates on a daily basis as well as graphs illustrating trends. This mass of data often creates panic, anxiety, and sombre feelings. There should be some attempt to provide more positive news as often as possible to evoke more positive thinking and hope by presenting other data to reveal for example the number of cases discharged from hospital, or the fatality rate per number of cases which is often minute. So for example, instead of revealing a depressing raw total of deaths over the month this could be stated as the percentage of deaths over the month in relation to the numbers of new cases in the month. An infected case to fatality death rate of 0.001% (1 in 10 thousand) sounds more reassuring than 20 deaths in the last 24 h. Many other percentages could be presented to give a more positive slant on the effect of the disease such as discharge numbers of recovered patients. Furthermore comparing some Covid percentages with other non-Covid events could add a sense of realism to the significance of the daily reports, such as the chances of being in a car accident, hitting a hole in one, winning first prize in Lotto. So presenting the statistics in a more friendly and positive message format can aid the dissipation of individual and group worry and offer increasing reassurance that progress on managing the disease is evident.

Rapid Antigen Test, Social Distance and Mask Wearing

Rapid Antigen Test (RAT) Problems

While polymerase chain reaction (*PCR)* tests are still available and remain the 'gold standard' for testing, many nations have turned to rapid antigen tests (*RATs*) out of convenience or as part of a requirement to return to work or school. They can provide results within minutes, don't require a healthcare worker or lab to process, and help to catch Covid cases that otherwise would have gone undetected. But with these benefits comes a range of limitations: the biggest one being that they can provide false negative or false positive results if instructions are not followed precisely.

With many people not testing, or relying on a negative *RAT* that may mislead many people they do not have the virus when in fact they do, it is all contributing to the November 2022 case surge. Mathieu et al. in Our World in Data (2022) shows the number of daily tests per 1000 people in Australia has noticeably decreased producing a negative correlation with the numerical increase in the number of cases. A not unexpected result! Moreover, the reliance on at-home testing has made it difficult for authorities to track case numbers with recent studies revealing that only between 7 and 10% of home testers even bother to report their results. Perversely, positive people tend not to report their result at all. RATs are a little expensive too, which added to the incorrect testing procedure and people fed up with testing and not testing when they should means *RATS* are not effective as a public health measure currently with the serious decline in testing.

Social Distance Issues

The concepts of social distance and mask wearing are two techniques that have been mandated in most countries from time to time in the efforts to minimise the spread of Covid. These two requirements need more clarification due to their worldwide ubiquity but serious potential misunderstandings and suspect effectiveness.

Social distance has been used as a major health defence against the spread of Covid. However, the term has been misappropriated and wrongly applied. What really is being meant is '*physical distancing*', that is keeping a certain distance away from others, usually a 1.5 m minimum.

Social distance has previously been used with a clearly different specific meaning in social psychology. It is the degree to which, psychologically and socially speaking, a person or group wants to remain separate from members of other different ethnic or social groups, or in the reverse sense, reflects the extent to which individuals or groups accept others of a different ethnicity, religion, nationality, gender/sexuality, age or other social background characteristic. Social distance is also involved in *ingroup–outgroup* distinctions and ethnocentricity.

Emory Bogardus (1947) created the *Bogardus Social Distance Scale* for measuring social distance by establishing the willingness of a person to interact with people from other groups. For example, an unwillingness to live next door to a family of a different ethnicity would indicate a high degree of social distance. On the other hand, willingness to marry a person of a different ethnicity would indicate a very low degree of social distance. Social distance is a cause of concern because it is known to foster prejudice, bias, hatred and even violence. The extreme social distance between Nazi sympathisers and European Jews was a significant component of the ideology that supported the Holocaust. Today, social distance as originally conceived fuels politically motivated hate crimes and school bullying and so *is really a very different concept to physical distancing*. But it probably is too late to get authorities and general public to use the term *physical distance* rather than *social distance* as the latter has become too well ingrained in daily life.

Moreover, use of the term '*social distancing*' might imply quite erroneously for some people that one has to cut off meaningful interactions with others (isolate yourself as much as you can). Physical distancing is preferable, because it allows for the fact that *social connection is perfectly allowable* and essential for emotional balance (e.g. by phone, email, SMS, Zoom) even when people are physically separated.

Mask Wearing and Aerosol Transmission

This requirement is related to the previous discussion on social (physical) distance in that the mask is supposed to prevent viral spread when people are close together. Linking mask and social distance is the fact that spread of Covid occurs via airborne particles (aerosols) and droplets. People who are infected with Covid can release particles and droplets of respiratory fluids that contain the virus into the air when they exhale (e.g. breathing, speaking, shouting, singing, exercise, coughing, sneezing), and these can of course be inhaled by others.

Experimental and epidemiologic data in the USA gives some support for community masking to reduce the spread of Covid among adults and children. Centers For Disease Control (CDC) Updated Dec. 6, 2021 recommends community use of masks as masks are primarily intended to reduce transmission in two ways:

1. The emission of virus-laden droplets by the wearer ('source control'), and
2. Reduce inhalation of these droplets by the wearer ('wearer protection').

The small prevention benefit of masking is derived from the combination of these two, source control and wearer protection. The relationship between source control and wearer protection is likely complementary reducing inward and outward flow, so that individual benefit increases with increasing community mask use. Mask use has been found to be safe and is not associated with clinically significant impacts on breathing, except for intense exercise. The limited available data indicate no decisive evidence that hiding the face of parents and teachers by masking impairs emotional or language development in children (CDC 2021).

But the effectiveness of imposed mask wearing is probably not that strong. Electron microscopy has revealed that the Covid virus ranges between 50 nm (μm) or 0.05 microns (nm), and 140 nm (μm) or 0.14 microns (nm) in diameter. As these incredibly small measurements are foreign to most people, they can better understood in relation to a millimetre as:

- 1 μm or micron (μm) is 1000 times smaller than 1 mm (mm).
- 1 nm (nm) is 1,000,000 times smaller than 1 mm (mm).
- 1 nm (nm) is 1000 times smaller than a micron (μm).
- 1 micron (μm) = 1000 nm (nm).

Material weaving gaps in standard cloth masks are up to 5000 times the diameter (0.005 mm or 5.0 nm) of the largest virus which is around 0.14 nm. Such small diameters are hard to comprehend so if we scale up the relative diameters we can compare a virus of 1.4 cm diameter to the cloth weave diameter of 500 cm or 5 m!! (Fig. 1.1).

Professor Colin Axon who advises the UK committee on airborne transmission compares the virus particles passage through the mask material like

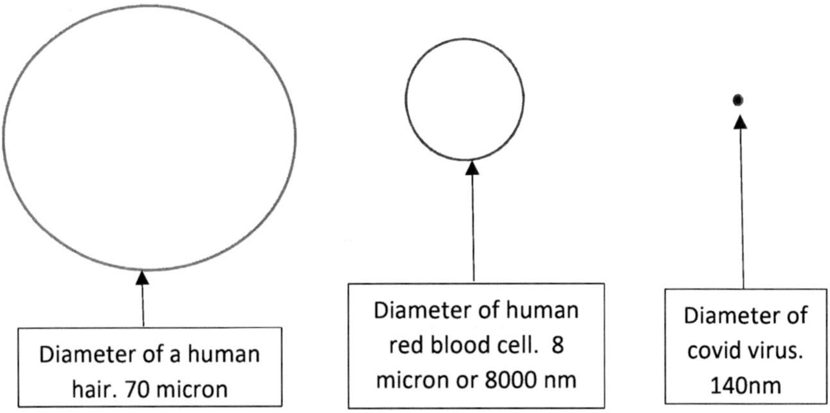

Fig. 1.1 Comparison diameter sizes of other body parts relative to the virus (not to scale)

firing marbles at builders' scaffolding reported in The Telegraph (17 07 2021). Public expression of such scientific evidence is avoided so as not to destroy the psychological effect of making people feel they have a comfort blanket for protection.

Once infectious droplets and particles are exhaled, they move outward from the source person, carrying the virus and transmitting infection. Indoors, the very fine droplets and particles transmitting infection will continue to spread through the air in the room, corridor or elevator and can accumulate where there was limited or no ventilation. This has been found to be a major cause of infection spread in quarantine hotels. The largest droplets settle out of the air rapidly, within seconds and these large droplets of mucus containing viral material often from coughs or sneezes are largely blocked by masks. The smallest very fine aerosol particles are small enough that they can remain suspended in the air for minutes and can also linger in the air after a person has left the room, remaining airborne for hours in some cases, and these are the one that masks cannot repel.

So the droplets of human mucus containing potentially thousands of viruses and aerosol particles do actually vary across a wide range of sizes, from visible to hardly detectable by electron microscope making the choice of mask very important. *N95* or *P2* masks are the gold standard but are costly and recommended one time use only. Cloth masks can only effectively block the largest droplets (i.e. 20–30 microns and larger), but cannot block the fine droplets and particles (aerosols) smaller than 10 microns or 10,000 nm, which increase in number and distance spread with the intensity of ejection, i.e. quiet speech versus a violent sneeze. Multiple layers of cloth with higher thread counts have demonstrated superior performance compared to single layers of cloth with lower thread counts. Some materials (e.g. polypropylene) may enhance filtering effectiveness by generating static electricity that enhances capture of charged particles while others (e.g. silk) may help repel moist droplets and reduce fabric wetting and thus maintain breathability and comfort.

The mask should form a tight seal around the face so there are no gaps and this can be helped by twisting the ear holders round the ear. A basic test to determine whether your cloth mask is working is to try and blow out a candle while wearing it. If air is getting through to extinguish the candle the reverse is also true. Cloth masks can go in the wash and be reused. You can reuse masks designed to be disposable, like the *N95* or *P2,* but you'll need to have a few on hand. When you take it off, place inside a paper bag for three days. This allows the mask to dry and after three days any germs will have died. Therefore have three, four or five masks and rotate them every day.

As a person can be exposed by an infected person coughing or speaking near them, scientists question if 1.5 m (4.5 ft) social distancing is enough to stop virus spread, as coughs/sneezes, depending on the strength of the expulsion, spread aerosols up to 4 m (12 ft) and air conditioners, depending on fan speed (wind blast), between 3 and 8 m. This implies the 1.5 m social distance standard is probably insufficient in many cases.

Though the risk of infection by breathing in particles carrying the virus generally decreases with distance from infected people but some circumstances increase the risk of infection:

- Being indoors rather than outdoors, particularly where ventilation with outside air is inadequate,
- Activities that increase emission of respiratory fluids, such as speaking loudly, singing or exercising in a gym,
- Prolonged time of exposure (e.g. longer than a few minutes),
- Crowded spaces, where it is difficult to avoid close contact as at football matches, check out queues, public transport, religious services, the cinema or local club, particularly if face coverings are inconsistently or improperly worn.

An additional issue with masks is that most countries don't have a national standard for masks that's regulated, and that puts the public and health industry at risk, with the possibility of fake and substandard masks being sold. There's been over 2000 products withdrawn from the Australian Therapeutic Goods Administration website alone that aren't compliant and these are just the ones sold into health care, not into hardware stores or small businesses. So there is limited confidence that many of the various masks being bought are actually fit for purpose. To be effective remember a mask must seal the face and the simple test for this is the blowing out of the candle test, and also note whether your glasses or sunglasses fog up, indicating air is escaping. If air can escape then it can also enter hopefully not delivering viruses. It is not just a problem with Covid but sectors such as mining, stonemasonry and asbestos removal where workers need protecting from inhaling dangerous particles.

Research is needed to develop and assess mask efficiency, particularly to identify the combinations of materials that maximise both their blocking and filtering effectiveness, as well as fit, comfort, durability, and consumer appeal. The concerns raised about effectiveness of physical distance and mask rules are part of the issues involved in the ethics of mandates (Chap. 10). Mandates for these requirements need to be judged in terms of ethical and bio-ethical principles and procedures to control the disease particularly principles of proportionality, autonomy and beneficence.

The purpose of this section is not an attempt to advocate that mask wearing and social distancing in terms of the relationship of expulsion of droplet velocity to social distance requirements is futile but simply to give some insight into the issues involved. In what circumstances you wear a mask or not is your choice, unless there is a government mandate, based on your assessment of the arguments and situation. You should really consider a mask in crowded inside contexts where you cannot use social distance as a protector. Many governments still require masks in hospitals and other health centres, public transport and airports. If you do wear a mask make sure it is fit for purpose as far as is possible, at least tight fitting with no air gaps and three layered. Single-layer cloth homemade masks to match your outfit may be pretty but are pretty useless.

References

Australian Government Department of Health. Health alerts. https://www.health.gov.au/health-alerts/covid-19. Retrieved 20 January 22.

Axon, C. (2021). The Telegraph. https://www.telegraph.co.uk/news/2021/07/17/cloth-face-masks-comfort-blankets-do-little-curb-covid-spread/. Retrieved 31 October 21.

Bogardus, E. S. (1947). Measurement of personal-group relations. *Sociometry, 10*(4), 306–311. https://doi.org/10.2307/2785570

Centers for disease control science brief: community use of masks to control the spread of SARS-CoV-2. Updated Dec. 6, 2021. https://www.cdc.gov/coronavirus/2019-ncov/science/science-briefs/masking-science-sars-cov2.html. Retrieved 18 February 22.

Madhi, S. A., Kwatra, G., Myers, J. E., et al. (2022). Population immunity and covid-19 severity with omicron variant in South Africa. *New England Journal of Medicine, 386*(14), 1314–1326. https://doi.org/10.1056/NEJMoa2119658

Mathieu, E., Ritchie, H., Rodés-Guirao, L., et al. (2022). Coronavirus Pandemic (COVID-19). Published online at OurWorldInData.org. Continually updated and retrieved from: https://ourworldindata.org/coronavirus

Reuters Fact Check. (16 July 2022). No evidence Omicron BA.5 is more infectious than measles or is 'the most infectious virus known'. https://www.reuters.com/article/factcheck-omicron-reproduction-number-idUSL1N2YW1T0. Retrieved 01 September 22.

US Covid Cases Today. Continually updated and retrieved from https://www.google.com.au/search?q=us+covid+cases+today&hl=en&source=hp&ei=VMKOY8zzGpyj1e8P6JOh0AQ&iflsigws-wiz

van Elsland, L., & O'Hare, R. (2020). COVID-19: Imperial researchers model likely impact of public health measures. https://www.imperial.ac.uk/news/196234/covid-19-imperial-researchers-model-likely-impact/. Retrieved 06 October 21.

WHO Coronavirus. (COVID-19). Dashboard. Continually updated and retrieved from https://covid19.who.int/

Wolter, N., Jassat, W., Walaza, S., et al. (2022). Early assessment of the clinical severity of the SARS-CoV-2 omicron variant in South Africa: A data linkage study. *Lancet, 399*, 437. https://doi.org/10.1016/S0140-6736(22)00017-4

Xinhua News Agency 08 07 2020. Editor: huaxia. Local infection number in Germany drops below critical mark after outbreak at slaughterhouse. http://www.xinhuanet.com/english/2020-07/08/c_139195441.htm. Retrieved 14 October 21.

CHAPTER 2

A Pandemonium of Pandemics and Epidemics

If you look into the seeds of time, and say which grains
will grow and which will not, speak them to me
Banquo to the three witches in Macbeth

Abstract A review of past pandemics/epidemics reveals their devastation on then powerful Empires. Quarantine, herd immunity, vaccination and statistical analysis are shown as developments of techniques from earlier contagions. The disputed origins of Covid-19 and government policies including the Swedish approach are reviewed. The chapter concludes with issues of transitioning from ICU and the Long Covid medical problems.

Keywords Past pandemics · Quarantine · Herd immunity · Omicron variants · Swedish approach · Long Covid

In the Past

We should not take the current Covid-19 pandemic lightly as history presents a warning picture of infectious diseases responsible for the greatest human death tolls in the past. For example, the bubonic plague killed approximately 25% of the European population in the mid-1300s AD. Devastating epidemics and pandemics hammered and brought doom to many flourishing early empires, civilisations and nations like Athens, the Roman Empire, the Byzantine Empire, the Mayan and Aztec, all of which were severely damaged by the decimation of populations and radically reduced ability to continue ruling large areas of the then known Earth or stop invaders. Thanks to the advances in epidemiology, pharmaceuticals and human behaviour management techniques, we are now able to exert immense control on disease spread, using

© The Author(s), under exclusive license to Springer Nature Singapore Pte Ltd. 2023

R. B. Burns, *The Human Impact of the COVID-19 Pandemic*,
https://doi.org/10.1007/978-981-99-1710-5_2

vaccination, effective quarantine, social distancing, mask-wearing and persuasive communication, so we no longer face the same mortality consequences as our ancestors once did when these terrible disease outbreaks threatened the planet, but we may well still face such economic political and social distress that governments could still be irreparably damaged.

While the distinction between pandemic and epidemic was emphasised as one of scale in Chap. 1, in the early historical episodes it is difficult to know how to categorise outbreaks as the known world was small and therefore disease spread was thereby limited. This limited spread was also a function of people not travelling far from their own cities and settlements. So what occurred several thousands of year ago would perhaps be more on the scale of local outbreaks nowadays, although the infections recorded then had invaded most of what in their experience was their known world.

The type of disease basis and underlying cause of spread of the epidemics/pandemics in the earliest events is not really known, and speculation is often all we have based on recent analysis of bodily remains. The number of infected and dying is also simply estimated. Some of the events were termed plagues too and most likely a result of infestation rather than viral based as now. What these earliest events show is evidence that disease spreading in pandemic-epidemic proportions in terms of the then population and known world are not just of recent origin but have impacted on many past civilisations which had no real knowledge of how to manage them.

Vengeance is mine, I will repay. (Romans 12:19)

In many ancient societies, people believed that spirits and gods inflicted disease and destruction upon those sinful persons and nations that deserved punishment. This was the basis of the Sodom and Gomorrah destruction, and Genesis flood myths. Many current religious cults still believe that pandemics, floods, droughts, fires and other scourges are sent by whatever God they worship to punish humanity for its sinfulness! In the past, such unscientific beliefs often led to disastrous responses to diseases that resulted in the deaths of thousands, if not millions, because if you believed some god destined this to occur then you could not stop it, so why take precautionary actions.

For example, in the case of Justinian's plague (see below), the Byzantine historian Procopius of Caesarea traced the origins of the plague (the *Yersinia pestis* bacteria) to China and north-east India, via land and sea trade routes to Egypt where it entered the Byzantine Empire through Mediterranean ports. Despite his apparent knowledge of the roles that geography and trade played in this spread, Procopius laid blame for the outbreak on the Emperor Justinian, declaring him to be a devil, invoking God's punishment for his evil ways. Some historians found that this event could have dashed Emperor Justinian's efforts to reunite the Western and Eastern remnants of the Roman Empire, and marked the beginning of the Dark Ages.

Luckily, humanity's understanding of the causes and spread of disease has improved, and this is resulting in a drastic improvement, albeit slow and incomplete, in the response to modern pandemics.

The Introduction of Methods to Control Disease Spread

Quarantine

The practice of quarantine began in Italy during the fourteenth century, in an effort to protect coastal cities from plague epidemics. Cautious port authorities required ships arriving in Venice from infected ports to sit at anchor for 40 days before landing. The word '*quarantine*' derives from the Italian '*quaranta giorni*', or 40 days.

Another early and successful attempt with quarantine on land occurred in 1665 at Eyam in Derbyshire, England, during the Back Death's final rampage in the UK. This plague provided the first historical examples of how effective quarantine could be in containing a disease by cordoning off the infected area. A bale of damp cloth sent to the village of Eyam, Derbyshire from London contained fleas carrying the bubonic plague. This spread rapidly through the village which made the remarkable decision to quarantine itself in an heroic attempt to halt the spread to nearby towns of Sheffield and Bakewell. The local Minister Rev Mompesson believed it was his duty to outsiders to prevent the plague moving on so he managed to gain the consent of the villagers to quarantine the settlement. The villagers refused to run and the Earl of Devonshire, who lived nearby at Chatsworth, sent food and supplies to the edge of the quarantine zone.

This showed a 'cordon sanitaire' was the most effective way of dealing with plague and other transmittable diseases. Eyam's mortality rate was higher than that suffered by the citizens of London as a result of the plague. In just over a year, 260 of the village's inhabitants, from no fewer than 76 different families, had died. The total population of Eyam has been estimated at between 400 and 700 before the plague struck. However, the courage of the village had probably saved thousands more in nearby towns. Plaques on many Eyam houses now show where the deaths occurred.

Statistical Analysis

The first instance of relying on plotting disease spread and statistical analysis to find answers appears to have occurred as in mid-nineteenth-century London, during a cholera outbreak. In 1854, Dr. John Snow, using a map to chart the spread of the cholera, came to the conclusion that it was spreading via tainted water. With a map displaying neighbourhood mortality data, he could demonstrate a large cluster of cases focussed around a specific pump from which people were drawing their water. Modern statistical approaches no longer rely on plotting what has leady happened but focus on modelling to predict how the pandemic will develop.

Vaccination

The Chinese employed smallpox inoculation (or variolation) as early as 1000 CE. It was practiced in Africa and Turkey as well, before it spread to Europe and the Americas.

Edward Jenner's innovations begun with his successful 1796 use of cowpox material to create immunity to smallpox, quickly made the practice widespread. His method underwent medical and technological changes over the next 200 years, and eventually resulted in the eradication of smallpox.

Louis Pasteur's 1885 rabies vaccine was the next to make an impact on human disease. And then, at the dawn of bacteriology, developments rapidly followed. Antitoxins and vaccines against diphtheria, tetanus, anthrax, cholera, plague, typhoid, tuberculosis, and more were developed through the twentieth and twenty-first centuries. The middle of the twentieth century was an active time for vaccine research and development. For example, whooping cough killed 290 babies each year in Australia in the early 1900s before vaccination which reduced the death rate to virtually zero by 1960. Methods for growing viruses in the laboratory led to rapid discoveries, including the creation of vaccines for polio, and other common childhood diseases such as measles, mumps, and rubella which reduced the disease burden greatly. Current vaccination by a number of approved Covid vaccines has significantly reduced the spread and lethality of the Covid virus.

Herd Immunity

Herd immunity is defined as the indirect protection from an infectious disease that happens when the vast majority of the population is vaccinated, or has developed immunity through previous infection. Even those who are not immune are considered protected because the likelihood of an outbreak is small. Herd immunity makes it theoretically possible to protect the population from a disease, including those who can't be vaccinated, such as newborns, those who have compromised immune systems, and even the few who object to vaccination. Chicken pox, measles, mumps, and polio are all examples of diseases for which most Western countries have achieved herd immunity due to vaccines. Similarly, the initial hope was that herd immunity promised a complete return to a world without Covid. Much like a bushfire that goes out when it runs out of fuel to burn, a pandemic begins to decline when the virus runs out of susceptible people to infect. But in reality this was probably a pipe dream and few people talk about it now as herd immunity has become progressively more mathematically impossible as variants emerge.

The percentage of a community that needs to be immune in order to achieve herd immunity varies from disease to disease. In early 2020, we were tackling the original *SARS-CoV-2*, which was much less infectious (estimated *R0* of 2–3) than current circulating variants. If we assume vaccines available had an effectiveness of 80%, this yields a herd immunity threshold estimate of 60–80%, i.e. we would have needed to vaccinate 60–80% of the whole population to see the epidemic decline. Mathematically, this was feasible.

However, new variants are far more infectious. *Delta* has an *R0* of about 5 and *Omicron* and its variants are in the ballpark of about 13–18, making it among the most infectious diseases known, theoretically increasing herd immunity threshold estimates up to 100–118%, and herd immunity via vaccination therefore mathematically impossible. There are other more practical limitations.

Vaccine hesitancy. Some people may object to getting a Covid vaccine because of religious objections, misinformation, fake news, fears about possible risks or scepticism about the benefits. Others display psychological reactance, '*I refuse to submit to your demands*'. If the proportion of vaccinated people in a community is below the herd immunity threshold, a contagious disease will continue to spread.

The geographical context of herd immunity. No community is an island, isolated from those around and it is the landscape of immunity that surrounds a community that really matters. Covid has occurred in clusters across most counties as a result of people's behaviour or local policies. Previous vaccination efforts suggest that uptake level will tend to cluster geographically, too. Localised resistance to the measles vaccination, for example, has resulted in small pockets of disease resurgence. Geographic clustering is going to make the path to herd immunity a lot less of a straight line, and it will turn into a game of whack-a-mole with Covid hotspot outbreaks. Even a country with high vaccination rates, such as Israel, is threatened by surrounding Middle East countries which haven't done the same and with populations able to mix, the potential for new outbreaks remains.

Protection questions. It's not clear how long the Covid vaccines will protect from Covid. Research suggests that Covid vaccines may have lower efficacy against some of the variants of the virus. New variants, which could be more resistant to vaccines, are still emerging.

Uneven vaccine roll-out. The distribution of Covid vaccines has greatly varied among and within countries. Vaccine roll-out is uneven across the globe. There are numerous countries in Africa, the Middle East and Asia that have low vaccination rates and limited supplies of vaccine. WHO has called for greater global equity in the distribution of and access to vaccines. Based on the current rate of vaccine roll-out, 109 countries missed the WHO's target for 70% of the world's population to be fully vaccinated by July 2022, and 36 nations had not even reached 10% vaccination cover with the average for the world being around 53%. Among severely ill patients worldwide, 90% were unvaccinated. A perfectly coordinated global campaign could have wiped out Covid, at least theoretically. If one community achieves a high vaccination rate and surrounding areas don't, outbreaks can occur if the populations mix. Israel began vaccinating its citizens in December 2020, and thanks in part to a deal with Pfizer–BioNTech to share data in exchange for vaccine doses, it began to lead the world in terms of roll-out. Meanwhile, Israel's neighbours Lebanon, Syria, Jordan and Egypt have yet to vaccinate even a small percent of their respective populations.

All this reflects the complexities and challenges of the pandemic and shouldn't overshadow the fact that vaccination is helping. But as new variants arise and immunity from infections potentially wanes, we will be still battling the threat with future surges and annual boosters as we do with flu. The conclusion is that given the challenges, it's not clear if or when any country will achieve herd immunity. At this point in the pandemic herd immunity is believed unlikely.

There Is No After Covid!

Many epidemiologists are theorising that the pandemic will end in an 'endemic'. a disease that's consistently present, but limited to a particular area. Malaria in sub-Saharan Africa is a good example where endemic disease spread and rates are predictable. Things will not go back to exactly the way they were before Covid because there is probably no 'after Covid'; it's always going to be there lurking in the shadows, continually requiring us to take measures when we gather, protect those that have risk factors for severe disease, and entertain annual or semi-annual boosters. However, the approved Covid vaccines are highly effective at protecting against severe illness requiring hospitalisation and lowering death rates. Even if it isn't currently possible to stop transmission of the virus, the vaccines are allowing people to better be able to live with it.

We are still learning about immunity to Covid. Most people who are infected develop an immune response within the first few weeks, but we don't know how strong or lasting that immune response is, or how it differs for people by age, ethnicity, etc. The general medical advice is that immunity from initial vaccinations that gave some protection from *Delta* need a booster support shot to raise protection levels for *Omicron* and its variants and boosters being given with a further booster needed in the July/Aug 2022 period. There have also been reports of people infected with Covid for a second time. Until we better understand Covid immunity, it will not be possible to know how much of a population is immune and how long that immunity last for, let alone make future predictions. These challenges should preclude any plans that try to increase immunity within a population by allowing people to get infected deliberately, despite plans to do so by letting *Omicron* run to create an epidemic of the unvaccinated, gaining added immune persons from this action. But this may not work because of the emergence of new variants and the need to get young children vaccinated.

Even if we don't reach herd immunity threshold, the greater the proportion of the population vaccinated, supported by other measures like mask wearing and improving ventilation, the more difficult it becomes for the virus to spread. Given the onset of winter flu in 2022, in both hemispheres, vaccination for both viruses was essential to reduce mortality rates.

Effects of Some Historical Pandemics

Disease and illnesses have plagued humanity since the marked shift to agrarian and metal working communities, and to overseas adventurers conquering new lands especially in the Americas. The scale and spread of disease increased dramatically with the growth of early trade in food, metal tools and weapons between communities and then between regions. The increasing widespread trade created new opportunities for human and animal interactions that sped up epidemics and pandemics as the world effectively became 'bigger', ushering in new diseases such as malaria, tuberculosis, leprosy, influenza, smallpox, cholera and others.

Epidemics more often developed into pandemics the more civilised humans became, with larger populations clustered together in towns and cities, more exotic trade routes, and increased contact with different populations of people, animals and ecosystems. While the interactions created through trade and urban life played a pivotal role in developing economies and political structures, it brought with it the virulent nature of not only old but newer diseases in the trajectory of pandemics.

A number of pandemics and epidemics (in the past brought nations and civilisations to their knees some examples below).

(a) Plague of Athens: 430–425 B.C

Athens experienced a five-year pandemic around 430 B.C., which commenced during a war between Athens and Sparta. Some estimates put the death toll as high as 100,000 people. The Greek historian Thucydides (460–400 B.C.) wrote *that 'people in good health were all of a sudden attacked by violent heats in the head, and redness and inflammation in the eyes, the inward parts, such as the throat or tongue, becoming bloody and emitting an unnatural and fetid breath'* (translation by Crawley, 1914).

No one really knows what this epidemic was but suggestions by medical scientists offer possibilities like typhoid fever and even Ebola. Many scholars believe that overcrowding caused by the war exacerbated the easy spread of the epidemic. The Athenians doing badly against Sparta's bigger army took refuge behind a series of fortifications called 'long walls' that protected their city, but encouraged the spread of disease in the crowded area. The war continued on, despite the epidemic, *but it ended Athens as a Mediterranean power as it was forced to capitulate to Sparta in 404 B.C.*

(b) Antonine Plague: A.D. 165–180

Roman soldiers returning home after a successful war against Parthia apparently brought back more than the spoils of victory. The Antonine Plague is believed to have been smallpox, decimated the army, and may have killed over 5 million people in the Roman empire (Pudsey, 2017). The epidemic contributed to the end of the Pax Romana (the Roman Peace), a period from 27 B.C. to A.D. 180, when Rome was at the height of its power. After A.D. 180, with a weaker army and disease spreading death throughout the Roman Empire instability grew and barbarian groups seized their opportunity to take over more and more of the Empire. Christianity became increasingly popular in the time after the plague occurred. *Thus as with Athens, an epidemic challenged the Roman Empire redirecting the course of history in Europe and Mediterranean.*

(c) Plague of Justinian

Bubonic plagues were due to a strain of the bacterium *Yersinia pestis* that is likely extinct today and was spread by fleas on infected rodents. *The Plague of Justinian of 541 A.D.* is named after the Byzantine Emperor Justinian (reigned A.D. 527–565) and wiped out an estimated 10% of the known world's population. Under Justinian's reign, the Byzantine Empire with its capital in Constantinople (Istanbul), reached its greatest extent, controlling territory that stretched from the Middle East to Western Europe. Gradually *his empire gradually lost territory following the plague and the Byzantine Empire gradually folded. Another example of the power of rampant disease to change history.*

(d) The Black Death 1346–1353

This was also a bubonic plague and perhaps the first recorded pandemic traversing both Asia and Europe, killing more than 75 million people in its wake. Some estimates suggest that it reduced Europe's population by half. The plague had considerable social and economic positive effects on Europe. The huge number of deaths produced difficulties in the labour market, with labourers and particularly serfs in short supply. This shortage forced an increase in wages as well as bringing to an end Europe's system of serfdom. Studies suggest that surviving workers had better access to meat and higher-quality bread. *Another significant historical and social change in the wake of a pandemic.*

(e) Moscow Plague 1770–1772

This led to government imposed quarantine. However, the terror of quarantine led to high levels of unrest and violence among the citizens. Rioting spread as fast as the infection did and Archbishop Ambrosius was murdered for encouraging crowds not to gather for worship. The empress Catherine the Great was so desperate to contain the plague and restore public order that she issued a hasty decree ordering that all factories be moved from Moscow. By the time the plague ended, as many as 100,000 people may have died. Even after the plague ended, *Catherine struggled to restore order and couldn't bring Russia back from the devastation caused with another example of a plague having severe political repercussions.*

(f) Epidemics in the Americas

European explorers brought a cluster of Eurasian diseases into America in the sixteenth century, including smallpox, and a form of viral haemorrhagic fever, killed 15 million inhabitants of Mexico and Central America, and *led to the collapse of the Inca and Aztec civilisations.* Some estimates suggest that 90% of the indigenous population was killed off.

Helped by the fact that disease had vastly reduced the size of any indigenous groups that opposed the Spanish forces, Cortés, conquered the Aztec capital of Tenochtitlán in 1519. Another Spanish force led by Francisco Pizarro conquered the Incas in 1532. The Spanish took over the territories of both empires. In both cases, the Aztec and Inca armies had been ravaged by disease and were unable to withstand the Spanish forces. *These are further examples of the power and impact of disease to change the course of history.*

(g) The Spanish Flu Pandemic (1918–1919)

This was the last pandemic before Covid hit us. The outbreak of the deadly *Ebola* and less deadly *MERS* and *SARS* were luckily only epidemics contained in small geographical regions Spanish flu was caused by an *H1N1* virus of avian origin. Although there is not universal consensus regarding where it originated, it certainly wasn't Spain, but it spread worldwide during 1918–1919. In the USA, it was first identified in military personnel in spring 1918. It is estimated that about 500 million people or one-third of the world's population became infected with this virus. The number of deaths was estimated to be at least 50 million worldwide with about 675,000 occurring in the USA. Mortality was high in people younger than 5 years old, 20–40 years old, and 65 years and older. The high mortality in healthy people, including those in the 20–40 year age group, was a unique feature of this pandemic. More people died during the 1918 pandemic than the total number of military and civilian deaths from World War I. Most deaths occurred in the 2nd and 3rd waves at the end of WW1 as mass troop movements especially demobilisation contributed massively to the global spread of flu with military personnel returning home around the globe. This is how it arrived in what were distant places then, like N. Zealand and Australia.

With no vaccine available then to protect against influenza infection and no antibiotics to treat secondary bacterial infections that can be associated with influenza infections, control efforts worldwide were limited to basic non-pharmaceutical interventions like isolation, quarantine, personal hygiene, disinfectants and limitations of public gatherings, all which were applied unevenly within and between nations.

COVID-19: The Current Global Culprit

COVID-19 is one of a number of known coronaviruses that have caused epidemics and pandemics recently. Coronaviruses are a large family of viruses that can cause diseases ranging from the common cold to the most serious as in the current Covid outbreak.

The current Covid epidemic apparently started in Wuhan China. Its origin is still in doubt with two competing theories:

1. ***Lab-leak Theory***. Was it a result of a virus escaping into the community from a government biological laboratory that experimented with viruses? This theory stemmed from a January 2020 paper by scientists from Wuhan Institute of Virology in the journal Nature, comparing the *COVID-19 genome* to that of its closest-known relative, a bat virus produced in the very same lab (Zhou et al., 2020). The lab-leak theory was grabbed by conspiratorial supporters that saw China as a deliberate creator of the pandemic moving the explanation from real science where it belongs to speculative global politics. An investigation by the World Health Organization in early 2021 ruled the lab-leak theory unlikely, but wasn't able to fully rule it out.
2. ***Wuhan wild life animal market***. The latest thoughts derived from the work of Australian University of Sydney Professor Holmes and colleagues who have debunked the lab-leak theory by mapping early cases of COVID-19 and pinpointed the Huanan seafood wholesale market in Wuhan as likely epicentre of the pandemic (Holmes, 2022; Worobey et al., 2022). Holmes had visited the Wuhan wholesale market in 2014 and noted the potential for transmission of viruses from animal to man, particularly the presence of racoon dogs that had been associated with the emergence of the SARS virus in 2002–04. Professor Holmes believes markets like these become engine rooms for disease emergence by putting humans and wildlife in close proximity to each other.

   Prof Holmes applied geographic clustering and spatial mapping (as had, in a simpler fashion, John Snow in seeking the source of cholera in London in 1854) and pinpointed the locations of more than 150 of the earliest reported COVID-19 cases from December 2019 with a very strong clustering around the market, a sort of epicentre that left him certain the virus originated in the Huanan seafood wholesale market. The alternative source, the Wuhan Institute of Virology, is more than 30 kms from the midpoint of the early cases, making it unlikely to be the origin. Prof Holmes is extremely confident that the virus is not from the laboratory, but which animal was case zero will never be known.

The jury is still out over three years later essentially due to obfuscation by Chinese authorities preventing thorough scientific investigation. Perhaps after this length of time, we will never really have the valid answer about the origin of Covid.

Covid Variants

There have been many variants over the last three and a half years as the Covid virus mutated. These have been given Greek alphabet letter names, e.g. *Beta, Delta, Omicron*. The most recent variant from which highly transmittable current subvariants have emerged is *Omicron* (Greek letter O in English, named by WHO). Ironically it should have been called *Xi*- the next letter on the alphabetical list, but WHO fearing Chinese retribution of some kind, refrained from this name as it is a common Chinese surname and graces even the Chinese president! However, many people like to regard the original emanation of the virus the *Wuhan Xi-virus* since it was the Chinese president's attempt to keep face that led to a disastrous delay by not admitting early enough to an outbreak that facilitated a massive epidemic and rapid transformation into a global pandemic through continuing international travel.

Most governments panicked by the fast-spreading Covid in 2020, threw out the existing rule book based on a hundred years of science and real-world public health experience as contained in a WHO SAGE report (2019). Instead, they generally implemented policies that:

- Used case numbers as the single metric to drive policy,
- Subordinated all other public policy goals in health, economic, social, educational areas to the imperative of crushing and killing the virus,
- Often accepted worst-case modelling scenarios based on flawed assumptions and faulty data as predictions,
- Ignored the age care segregation threat of Covid, with people over 75, being 10,000 times more at risk than those under 15, and
- Applied restrictive health orders supported by law enforcement professionals to thwart resistance, some examples of which are listed in Chap. 3.

Luckily it worked with social distancing, selective isolation, venue density numbers and strong vaccination rates now permitting the most drastic elimination strategies of mandated quarantine/isolation and travel bans to be abandoned apart from in China, and the general reset strategy is focussed strongly on high vaccination rates and encouragement of mask wearing, social distancing and sanitation.

One reason that Covid has riveted global attention is that, this time, those with more social capital have had their lives disrupted. For example, the Ebola virus, far more contagious and deadly than Covid, with very young children the most vulnerable group, was concentrated and restrained within West Africa and did not affect huge numbers of people worldwide like Covid (Dhama et al., 2020).

The brief historical resume summarised earlier poses the intriguing question of whether the current pandemic will change the future as earlier ones did from what it might have been by imposing global economic and social distress, unrest through high inflation, as well as altering the balance of world powers. The high level of contagion in China caused prices to surge and is continuing to impact global and national supply chains. The virus has come back to bite China whose government placed over 600 million living under restrictions (and rising), including 400 million under full lockdown in April 2022 in its huge economic/business heart and port of Shanghai, and 21 million in Chengdu August 2022 (Mathieu et al. Our World in Data 2022). The economic effect is already being felt severely within China, as the services sector takes its biggest hit since the pandemic first emerged in Wuhan. Factories have shut and the logistics sector is suffering disrupted trucking capacity due to increasingly strict rules on movement. This will also affect supply chains internationally with knock on inflationary effects globally. The Chinese Government *COVID-ZERO* strategy is like the crock of gold at the end of a rainbow, an unattainable goal, never a valid strategy and no longer a scientific policy, but an impractical non-negotiable authoritarian political dogma. It is the only country with a Covid-zero aim.

The Age of Omicron: The Route to Normal? (Whatever that May Be)

Initial Strategy

The Age of Omicron sounds like the title of a space age horror movie. Perhaps that description is not far off the mark as this highly contagious scourge with its many variants ravages country after country with authorities getting first-hand lessons in exponential mathematics in 2022. A few examples will suffice: in the first week of 2022, London had a 1 in 10 infection rate, Wales and Scotland 1 in 20, France had over 300,000 infections per day with 70% of those in intensive care units in Paris public hospitals being unvaccinated, and Ireland over 17,000 infections per day while Australia was topping 106,000 infections per day and the USA had increased infections by 36% over the last week of 2021. The peaking of *Omicron* in the first quarter of 2022 in most countries caused massive increases in case numbers but hospitalisations dropped significantly as a ratio to cases due to much decreased severity. After almost two years of '*Covid-control*' mind-set, few expected that Australia would find itself recording around 100,000 cases a day in early 2022. Data above is a selection from Mathieu et al. Our World in data (2022).

When the *Delta* variant first arose in late 2020, its *R0* ranged between 3 and 8 with a mean of 5. But at the end of 2021 Omicron *RO* exploded to 15 with a mean of 12. Remember the caveat is that *R0* assumes the population is unprotected but that is irrelevant in countries with two dose vaccinations plus first booster like those in Europe and in Australia though the *Rt* remains high for those who have not had the booster as evidence in the UK suggested the standard two dose vaccination may only offer protection of around 19%. A better estimate of risk is that based on research from S.Africa and the USA where the risk of severe disease is 70–80% less than that when *Delta* was roaming around, evidence of the benefit of vaccination which is being amplified with two boosters in 2022.

WHO on 7 January 2022 warned that the tsunami of *Omicron* cases was so huge and quick that it is overwhelming health systems around the world and its chief Dr Tedros said a record 9.5 million cases of the coronavirus were tallied around the world over the 2nd week in January, 'the highest number' reported so far in the pandemic. WHO was certain that was an underestimate because of a backlog in testing around the year-end holidays.

Given the much lower severity level of *Omicron*, governments globally have continued with variations of reduced restrictions and mandates like those earlier applied to *Delta* which had brought critical success and time for many nations before high levels of vaccination could be achieved. However, even these lighter touch policies were at a cost to their populations causing further ongoing massive economic, social and psychological distress due to contact isolation rules and limited density for venues. A further crucial reset must be invoked to restore a semblance of sanity to the pandemic rule book and rebuild confidence that we can once again live with the *Omicron* and it spawned subvariants. The developing theme now is that the new variants should be treated as an endemic virus like flu and a focus change to managing the disease, not elimination. Massive costly testing, tracing and isolation programs are like sticking a finger in the hole in the dyke after the village is already submerged, according to Dr Clive Dix, former head of Britain's vaccine taskforce (The Guardian report 08 01 2022).

Another way of looking at evaluating the severity of Covid is to compare it with some of the major pandemics and view the death rates as a percentage of the estimated world population at the time (Table 2.1). Remember these are all estimates.

These figures suggest that not only is Covid not as lethal as many previous diseases but the extremely low mortality rate is due to high vaccination rates, high levels of heath care and sanitation, and appropriate use of mandated social restriction measures like quarantine. But where vaccination rates remain in the low 60% and other restrictions loosened as in the USA, *Omicron* is powering through the population leaving over 1 million Americans for dead. After two years, people generally worldwide were also becoming immune to the messaging about Covid and more relaxed in their daily behaviour. But is has not gone away.

Table 2.1 Death toll as % of world population. Data collated by author from many historic accounts and documents. Note the figures are estimates and rounded

Pandemic	*Death rate % of world population estimate (%)*	*Death toll estimate (M)*	*World population estimate*	*Year of estimate*
Plague of Justinian	19.1	40	210 M	500
Black Death	51	200	390 M	1300
Smallpox	12.1	56	460 M	1500
Antonine plague	2.6	5	200 M	200
Spanish Flu	2.5	45	1.82B	1919
Third plague	1.0	12	1.26B	1850
HIV/AIDS	0.7	30	4.46B	1981
Covid-19	0.0084	6.59	8.00B	2022

Despite the obvious success of government mandated health policies reflected in the low Covid death rate of 0.0084% of world population, the current pandemic has exposed some ethical issues in the inadequacy of our systems and responses to produce disproportionate, inequitable tragic consequences for health and livelihoods for some individuals, their communities, and even whole societies. As noted in later chapters there are considerable ethical and moral implications arising from institutionalised forms of discrimination in individual nations and globally, located for example,

- In age (the aged care group in particular),
- In ethnicity/class (with lockdown, and job loss particularly hitting working class and poor persons and immigrants),
- In gender (with women dealing with home education duties as well as normal homemaking),
- In the digital divide, and abilities (with those with inadequate English unable to follow health instructions and special needs children being massively disadvantaged by missing school).

Even as vaccinations are being rolled out, it is obvious that there are '*haves*' and '*have nots*' in most countries and between countries, with practices/ policies that serve to perpetuate bias and exclusion. Grappling with Covid has made it clear that mental and physical health are indivisible and in the aftermath of the pandemic, societies worldwide will have to improve linkages between mental and physical health support services, particularly for marginalised and vulnerable groups.

Sweden Did Their Own Thing

In March 2020 as the pandemic spread through most of the world, Sweden took a path no other nation did and became a many millions strong control group set against an almost global experiment of mandated close down, restrictions and behavioural control (e.g. China, Victoria Australia). This global action of closing down societies to prevent the spread of a virus had never been tested before and was implemented without any cost/benefit analysis as to economic and social impacts. For most of 2020, Sweden imposed no movement restrictions, no school closures, no mask wearing. From November 2020, a few modifications were made on density limits for public gatherings and restaurants (Anderberg, 2022).

As 2020 passed and 2021 progressed, many countries like the UK, USA, France, Spain, Argentine that had even gone as far as fining people for going fishing alone, eating a sandwich on a park bench and using surveillance drones over children's play grounds, started to exceed Sweden's death rate. When the Eurostat agency issued excess mortality rates for 2020 (excess deaths over mean number normally expected), Sweden was in 22nd place out of 30 European countries. By December 2021, 56 countries had more deaths per capita than Sweden. In fact between Jan 20 and June 21 Sweden registered an excess mortality of minus 2.3%, i.e. less death than expected normally indicating that Covid had no impact on death rates there (Anderberg, 2022). This was achieved without the devastation of economy and society as in other countries. There was never any route guaranteed to stop Covid deaths, only a set of alternatives that each carried different risk levels, as even in Sweden, winners and losers were created as a child could go to school and be with their friends while the elderly were advised to stay home as far as possible, an age group where death rates were as high as elsewhere.

An official government enquiry into Sweden's Covid response was issued in February 2022 and concluded that the no lockdown strategy was fundamentally correct but noted countries that employed lockdowns experienced worse outcomes than Sweden.

Is Covid as Deadly As Feared? The Australian Experience

The Australian Health Department data also revealed that earlier in the pandemic, lockdowns and strict Covid protocols saved fewer lives than expected. This suggests that the lives saved from preventing Covid infection were offset by other causes of death, and quite possibly the longer-term cumulative effects of social and care deprivation under Covid policy such as insufficient staff availability in aged care homes impacting levels of care and attention over such basics as maintaining pill delivery schedules and blood sugar checking for diabetic patients.

A realistic assessment can be obtained from the knowledge that Australia's normal annual death toll is around 160,000, so that from March 2020 to Jan 2022 the average total deaths would have been around 307,000, however, the total number of Covid deaths in that period was 3835 or 1.2% of all deaths over the 22 month period (Australian Government Department of Health and Aged Care. Health Alerts. 2022). In fact, the main 'killers' were the usual suspects: cancers, heart disease, dementias and strokes. In the 23 months to 1 Feb 2022, the recorded number of suicides in Australia was 73% more than Covid deaths. Flu virtually vanished over the winters 2020 and 2021 but normally contributes on average around 1000 deaths per year or 0.65% of the normally expected deaths over the 22 months used above for the Covid calculation.

We certainly have never even considered making citizens suffer the crippling social, psychological and economic effects of lockdowns which can cause more harm than good when managing the annual flu nor do we restrict exercise and social interaction, causing increased alcohol dependency, loneliness, forcing families apart, and decreasing possibilities of bonding at birthdays, weddings and funerals, all leading down a pathway of declining public health. Neither do we panic the public by reading out the number of flu deaths each day either. Covid had not by the end of 2021 turned out to be the 'killer' impact expected but the highly restrictive government policies did.

Sceptical voices having noted the futility and collateral harms of lengthy lockdowns and movement restrictions applied generally, argue for targeted policies to protect the vulnerable, while keeping the rest of society functioning, finally insisting on endemic disease management with recommended sanitation, social distancing and vaccination policies emphasised. The compensating feature now is that the Omicron variants while more contagious, apparently are less severe than the Delta variant that preceded them affecting the nose and throat more than the lungs, and therefore not as deadly. For example, in New South Wales in October 2021, 184 patients were on ventilators 0.67% of the 27,259 known infected *Delta* cases. By mid-January 2022, there were 102 on ventilators, just 0.014 of the 723,137 known cases of *Omicron*, evidence of its far greater transmissibility but far lesser lethality (Australian Government Department of Health and Aged Care. Health Alerts. 2022).

The Reset Strategy

So, *Omicron* and its variants have now repainted how many nations are living with Covid. Since many developed countries are now around the 90% level of double vaccination, most government health policies around the world have redirected focus away from elimination to allowing Omicron to 'run' eventually creating an endemic situation where small flare-ups can be strongly controlled and contained, relying on the high level of vaccination to protect nearly all citizens. In discussing herd immunity above, it was noted this was an unlikely prospect, so the current aim would be to depress the contagion into endemic proportions.

The evidence of the utter pointlessness of the previous over-reach theatre in the regulatory environment during 2020/21 is highlighted by the inability to prevent two-thirds of 25 staff at Princess Elisabeth Polar Station, an extremely isolated Belgian scientific research station in Antarctica, catching Covid from a single positive case detected on December 14, 2021. Based in one of the world's remotest regions, all were fully vaccinated, passed multiple PCR tests and were quarantined before entry to the station. Yet Omicron still emerged there!

The set policy changes permeating actions by many governments now have involved bringing an end to the massive deployment of staff time and energy in contact tracing and attempting to stop excessive testing of large numbers of people who only '*suspect*' they may be infectious. Casual and close contacts have been redefined to prevent isolating large populations in quarantine which had already started to bring economies to a halt, supply chains broken, with produce and goods simply not making it to market. Lockdowns and border closures have become a thing of the past. These changes have started a massive surge in infections but vaccinated persons only appear in general to have mild symptoms while it is the unvaccinated and medically compromised very elderly that are severely at risk, the latter reflecting a disgrace with neglected aged care patients not having received vaccinations.

National policy objectives in most countries are now designed to balance the need to keep people at work and to protect the capacity of hospitals to cope, with further changes enabling workers in the transport, freight, logistics, emergency services, energy, water, waste management, food, beverage, telecommunications, data, broadcasting, media, education and childcare industries to return to work immediately and stop the pandemic of human distress. That is a pragmatic approach to open up nations around the world, dissipate the economic, social and educational disasters, and live with a disease that will always be floating round the world for the long haul. In the same way as Australia accepts around 1000 flu deaths each year, the number of Covid deaths will have to be '*accepted*'. From 2022, personal responsibility will hopefully replace government mandates in most nations, which means most people can decide to what risks they are comfortable exposing themselves, moving well away from the emergency mentality of the last two years. Alert but never complacent.

The reset does possess the double advantage of high vaccination immunity and virus induced immunity. There will be so many immune that the virus will eventually struggle to find any more susceptible hosts to infect. It will burn out and crash quite quickly; that was the rationale. But new variants causing the latest burst of infection in late 2022 and early 2023 will be the most challenging of the last two years. Most of the serious cases will be among the unvaccinated, and for them, immunity will be their consolation prize. Currently in Australia, unvaccinated people are 24 times more likely to be admitted to an ICU than those who are triple vaccinated.

UK Experience a Warning for Other Countries

When Australia debated whether to end quarantine requirements for close contacts of Covid cases, and reduce quarantine period for cases, the UK and Europe had already begun to unwind restrictions and offer a reveal into how post-pandemic life works and what lesson could be learned. The last of England's remaining mitigation strategies were abandoned at the beginning of March 2022: anyone testing positive was no longer legally required to isolate at home; residents did not have to keep testing or tell employers that they had virus; no mask mandate for most public spaces; and free mass symptomatic and asymptomatic testing for the general public ended.

The UK was learning to live with Covid but by no means virus-free. The danger of contracting the virus still lurked everywhere and cases soared, with a record number of more than 4.1 million people infected with the coronavirus mainly *Omicron* across England by the end of March one month after abandoning restrictions in February, and recording as an example, 19,950 new cases on 14th April. In the UK, managing Covid is now an exercise in personal responsibility. Some people still feel trepidation about learning to live with the coronavirus after two years of anxiety and disruption and are understandably cautious about a return to normal, particularly with the emergence of the new Omicron variants. '*Living with COVID*', will mean different things to different people; to many, it means doing nothing but for others it means responding sensibly to the change and minimising its potential effects, yet others will be fearful unable to adapt and may even become housebound.

The pandemic is not over yet in the UK as infection and reinfection pose continued threat to the economy and its health systems. The unwinding of all restrictions meant that the aged and clinically vulnerable people like the immunocompromised had to increase their own precautions to protect themselves pushing them further into self-shielding. For them with so many people infected in England, going anywhere meant assuming that any indoor or outdoor environment, in fact any public space will have infected people in it. A model of learning to live with Covid like the UK isn't simply just '*ignoring the virus*', but providing safe environments for everyone including the aged and immunocompromised to exist with it, a strategy which unfortunately Australia only took minimal notice of. A more appropriate model of learning to live with the virus requires not just high vaccination levels but also ventilation standards in all public buildings and workplaces, public education about airborne transmission, people wearing masks and social distancing, particularly in indoor high-risk environments and sanitising hands.

The UK's experience in unwinding restrictions also has further lessons for the world. There, public debate has jolted medical authorities to start offering a fifth booster jab before winter 2022 to keep a lid on the new variants and is probably something that everybody right around the world is going to have to do.

The Australian Approach

A similar pattern of increased transmission during 2022 has developed in Australia. On July 31, 2021, various Australian states were in deep lockdown with contact tracing. That day, in the previous 24 h, 7 new cases were recorded. The pandemic's total cumulative cases in Australia had reached just over 34,000 infections with the cumulative deaths of 924 persons. The CFR was 2.7. (https://www.covid19data.com.au). State premiers were giving daily media reports each morning with detailed Covid updates on cases and deaths to a panicked population. The goal then was no new cases and no deaths with severe isolating lockdowns mandated masks and for some professionals in health, education and police services mandated vaccination.

Fast-forward a year and on Friday 30 July 2022, Australia recorded just over 45,000 new cases of Covid in the previous 24 h with 5000 admitted to hospital, the nation's total cumulative pandemic caseload nudged 10 million, with the saddest statistic of all being the deaths of 157 people across Australia that day. These July 2022 drastically compare with the low figures a year earlier, and testify to the current surge by Omicron and especially its variants *BA.4* and *BA.5*; more contagious but less lethal with a *CFR* around 0.08. In hindsight, public health mandated regulatory over reaction to such low figures in 2021 with its quarantine, movement restrictions and contact tracing, when compared with the current 2022 situation of burgeoning cases and deaths appears well overblown (Mathieu et al., 2022).

What has changed? The answer lies in:

1. Partly as noted in Chap. 1 from *Rt* data, that current *BA.4* and *BA.5* are more transmissible than previous variants and subvariants, and are better able to evade immunity from vaccines and previous infections, and
2. Partly from the current cavalier approach of authorities having no wish to re-arouse public backlash by imposing mandates but simply offer encouragement and advice for people to take responsibility and sensible precautions which apparently some didn't.

In the age of *Omicron*, personal responsibility has become the mantra as Western societies move somewhat clumsily towards reclaiming personal freedoms lost in the name of securing public health but this can be a double edged sword. The freedom is not total freedom but has to be a *responsible* freedom; it means being sensible, heeding health advice to be applied in terms of personal lifestyle, age, gender, etc. Every person has the right to ignore medical advice and refuse medical treatment but must accept responsibility for the implications and these are shaping up to be quite devastating for the unvaccinated and partially vaccinated among young people and aged care persons.

While many have been pleased at this opening up, there has been considerable criticism that vulnerable people would be hit hardest as the changes infer social mixing is acceptable. Rather than a removal of restrictions, it actually presents *a removal of protection* allowing those who want to do what they want freedom to do so without consideration of others. In most democracies the emphatic notion is that individual responsibility is good and collectivism bad. The reverse is probably more relevant in dangerous situations. Thinking of ourselves as a collective in pandemic times increases community involvement, more democratic decision making rather than imposed decisions, facilitates mutual aid groups with a thrust towards shared identity and shared responsibilities increasing the resilience of the community and slows down the spread of the virus. Thus restricting our thinking and policy to individual and personal responsibility may seem like sound politics but in public health terms maybe not so bright, and ignores consideration of the more vulnerable such as the aged, the impoverished, the mentally ill, the disabled and their range of care workers.

Worldwide, there has been a considerable loosening of restrictions during mid-2022. Despite covid cases tripled across Europe in the six weeks prior to the end of July, as travel and tourism has returned in full swing accounting for nearly half of all infections globally, according to the World Health Organisation. For example, health authorities in Greece a major tourist destination, announced 136,077 new cases of Covid and 271 virus-related deaths during the week of July 18 to 24. While Italy did away with the health pass that had been required to enter restaurants, cinemas, gyms and other venues. People who catch Covid are no longer required to go into self-isolation in Spain. In Germany, travellers no longer have to prove their vaccinated to enter the country. In May, the European Union dropped its mask mandate for passengers on flights. In the same month, Greece lifted Covid restrictions on foreign and domestic flights. Even as Europe has come to rely on a vaccine-only strategy, there not enough people have taken up the three or four jabs necessary to prevent the spread of Omicron. The WHO encouraged European governments to increase vaccine uptake in the general population ahead of 2022 winter when other respiratory illnesses were likely to circulate. People's behaviour, however, remains a challenge.

To those exploring the possibility of a European holiday all appears to be normal. But people will need to evaluate their own risks before leaving the house or travelling abroad. That includes all the usual considerations like where you are going, who you are meeting with, whether you are meeting indoors, how long you will be indoors, whether you will be wearing a mask and do a *RAT* test if you get a sniffle or other indication. While vaccines have put us in a better position than two and half years ago, the path out of the pandemic depends on striking the right balance between complacency and constant vigilance. Good news is that countries where mask-wearing is a cultural norm, particularly Japan, South Korea, Singapore, are having success against the persistent *Omicron* subvariants offering a policy to lower transmission. Underlying the widespread acceptance of masks in these counties is a sense of personal responsibility to protect others.

People are on the move again, with personal and public reactions towards the pandemic totally changed. The sense of unity people felt at the start of the pandemic has given way to individual responsibility or is it irresponsibility? Authorities are responding to the public wave. Instead of treating the surge in cases as an emergency, most nations now appear to be committed to living with the virus, free from lockdowns and mandates and with borders wide open. Yet, as the virus has changed, so too have our personal risk acceptance levels.

Depending on future evidence the reset that populations around the world are enjoying may have to be short lived with minor levels of mask wearing and social distancing strongly recommended as new variants keep emerging. *XBB* and *BB1* are starting to move round the globe with perhaps an ominous outcome at superspreader events for the Xmas/New Year festive season 2022/23. It is unlikely lockdowns and international travel will be reimposed except China. Lockdowns and long isolation for contacts created havoc economically, socially and emotionally in most nations and as Chap. 10 indicates were originally imposed without any cost–benefit analysis.

Now the messaging in western nations has become somewhat confusing, with no clear signals on mask-wearing and other precautionary measures, and booster shot being ignored. In 2021 on 7 April Victoria with only 8 cases the state government imposed over 70 days of extremely strict quarantine/isolation. April 2022 there were around 9000 cases, but no action from the state government. This inaction represents not a positive policy but a general lackadaisical approach with authorities fearing to reignite the anti-establishment furore of the earlier severe mandates (Chap. 3).

Health bureaucrats should only be a source of advice. Elected politicians should make the decisions (and can be held responsible). Every nation now needs to realise the goal to eliminate war against Covid is over, with *Omicron* and its variants imposing an acceptance of reality that the original approach must be diluted and realigned with what we now know. That is a sensible wariness of infection, with isolation of the symptomatic, an unremitting focus on vaccinations, application of current and evolving treatment practices based on valid and reliable research, and better health resourcing particularly to those who are clearly now identified as the most vulnerable like the aged, and the drastic reframing of strict isolation rules that were destroying the economic bases of countries particularly in respect of supply chains and hospital staff. It must be accepted that even triple or quadruple vaccination won't stop some from getting the disease or even reinfection and passing it on.

The lowering of booster vaccination levels (Table 2.2), along with the risk posed to vulnerable people, experts say allowing the virus to run unchecked gives it more opportunity to develop new mutations that evade immunity. As new variants and subvariants continue to emerge, it already feels as if we have become locked in a vicious cycle with more transmission spurring more variants and more variants driving more transmission. Comparing Covid with influenza was a fallacy too. If you get the flu, it's bad for you in that period when you have it. Once you're out of it, you're out of it. Covid is not that simple. It has a number of long-term complications which seem to increase every time you get it plus the ongoing saga with Long Covid. We still don't know how long these complications linger after infection, so it was unclear how harmful repeat infections could end up being. We are only at the beginning of a long journey involving both Covid and Long Covid.

Table 2.2 Booster per 100 persons of population various dates in Oct 2022

Country	*Boosters per 100 persons in population*
Chile	139.3
Singapore	78.8
Italy	75.4
France	64.4
UK	59.8
Australia	54.5
USA	42.0
India	15.5
Russia	13.2

Data does not discriminate between having one or two boosters, e.g. Chile. (specific items culled from Mathieu et al. Our World in Data—Covid based on Johns Hopkins University COVID-19 Data Repository)

The overall picture reveals that in many Western nations there has been a massive failing of leadership in public health, abandoning health and science, that is impacting not only lives but the economy. An unfettered epidemic is essentially running with a vaccine-only strategy that is insufficient. A multilayered approach is essential and the more layers you stack together the better to reduce transmission. The time has come for a new Covid campaign to refresh people's understanding of how additional behaviours to vaccines, like masking, physical distancing, hygiene, testing can influence their and others' risk of new or reinfection.

The Pandemic of Reinfection

Much early thinking was that full vaccination would be the saviour. However, research now begs to differ. Reinfection is now a growing problem globally, as with every reinfection you get cumulative health impacts, with increased risk of significant cardiovascular complications.

The level of protection you have depends on factors such as:

- Age/immunocompromised status: This means you are less likely to produce a robust response to vaccination, thereby increasing a your risk of reinfection.
- Vaccination: There is a lower reinfection rate in those who have been vaccinated.
- Time: Antibodies to viruses wane over time, so you're more likely to be reinfected from the 28-day mark.

It all comes down to how many antibodies you've got left in your system when you next get exposed to the virus. The Omicron mutated subvariants in mid/late 2022 have a higher level of immune escape and are able to sidestep around the antibodies produced in the initial infection. Generally, reinfections are likely to be less severe than primary infections.

In June 2022, US researchers published preliminary results of a study looking at the impacts of Covid infection and reinfection using health records of more than 5 five million American veterans, of whom 250,000 people had been infected once, 36,000 who had been infected twice, and 2000 people who had been infected three times. For every health outcome measured, the hazard ratio (a measure of how often something happens in one group compared to another) *increased with each infection.* (Al-Aly et al., 2022). The risk of cardiovascular disease, for example, increased after one infection, but doubled in people who had two infections, and tripled in those who had been infected thrice. Similar cumulative risks with successive reinfection were also shown for pulmonary disease, clotting and blood disorders, neurological disease, mental health problems, kidney disease, musculoskeletal disease, fatigue and so on. The message from the data is clear: Covid is not just a bit of flu, and having it once doesn't 'get it over with'.

Real-world data from the UK Health Security Agency report week 19 (May 2022) showed the ability of current vaccines to stop people getting infected or reinfected has been dramatically reduced in the face of the newest and most immune-evasive variant. Among people who received two *AstraZeneca* doses and a *Pfizer* booster, protection against infection (10–14 weeks post-vaccination) had fallen from 95% against *Delta t*o just 45% against *Omicron.* For people who received two doses of the *AstraZeneca ChAdOx1-S* vaccine and then a *Pfizer BNT162b mRNA booster*, by week 20 the data from the UK Health Security Agency indicated zero protection against infection with Omicron. Ditto for the *Moderna* booster if you received *Pfizer* for your first two shots. You should assume you have less protection now, and while it's essential to get your boosters, don't make the mistake of ditching masks or social distancing permanently. .

Covid and Pregnancy

Recent US research from Centres for Disease Control has revealed that Covid infection during pregnancy increases potentially dangerous health issues compared to non-pregnant women, with 10% higher risk for severe infection, 4% of being admitted to ICU and 3% for ventilation. Not only were pre-term births and neonatal deaths higher, one-third of babies born to covid infected mothers required admission to neonatal ICU. Thus, unvaccinated pregnant women add to the list of covid compromised.

For a pregnant woman, Covid vaccination does NOT increase the risk of or cause miscarriage. Numerous peer-reviewed articles in respected medical journals include many tens of thousands of pregnancies in all, and come from many countries. For example, the Nordforsk study in Norway and Denmark (2021–2022) looked at 160,000 pregnancies between May 2021 and January 2022. The researchers examined whether the pregnant women were at a higher risk of complications such as premature birth, stillbirth and low foetal growth. No increased risk was found for any of the pregnancy complications examined. Miscarriage is unfortunately a relatively common pregnancy problem, occurring in approximately 25% of all pregnancies, so there will be cases of women experiencing miscarriage around the time of receiving their Covid vaccination. However, this association is coincidental, not causal, with published data indicating the risk of miscarriage is similar in both vaccinated and unvaccinated women. The conclusion is that pregnant women should not avoid vaccination.

COVID Isn't Over When You Stop Coughing; Beware the Coffin They Carry You off in!

Transitioning from Intensive Care

Through the course of the pandemic, there have been thousands of intensive care unit (ICU) admissions around the world. A large number of these were older individuals, but a remarkable number were also younger, formerly healthy individuals. For all patients, the shock of being admitted to ICU and their experiences while being treated are extreme, and for many can make readjusting to everyday life a struggle. In fact a new syndrome, post-intensive care syndrome has been postulated as a crisis after a crisis. Cognitive deficits and mood disorders are common in those who survive the ICU, with 47% suffering from depression or anxiety even two years post-ICU. Adding to the stress for some are financial difficulties and social dislocation after a long stay in ICU (Guck et al., 2021).

Though research in this area with regards to Covid is still somewhat limited, Guck et al. (2021) have drawn from extensive existing literature on the psychological consequences of ICU stays with other diseases to create a probable list of psychological issues Covid patients may face post-ICU. Using existing publications on medical interventions for other breathing infections like *SARS* and *MERS*, the team identified five broad areas of issues that commonly occur in post-ICU patients: medical trauma and post-traumatic stress, cognitive deficits, fatigue and depression, social stress and readjustment, and illness anxiety. The authors argue that each of these may need treating in different ways according to individual differences in intensity, some involving cognitive behaviour therapy and some diaphragmatic breathing exercises, with emphasis on those that can be delivered as outpatient or telemedical interventions.

Long Covid

There are also serious medical and psychological problems for former Covid patients worldwide who had not required ICU treatment. These former patients report experiencing a wide array of extended symptoms, which have collectively been dubbed *Long Covid*. It is turning into a mass casualty event in many nations, and a significant cause of long-term disability, given its 1 in 10 to 1 in 30 presentation after the main Covid event.

Long Covid bundles up a wide range of conditions in different combinations from person to person and there is no diagnostic test for who may or may not develop it. Health professional involvement can be anything from cardiologists, to respiratory physicians, to endocrinologists and urologists because there's more than 200 potential symptoms in total that sufferers have singly or in combination that need addressing. The problem arises in making sure people are triaged appropriately to the right destination person. Many of these symptoms are neuropsychological, and while theories exist as to what may be causing these symptoms no single mechanism has been agreed upon yet. Describing it as a '*post-Covid condition*', the WHO can still only define Long Covid vaguely as an occurrence in people with a history of probable or confirmed infection usually three months from the onset of Covid with symptoms that last for at least two months and that cannot be explained by another diagnosis.

Around the world about 10 to 30% of people infected with the coronavirus are developing Long Covid symptoms the most enduring of which include crippling fatigue, brain fog, headaches, loss of smell and hair loss, along with other physically debilitating symptoms like shortness of breath, vertigo, pain and numbness, sleep disruption, and scarring of the lungs. Of most severe patients, some become bed-bound. Symptoms may fluctuate, disappearing then return over time. Surprisingly, it is hitting many extremely fit people across the world who did not experience a prior severe Covid infection. All of a sudden a few weeks after their last acute Covid-like symptoms resolved, these Long Covid symptoms emerge.

What we do know is Long Covid produces many signs and symptoms that are consistent with autoimmune disorders, and that suggests that it may be immune suppression or immune activation or even hormonal manipulation. Covid is not just any virus. It is a very inflammatory virus causing systemic inflammation and via the blood vessels with the inflammation transported round the body everywhere with the blood circulation. In that way the virus may inflame a variety of organs such as the liver, the heart, the kidneys, and the brain.

Long Covid funding is being provided by many health authorities around the world, such as the USA ($1.5 billion) and the UK (£50 million) spending heavily on tackling it with innovative research projects for new treatments and comprehensive patient support. In the UK nearly 2 million people are suffering Long Covid and 1.4 million of these, according to the UK Office for National Statistics (Census Report April 2022), report that Long Covid affects their day-to-day lives, and unfortunately felt Long Covid was not taken seriously because many of the symptoms of Long Covid mimic other illnesses and disorders. This led to diagnosis and treatment delay as the first task of doctors is to ensure that the patient does not have another illness or infection before assuming it must be Long Covid. It was noted that this scepticism in now declining in the UK with wider awareness of the numbers of sufferers involved.

Research into Long Covid

Research from Leicester University UK into the impact of Long Covid involving a 2,000 strong sample from 39 NHS hospitals who had been admitted after contracting Covid found that only 25% of people who had been hospitalised had fully recovered five months after they had been discharged, which increased only slightly to 29% after a year. Being female, or obese or having had mechanical ventilation while in hospital were all associated with even poorer rates of recovery. Among the symptoms reported by these patients a year after their initial infection were fatigue, muscle pain, poor sleep and breathlessness.

In a very recent study in the UK comparing 46 severe Covid patients with 460 matched controls, researchers found the cognitive impairment is the equivalent to ageing 20 years, going from 50 to 70 years old, or losing 10 IQ points. The specific neurological brain changes presented a distinctive pattern different from those seen in early dementia or general ageing (Hampshire, 2022). Given that more than around 2 million people have been hospitalised in the UK with Covid over the past two years, it is clear from such findings that the legacy of this disease is going to be huge not just in the UK but globally. The limited rate of recovery in terms of improvements in brain function, mental health, organ impairment and quality of life demands urgent development of ways to tackle Long Covid is becoming a highly prevalent long-term condition.

In another UK large sample study, those experiencing Long Covid have reported a wider set of symptoms than previously thought, including hair loss and sexual dysfunction. Electronic health records of 2.4 million people in the UK from January 2020 to April 2021 were analysed (Subramanian et al., 2022). The cohort included 486,149 people with confirmed SARS-CoV-2 infection who were not admitted to hospital, matched with a control group of 1.9 million people with no recorded evidence of coronavirus infection. People who tested positive for the virus reported at least one of 62 symptoms more frequently 12 weeks after initial infection with Covid than those who had not contracted the virus. The frequent symptoms were loss of sense of smell, hair loss, sneezing, ejaculation difficulty, reduced libido and shortness of breath. Other common symptoms were chest pain, a hoarse voice and fever.

An extremely large sample UK study (Thompson et al., 2022) reviewed data from nearly 7000 people in health surveys plus electronic health records of more than 1.1 million people diagnosed with Covid. They found symptoms of Long Covid more frequent

- in females, with the odds 50% higher in women than men.
- in those with poor health before the pandemic, asthma particularly increases chances of getting the post-viral illness, but no strong evidence

of associations of Long Covid with a previous medical history of diabetes, high blood pressure or high cholesterol was evident, and
- in those aged 50+, with the likelihood of developing Long Covid increasing up to the age of 70.

A British innovation in the Long Covid saga is a Living with Covid Recovery app that a clinician can recommend to a patient for self help. It includes topics like breathing, nutrition, anxiety, mindfulness, fatigue, brain fog, depression and sleep which patients have singly or in various combinations. Patients work through the interactive programmes, which clinicians can monitor and offer feedback. It has been instituted in 42 clinics so far with 410 clinicians supporting 6500 patients. It is not a randomised control trial, but trajectories can be discerned and the programme appears successful for most who use it and evaluation is ongoing.

A variety of large-scale studies are ongoing in US public and private health sectors, including the National Institutes Of Health (NIH) and Veterans Affairs (VA). For veterans alone, more than 620,000 have been diagnosed with Covid, more than 22,000 have died, and nearly four percent have died from related health conditions, roughly twice the rate of the general public in the USA. There are currently 17 VA sites around the country, studying veterans who are feeling the lingering effects of Covid. An estimated 4,300 patients, of the more than 23,000 officially diagnosed with Long Covid are taking part in this research, will actually serve to provide clear directions for treatments and strategies moving forward. The VA is uniquely qualified to take part in such a research study, given the care, education and research it's provided for so long to so many veterans on a laundry list of debilitating diseases. The VA is also be part of a wider-ranging collaborative NIH study, that is focussing on those with and without long-term Covid symptoms using sample of 40,000 people, which hopefully will provide some answers in this complex puzzle of an evolving virus. But even addressing some of the comorbidities that accompany Long Covid such as depression and PTSD has not been shown to be helpful in reducing the underlying main effects of Long Covid such as fatigue, brain fog, pain and numbness.

Most of the patients at St Vincent's Hospital new Covid clinic are young people. This clinic was opened in late March 2022 and April 2022 saw another open in the Australian Capital Territory as its deleterious effects on many former Covid patients come to light. Other studies have shown that patients who are at higher risk of post-Covid conditions are those who have other existing chronic illnesses such as respiratory disease, diabetes, hypertension, also, those who are of older age.

Long Covid is now impacting ability to work, with up to 4 million Americans with serious debilitations and many bed bound contributing to the labour shortfall there. Similarly in the UK, the Trades Union Council estimate 20% of Covid patients have left the workforce. Long Covid is affecting the ability of sufferers to remain employed but many are unable to obtain short workers' disability and workers' compensation with Long Covid still not recognised as a medical condition. With around 6 million Australians having contracted the virus, with an average of around 20% depending on sample getting Long Covid, that could mean up to 1.2 million are likely to be affected by a burden of multiple mild to serious Long Covid symptoms, which could have a significant impact for the healthcare system and even the workforce. The Australian Government estimates that it has already cost the Australian economy 3 million working days in 2022 alone seriously affecting the labour market with 12% of Covid-related absenteeism attributed to Long Covid.

Cardiovascular and Diabetes Risk

In Australia, two medical research bodies are delving into the long-term effects of Covid. The Busselton Population Medical Research Institute holds some of the most detailed community-health data in Australian derived samples on volunteer baby boomers at different stages of their lives, to help identify chronic disease patterns and risk factors. These samples are sent to Murdoch University's Australian National Phenome Centre (ANPC) and compared with data all over the world to try to determine the long-term impacts of Covid. The investigation to date shows that a year after a Covid episode, there is a much increased cardiovascular risk, and its severity is strongly correlated with the severity of the initial infection. There's also evidence of new onset diabetes and increased diabetes risk in the general population that's been exposed to Covid.

Erectile Dysfunction

When you get Covid, it can affect the lining of the blood vessels, and this can create difficulty in getting blood flow from one part of the body to the other, including blood flow to the penis. Getting Covid can make men at five times higher risk of erectile dysfunction according to US research, and some men are also experiencing penis shrinkage after battling Covid (Harirugsakul 2020).

Brain Fog

One of the more widespread cognitive consequences of Long Covid is '*brain fog*' manifesting variously as extremely low energy, confusion and poor memory. Two years after having Covid, diagnoses of brain fog, dementia and epilepsy are more common than after other respiratory infections (Zhao et al., 2022). Studies at Harvard University estimate 22–32% of recovered Covid patients develop brain fog. While brain fog (or difficulty concentrating) isn't a medical term, it's generally used for certain symptoms that can affect ability to think and is one of the most common symptoms with many post-Covid patients unable to perform their usual activities including work and study due to their post-Covid neurological effects. But there is a spectrum with some mild change in cognition that is barely noticeable while others are unable to work at all.

More brain fog, neurological and psychiatric disorders were seen during the *Delta* variant wave than with the prior *Alpha* variant. The *Omicron* wave was linked with similar neurological and psychiatric risks as Delta. It is still not known how severe, or how long-lasting, the disorders are. Nor is it clear when they began, since problems may be present for some time before a diagnosis is made.

In June 2022, researchers at La Trobe University found 'toxic clumps of protein', or amyloid assemblies, appearing in the brain after a Covid infection appeared to be similar to those found in Alzheimer's disease and dementia. These may have been responsible for the brain fog neurological symptoms of Long Covid. The good news is that the study shows children are not as severely affected on the whole and tend to recovery over a finite time (Charnley et al. 2022). Another Australian study, the collaborative ADAPT study, an ongoing observational study involving St Vincent's Hospital Sydney and University of New South Wales has found similar effects with about 20% of those suffering from Long Covid experiencing brain impairment for at least 12 months without improvement after analysing 128 patients over 12 months. Importantly, the researchers have identified a nerve toxin in a particular pathway in the brain that causes cognitive impairment. This explains why the symptoms have been likened to a traumatic brain injury. This provides the possibility of repurposing existing drugs to modulate this toxin, potentially offering a treatment.

A recent Swedish study of Long Covid (Hedberg et al., 2022) also supports the autoimmune/brain toxin disorders hypothesis with evidence that some Covid-recovered people may harbour pockets of SARS-CoV-2 somewhere in their body just enough to activate the immune system. This is similar to shingles developing derived from Chicken pox virus after many decades, but in the case of Covid the viral activation of the immune system occurs soon after initial recovery. Such infection may also reawaken latent viruses such as the Epstein–Barr virus to create problems for the bearer. Two non-structural proteins, produced during SARS-CoV-2 replication, have also been detected that can form amyloid clumps, which are toxic to brain and nerve cells. Amyloid is a molecular hallmark in some neurodegenerative diseases like Alzheimer's and Parkinson's which probably causes the common brain fog conditions in Long Covid. So focus is being extended in future research onto the interaction of viral protein relics with the autoimmune and nervous systems.

To illustrate the difficulties faced by those suffering from post-Covid brain fog, researchers based at Oxford University recently published a qualitative study which takes a detailed look at brain fog sufferers' lived experiences (Zhao et al., 2022). Recruiting via online support groups, the discussions participants had during small focus groups detail the life-changing impacts of cognitive impairment, from difficulties completing the weekly shop to extensive struggles with dismissive healthcare professionals. Many experienced issues conducting their jobs, and while some recovered over the course of the study, but many did not, suggesting this may become another widespread long-standing post-Covid issue for both patients and healthcare professionals in the future.

Further studies using brain imaging at Oxford University, University College London and the US National Institute of Health reveal Covid has caused even worse brain damage and shrinkage than was originally thought in patients who have only had mild respiratory illness from the virus. This neurobiological harm showed shrinking of the brain in areas processing smell, memory, thinking and emotion which can manifest as mood, anxiety and cognitive symptoms (Douaud et al., 2022). Long-term follow-up is planned to see if the effects reverse over time. As research suggests that around 81% of those with Long Covid may experience brain fog, there is an urgent need for specialised health and support services that are easily navigable by those suffering from the symptoms.

To help reduce and even clear brain fog, the following are recommended to boost thinking and memory:

- Exercise. Start slow, perhaps just two to three minutes a few times a day. While there is no established 'dose' of exercise to improve brain health, 30 min a day, five days a week is generally recommended.
- Eat a Mediterranean-style diet including olive oil, fruits and vegetables, nuts and beans, and whole grains has been shown to improve thinking, memory and brain health.
- Avoid alcohol and drugs. Give your brain the best chance to heal by avoiding substances that can adversely affect it.
- Sleep well. Sleep is a time when the brain and body can clear out toxins and work towards healing. Give your body the sleep it needs.
- Participate in social activities. We are social animals. Not only do social activities benefit our moods, but they help our thinking and memory as well.
- Pursue other beneficial activities, like listening to music, practising mindfulness and keeping a positive mental attitude.
- Break tasks into sequential units and tackle each in turn.

Note that this is general advice; as yet there are no specific proven, medically prescribed therapies or time line to treat 'brain fog'. Pace yourself and give yourself time to recover. Everybody's journey is different. Don't be too hard on yourself if you are not meeting your expectations for recovery. Consider specialist referral if there are 'red flag' symptoms that could be new-onset dementia or epilepsy. With still limited understanding of all the ramifications of Long Covid, it is apparent that it will pose a serious, health, economic and social impact worldwide over the next few decades. There is an urgent need for dedicated Long Covid clinics globally.

For a very recent book detailing the Swedish 'experiment' check out *The Herd: How Sweden Chose its Own Path Through the Worst Pandemic in 100 years,* by Anderberg (2022) Scribe Press.

For readers who wish to read more detail on some of these historic pandemics try Wright, J. (2017) *Get Well Soon.* Holt and Co. New York.

References

ADAPT Study. St Vincent's Hospital Sydney. Retrieved 23 September 22 from https://www.svhs.org.au

Al-Aly, Z., Bowe, B., & Xie, Y. (2022). Outcomes of SARS-CoV-2 reinfection. *Research Square*. https://doi.org/10.21203/rs.3.rs-1749502/v1

Anderberg, J. (2022). *The herd: How Sweden chose its own path through the worst pandemic in 100 years*. Scribe Press.

Australian Government Department of Health and Aged Care. Health Alerts updated weekly. https://www.health.gov.au/health-alerts/covid-19/case-numbers-and-statistics

Centers For Disease Control (2019). Retrieved 27 September 22 from (https://www.cdc.gov/coronavirus/2019-ncov/cases-updates/special-populations/pregnancy-data-on-covid-19/what-cdc-is-doing.html)

Charnley, M., Islam, S., Bindra, G. K., et al. (2022). Neurotoxic amyloidogenic peptides in the proteome of SARS-COV2: Potential implications for neurological symptoms in COVID-19. *Nature Commun., 13*, 3387. https://doi.org/10.1038/s41467-022-30932-1

Crawley, R. (1914). *The history of the Peloponnesian war*. Dent.

Dhama, K., Khan, S., Tiwari, R., et al. (2020). Coronavirus disease 2019–COVID-19. *Clinical Microbiology Reviews 33*(4). https://doi.org/10.1128/CMR.00028-20

Dix, C. (2022). The guardian report. Retrieved 15 April 22 from https://www.theguardian.com/world/2022/jan/08/end-mass-jabs-and-live-with-covid-says-ex-head-of-vaccine-taskforce

Douaud, G., Lee, S., Alfaro-Almagro, F., et al. (2022). SARS-CoV-2 is associated with changes in brain structure in UK Biobank. *Nature, 604*, 697–707. https://doi.org/10.1038/s41586-022-04569-5

Freiesleben, N., Egerup, P., Hviid, K. V. R., et al. (2021). SARS-CoV-2 in first trimester pregnancy: a cohort study. *Human Reproduction, 36*(1), 0–47. https://doi.org/10.1093/humrep/deaa311

Guck, A., et al. (2021). Psychological complications of COVID-19 following hospitalization and ICU discharge: Recommendations for treatment. *Professional Psychology: Research and Practice, 52*, 318–327. (2021) https://doi.org/10.1037/PRO0000402

Hampshire, A., Chatfield, D. A., Jolly, A., et al. (2022). Multivariate profile and acute-phase correlates of cognitive deficits in a COVID-19 hospitalised cohort. *EClinicalMedicine, 47*, 101417. https://doi.org/10.1016/j.eclinm.2022.101417

Harirugsakul, K., Wainipitapong, S., & Phannajit, J. (2022). Erectile dysfunction after COVID-19 recovery: A follow-up study. *PLoS ONE*. https://doi.org/10.1371/journal.pone.0276429

Holmes, E. (2022). University of Sydney Media Office. 18 August 2022. How do we know the origins of covid came from a market? Retrieved 30 September

22 from https://www.sydney.edu.au/news-opinion/news/2022/08/18/how-do-we-know-the-origins-of-covid-came-from-a-market.html

Hedberg, P., Granath, F., Bruchfeld, J., et al. (2022). Post COVID-19 condition diagnosis: A population-based cohort study of occurrence, associated factors, and healthcare use by severity of acute infection. *Journal of Internal Medicine.* https://doi.org/10.1111/joim.13584. https://www.covid19data.com.au. Creative Commons Attribution 4.0 Int. Lic. Retrieved 04 September 22

Leicester Biomedical Research Centre. Press release 16 12 2021. People with Long-COVID after hospitalisation face limited recovery after one year. Retrieved 03 March 22 from. https://www.leicesterbrc.nihr.ac.uk/phosp-covid-one-year/

Living with Covid Recovery App. https://www.ucl.ac.uk/healthcare-engineering/covid-19/covid-19-engineering-research/living-covid-recovery Retrieved 20 September 22

Mathieu E., Ritchie, H., Rodés-Guirao, L., et al. (2022). Our world of data—Covid. Published online at OurWorldInData.org. Retrieved 24 October 22 from https://ourworldindata.org/coronavirus Online Resource

Murdoch University Western Australia. Retrieved 11 October 22 from https://www.murdoch.edu.au/news/articles/anpc-delivers-breakthrough-in-understanding-the-effects-of-covid-19

National Institutes of Health and Veteran Affairs. News briefs. https://www.research.va.gov/covid-19.cfm. and https://covid19.nih.gov/covid-19-topics/long-covid Both provide regular updates.

Nordforsk Studies on pregnancy 2021–2022. Retrieved 07 September 22 from https://www.nordforsk.org/news/key-findings-two-nordic-covid-19-studies

Pudsey, A. (2017). *Disability in antiquity chapter 2.* In C. Laes (Ed.), London.

Subramanian, A., Nirantharakumar, K., Hughes, S., et al. (2022). Symptoms and risk factors for long COVID in non-hospitalized adults. *Nature Medicine, 28*(8), 1706–1714. https://doi.org/10.1038/s41591-022-01909-

Thompson, E. J., Williams, D. M., & Steves, C. J. (2022). Long COVID burden and risk factors in 10 UK longitudinal studies and electronic health records. *Nature Communications., 13*(1), 13528. https://doi.org/10.1038/s41467-022-30836-0.3528

Trades Union Council, UK. 20 Jun 2021. Retrieved 17 August 21 from https://www.tuc.org.uk/research-analysis/reports/workers-experiences-long-covid; https://www.bbc.com/worklife/article/20220616-the-workers-battling-long-covid

UK Health Security Agency: COVID-19 vaccine surveillance report. Retrieved 26 October 22 from (https://www.gov.uk/government/publications/covid-19-vaccine-weekly-surveillance-reportsweek19)

UK Office of National Statistics (ONS). Census 2021. Published April 2022. Prevalence of ongoing symptoms following coronavirus (COVID-19) infection in the UK. Retrieved 3 December 22 from https://www.ons.gov.uk/peoplepopulationandcommunity/healthandsocialcare/conditionsanddiseases/bulletins/prevalenceofongoingsymptomsfollowingcoronaviruscovid19infectionintheuk/1december2022

WHO Sage Report. (2019). Retrieved 19 April 21 from https://www.who.int/groups/strategic-advisory-group-of-experts-on-immunization

Worobey, M., Levy, I., Serrano, M., et al. (2022). The Huanan seafood wholesale market in Wuhan was the early epicentre of the COVID-19 pandemic. *Science.* https://doi.org/10.1126/science.abp8715

Zhao, S., Shibata, K., Hellyer, P. J., et al. (2022). Rapid vigilance and episodic memory decrements in COVID-19 survivors, *Brain Communications, 4*(1). https://doi.org/10.1093/braincomms/fcab295

Zhou, P., Yang, X. L., Wang, X. G. et al. (2020). A pneumonia outbreak associated with a new coronavirus of probable bat origin. *Nature*. 579, 270–273. https://doi.org/10.1038/s41586-020-2012-7

CHAPTER 3

Impacts of Fake News and Conspiracy Theory

The greatest enemy of knowledge is not ignorance, It's the illusion of knowledge'
Daniel J. Boorstin
The problem with the world is that intelligent people are full of doubts, while the stupid ones are full of confidence'
Charles Bukowski
Real knowledge is to know the extent of one's ignorance'
Confucius

Abstract This chapter investigates the rapid spread of conspiracy theories, fake news and misinformation. The perpetrators were a heterogeneous grouping from those who genuinely felt aggrieved with the removal of personal freedoms by public health orders rather than by elected government, to long-term convinced anti-vaxxers, 'sovereign citizens' who argued no laws apply to them and even Doomsday preppers. Rallies and convoys blocking roads and bridges occurred in many world cities. The major focus was mandated vaccination. The impact of denialism, artificial confirmation bias and paranoia in creating this tumult is discussed. Miracle cures like Ivermectin became a popular online topic. The use of debunking, prebunking and the 'Bad News' game to thwart the conspiracy theories and fake news is discussed and shown to be effective.

Keywords Conspiracy theories · Fake news · Mandated vaccination · Denialism · Confirmation bias · Debunking

© The Author(s), under exclusive license to Springer Nature Singapore Pte Ltd. 2023
R. B. Burns, *The Human Impact of the COVID-19 Pandemic*,
https://doi.org/10.1007/978-981-99-1710-5_3

Introduction

The outbreak of the *SARS-CoV-2* novel coronavirus has been accompanied by another contagion, that of a plethora of misleading and false information, especially on social media, leading to an outflow of rage in street protests in many cities worldwide. Pandemics involve not only medical issues but equally evolve into socio-psychological issues encompassing human behaviour, attitudes and emotions as it is people who determine the spreading and containment of diseases by their behaviour and who can generate socially disruptive, divisive and potentially harmful actions like protests against mitigation restrictions, become panic buyers, manifest increasing domestic violence and descend into drug/alcohol abuse and mental stress.

The Conspiracy Theories, Fake News and Misinformation Virus

About 70 years ago, Dr Jonas Salk released the vaccine that prevented the scourge of polio round the world. There was barely any voice raised then, virtually all children were vaccinated, and no child eventually died needlessly through a disease that was entirely preventable nor did those vaccinated have to endure a lifetime of hobbling in callipers. Similar positive stories can be told about measles, mumps and chicken pox vaccinations and the disastrous impairments they have prevented. Yet despite this completely accessible history of fantastic medical successes, we now even have several rogue politicians leading an attack, opposing vaccine mandates, lockdowns, border closures and quarantine, one appearing on an inflammatory far right US TV programme InfoWars during which he urged people abroad to rise up and protest at Australian Government offices overseas. The programme host also compared Australian quarantine facilities with Auschwitz. A newly named Australian political party, the United Australian Party, was born to contest (rather unsuccessfully) the May 2022 general election, with anti-vaccine mandate manifestos like '*Freedom for all Australians*' and '*Equal treatment for all Australians*' to appeal to the mind-set of anti-vaxxers et al. This is clearly indicative that there has been and still is an increasingly obvious and concerning trend that the Covid virus is not the only pandemic sweeping the globe.

Conspiracy theory is not new. One of the earliest modern ones was the fake Russian *Protocols of the Elders of Zion* which as a classic of anti-semitism claimed the Jews were aiming to erect a secret world government. This was followed later by other deemed conspiracy events, such as Princess Diana faked her own death to escape the Royal family; that the CIA assassinated President Kennedy; and that the Port Arthur massacre in Tasmania was faked to give the government a solid argument for banning guns. Several important movies have given credence to conspiracy theories such as *The Da Vinci Code* with the falsehood of Christianity the focus. So too *The Matrix* that destroyed the idea that reality is reliable. It is not just the right wing involved, but also left wing post-modernism engaged with its narrative that there is no absolute reality only the interpretation of what each individual perceives.

Psychologists suggest three reasons why people are easily led into the conspiracy mind-set.

- Firstly, in a complex world, people really do want to know the truth about what is going on. Such as why are interest rates rising rapidly, and is the world actually heating up and if so is the real culprit carbon dioxide?
- Secondly, many people feel the current complexities of living that prevent them having control over their lives and believe external control of their lives is rampant, almost a form of delusional paranoia.
- Thirdly ,humans need social relationships and in-group cohesion with others who feel the same way is a major source of this, almost a magnetic attraction providing support and validation of one's beliefs especially for those more credulous than others and needing to boost their self-esteem.

But Covid, with the aid of the internet universe, ramped up conspiracy theory and mind-sets with the increasing incursion of government and its agencies into the everyday lives of every citizens. And many were uncomfortable with all or some of the mandates particularly compulsory vaccination. Conspiracies do occur from time to time and its quite reasonable to hold and debate issues about the efficacy of vaccines for example, as long as it is based on valid research evidence and a willingness to disagree peacefully.

Political Polarisation

One psycho-sociological barrier to positive national coordinated action to manage serious problems within countries is political polarisation. '*Attitudinal polarisation*' concerns groups that have opposing issue positions common in democratic countries, whereas '*affective polarisation*' implies groups really hate and distrust those from the opposing party(ies). Affective polarisation involves decreasing trust with dangerous political consequences, as in the recent US political scene, and in many nations, the conspiracy theories brigade, privileging partisan beliefs and misinformation over government policy information can undermine social and economic conditions and impair public health (van Bavel et al. 2018, 2020).

Polarisation is dangerous during a pandemic, as it can lead different segments of the population to arrive at different conclusions about the degree of threat and appropriate actions. Polarised group members and mainstream community receive different news and promoted beliefs as individuals self-select mainline news and social media sources or partisan '*echo chambers*' (Bakshy et al., 2015). Less cross-partisan interactions and information sharing have developed over the Covid issue due to isolation restrictions effecting a decrease in personal contact, reducing opportunity for cross-partisan communication that is essential to produce a shared understanding.

However, there are actionable steps that could reduce polarisation. First, the pandemic not only highlights a common identity with individuals all facing the same risk, but also fosters a sense of shared fate. By highlighting an overarching identity, politicians, the media and opinion leaders can reduce political division around the issue (see Chap. 4). Second, a growing body of work shows that misperceptions of the other side underlie polarisation (Lees et al., 2020). Therefore, it is vitally important to combat any misinformation that could generate partisan motivated reasoning and inaccurate beliefs (see 'Thwarting fake news and misinformation' below). Finally, leaders can highlight bipartisan support for Covid-related measures, when they exist, as such endorsements in other contexts have reduced polarisation and led to less-biased reasoning.

The Heterogeneity of Virus Restrictions Opposition

This rather insidious and dangerous *infodemic virus*, hanging onto the Covid coat tails, is a cacophony of conspiracy theories and false information infecting many credulous people around the world promoting 'sick' response behaviours that could lead some adherents, and worse still, innocent casual contacts into serious illness and even death. For example, one despicable person in Australia has been pretending to be an Aborigine and contacting other Aborigines to persuade them not to get vaccinated as it is a 'whiteman's ploy'.

The Australian convoy to Canberra displayed a heterogeneity of subgroups that showed up with diverse goals, overlapping motivations and some familiar calling cards of parallel recent Canadian and USA rallies and conflicting views within the groups about how they should make their stand (Crikey, 2022). Their sole bond was an emotional connection and general rejection of government and politics as a solution to their problems; strangers became friends as this passionately held tenet of belief found approving ears. In effect they'd found their community and people that were like them. It provided a sense of a shared community, for many, replacing loneliness with belonging.

The mobs that rampaged in rallies and convoys though the streets of many world cities, from Ottawa, Paris, Amsterdam and Canberra just to name a few, consist partly of the sad and the mad with deluded beliefs about the virus, unbacked by any scientific facts, plus another demographic, people distraught and angry that they have or were about to lose their jobs and other entitlements of democratic-free society such as freedom to cross borders, comfort sick and lonely elderly relatives and enjoy evening entertainment at club and pubs and not to be locked into their homes. This group who generally were not anti-vax or conspiracy devotees are perhaps people who may well possess and argue some ethical justification for their protests against governments' over-reach as will be noted in Chap. 10 where the ethics and moral judgement issues concerning over-reaching mandates and public health regulations are discussed. A perhaps unexpected group joining in were some extremist

Christians with an '*end of time*' rhetoric flowing on social media with the black hand of the Devil at work articulating the virus and the decision making of politicians and scientists as they lurched towards an apocalyptic finale with the 'Second Coming' imminent.

A far more insidious group infesting the rallies were '*sovereign citizens*' who believe that no law applies to them, refuse to pay income tax in many cases, as well as ignoring such things as driving licences, car insurance and of course public health requirements. They consider themselves to be '*natural*' persons, born with their own natural rights that are unable to be constrained by governments. They oppose the very foundations of democracy and rely on incorrect pseudo-legal language to assert their independence. How many of the rally groups feel about government edicts is reflected in the quote '*A plague on both your houses*' (of parliament) adapted from Shakespeare's Romeo and Juliet, Act III, Sc. 1; they forget that the prescient Shakespeare added the pun, '*Ask for me to-morrow, and you shall find me a grave man*'. Surprisingly, one small element that surfaced among the Canberra 'mob' was an anti-paedophile group. It looks as if any section of the populace with a grievance or mission adhered together as one protest.

Anti-vaxxers

Anti-vaxxers are not all stereotypic uneducated, unsophisticated laypeople from the lower socio-economic strata. The anti-vaccination proponents are also a heterogeneous group; some refuse all vaccination '*the vaccine resistant*', while '*the vaccine hesitant*' consists of many subgroups, with a variety of reasons offered.

Vaccine hesitants: Some want to avoid certain specific vaccinations or reduce or delay the overall number of vaccinations. There is also a naturalist bias in some communities, which maintains that since vaccines are manmade and therefore unnatural, they may confer an immunity inferior to natural immunity and have refused for a number of generations to get their children vaccinated. Among the hesitant are also those that may have had bad reactions to vaccines or medications in the past. Some may have underlying health issues or be undergoing treatment for other conditions and be worried about any side effects that a Covid vaccine might cause. In the vast majority of cases, doctors argue their fears are unfounded.

Misinformation about vaccine safety drives reluctance to vaccinate children an open-access study finds. Romer et al. (2022) reported nearly 78% of US adults but only 31% of children ages 5 to 11 had completed the primary set of vaccinations against COVID-19. They attributed that dramatic discrepancy to the acceptance of misinformation about the safety of vaccines for young people in general and the COVID-19 vaccines in particular. The researchers found that hesitancy to have children vaccinated against Covid was associated with misbeliefs, such as that vaccines contain toxins like anti-freeze, and about specific vaccines, such as the flu vaccine increasing the chances of contracting

Covid (no evidence exists for this). There are also still unfounded assertions from all over the world associated with the fears that the measles, mumps and rubella (MMR) vaccine cause autism spectrum disorder or neurological disorders thanks to the massive publicity given to the erroneous and invalid research of Dr Andrew Wakefield.

The latest attempt to thwart the real value of Covid vaccination to create more hesitants is an anti-vax conspiracy film *Died Suddenly* baselessly alleging that Covid vaccines are causing large numbers of deaths, particularly in young people (CheckMate ABC News investigation 02 Dec 22). It has been viewed more than 10 million times in 10 days. The nasty suggestion is that Covid vaccines have been deliberately designed as a depopulation tool. The CheckMate investigation revealed that the claims are incorrect, lack any evidence or have been taken out of context.

Many other hesitants are pregnant ladies, with concerns up to a third of pregnant women could be unvaccinated. President of the Royal Australian and New Zealand College of Obstetricians and Gynaecologists, Dr Bopp, believes that a third of pregnant women are fully vaccinated, a third have had one dose, and a third have had no doses whatsoever in Australia and N. Zealand. Misinformation, largely circulated through social media, claims there has not been enough research done on the effects on pregnant women. A recent study from Scotland, published in Nature Magazine (Stock et al., 2022), offers perhaps the clearest view of the scale of hesitancy among pregnant women. Analysis of data relating to more than 87,000 women between the start of vaccination uptake in December 2020 and October 2021 found that just 32 per cent of women who gave birth in October 2021 were fully vaccinated, compared with 77 per cent of the general female population aged 18 to 44. This is reflected in data from the UK Department of Health that showed 98 per cent of pregnant women critically ill in hospital with Covid were unvaccinated.

Demographic data finds that vaccine hesitants are more likely to be educated, older mothers with higher socio-economic status. Vaccine hesitancy is a worldwide phenomenon, but hesitant sentiments are still greatly in the minority, with estimates suggesting that about 80% of the world population agree that vaccines are safe (Franklin et al., 2019).

The Complacent Young: Another large proportion of the remaining unvaccinated can be broadly and crudely separated out into a category labelled 'the complacent young'. Currently, 85.2 per cent of 20 to 24-year-olds and 87 per cent of 25 to 29-year-olds are fully vaccinated (two vaccinations), in Australia which has an overall vaccination rate of one of the highest in the world, but there has been a lethargy towards getting the first booster. Lower rates for some younger age groups mean that about one in seven is unvaccinated, and these are the people that have been overwhelmingly the conduit for the recent surge in *Omicron* as their active mingling lifestyle provides a huge potential to spread the virus. While some young people are espoused to the conspiracy and anti-vaxxer beliefs, many are just apathetic assuming they are fit and bulletproof therefore less likely to get seriously ill or die from Covid.

The vaccine resistant real activists: Real activists are a tiny but vocal minority, strong in their views, diverse in their reasoning including those who have been converted online through conspiracy theories and misinformation. Their approach is '*psychological reactance*', a negative response to the imposition of rules, regulation or attempts at persuasion that are perceived as a threatening attack on autonomy and freedom of choice. Psychological reactance has been a common feature of many public health campaigns, e.g. fluoridation of water for dental hygiene and smoking. While these psychologically reactive people are a minority, they are vocal and determined.

In a longitudinal cohort study of psychological reactance in Poland (Waszkiewicz et al., 2022) on the public acceptability of Covid vaccination and real vaccination levels among a representative sample of adult Polish citizens conducted June 2020 and, one year later, the same group was approached to compare the hypothetical declarations with the real vaccination decisions. A significant part of the group that declared reluctance and hesitation towards Covid vaccination before it was available actually got vaccinated or planned to get vaccinated. Among the previously vaccine-reluctant individuals, the main reasons included concern about their health and safety (69%) and their desire to travel (26.6%) as well as the pursuit of herd immunity and a notion of common social safety (12.6%). The main factors helping to increase vaccination acceptance apparently in this group are based on a self-centred pursuit of safety and freedom from restrictions. A focus on these issues may help public health professionals to develop a more effective vaccination campaign.

It was Mark Twain who once said '*facts are stubborn things, but statistics are pliable*'; online poll results concerning vaccination should be taken with a grain of salt as they can be and have been easily manipulated. The Australian Broadcasting Corporation (ABC) 8 10 2022 underscored Twain's point by reporting a RMIT fact-check, concerning a set of responses to online questions that indicated half the respondents regretted getting vaccinated against Covid or were happy with their decision to remain unvaccinated. The survey also showed 'only 35 per cent out of more than 45,000 people said they were vaccinated and would make the same decision again'. Since more than 97 per cent of Australians over the age of 16 have had at least one dose of a Covid vaccine and more than 95 per cent have had two, the reported survey data obviously does not reflect reality. About 44 per cent of respondents claimed they had not received any doses of a COVID-19 vaccine, while the Federal Health Department reports that just 2.7 per cent of Australians aged 16 and over are unvaccinated.

Detailed analysis identified dozens of instances of the poll being shared in online groups populated by anti-vax activists, some with direct callouts encouraging manipulation of the results. '*come on folks get to it. Show them the results we want them to see*', one such post on Telegram reads. Another reads, '*keep voting and share far and wide*'. Links to the poll have also been shared outside Australia, including a Croatian Facebook user with more than

50,000 followers. Dr Kruger, director of the Asia Pacific division of the Information Futures Lab, indicated that in this example, the poll has been shared by groups that track back to anti-vaccine websites with a particular focus on Covid. These online poll results were certainly invalid as they typically reflect biased opinions of people who frequently 'used' social media to create certain false implications.

The take-away from those examples of mandate opponents above strongly indicates that it is an erroneous, uninformed and inadequate policy by governments and public health officials worldwide to lump all these subgroups together as this does not bring understanding of their different perceptions and motives which would facilitate the development of focussed attempts to try to alleviate the different concerns of the various subgroups. Despite this, there is much psychological evidence that what people say about their beliefs and attitudes in surveys is often different from what they actually do when faced with the real situation (e.g. this also occurs in ethnic or religious issues), and this holds for vaccination too as demonstrated in the Polish study above. Studies before vaccination was commenced generally predict a lower take-up than what eventually takes place when people are faced with a lethal pandemic. This is an optimistic sign that as the *Omicron* and other variants amplify case numbers and with unvaccinated persons' deaths on the rise, available vaccines are perceived as overwhelmingly safe and highly effective, with hesitancy and reactance considerably weakened.

Unfortunately, anti-vaccine viewpoints and arguments are more compelling and very widespread in social media like a magnet drawing in waverers. Yet, the general attitude of government and scientific literature towards all anti-vaxxers may appear hostile and strengthen their in-group bonding and generate unquestioning allegiance, a powerful example of psychological reactance (see Chap. 4).

Denialism

Denialism is also involved in maintaining belief. It is defined as rhetoric employed in order to give the appearance of legitimate debate where there is none, with the goal of rejecting an argument for which there is a consensus of expert opinion. A large subpopulation of the anti-vax movement are '*denialists*', typically motivated by ideology, eccentricity and idiosyncrasy. There are certain ground rules of scientific debate:

1. The ability to critically evaluate one's own as well as the opposing viewpoints,
2. The ability to consider all of the evidence rather than just portions of it,
3. The application of logic to making arguments. However, denialists do not employ these ground rules and render it impossible to debate a topic rationally.

Diethelm and McKee (2009) assigned central themes to denialism: these are conspiracy theories, 'fake' experts, selective consideration (or exclusion) of evidence, impossible expectations of research and misinterpretation of data and other logical fallacies. These elements obviate rational debate. To overcome these, Diethelm and McKee (op cit) suggest that pro-vaxxers change the subject from vaccines to the tactics that are being employed. If one could demonstrate that the anti-vax argument is unfair, biased, lopsided or distorting, it might help reveal that the arguments are not valid. Furthermore, by discussing 'how' the arguments are made rather than the arguments themselves, it may gradually sensitise denialists to the nature of scientific discussion. In other words, if denialists could be made to see, for example, that they are not considering all of the evidence but only a portion of it, it might help facilitate a more reasonable conversation.

Scientists are committed to truth and object to false or misleading information, and this necessitates a willingness to hold open discussions with people who hold opposing points of view. There is no other way to work through information and reach valid conclusions based on facts. For that reason, scientists must encourage frank, open and frequent discourse with denialist anti-vaxxers, but it is important for scientists to understand the different anti-vax viewpoints for the most productive and mutually beneficial conversations. Creating narrative stories can be a helpful tactic, as much as scientists tend to prefer data and dry facts. The anti-vax narrative is replete with extravagant anecdotal evidence and storylines which have the tendency to be misinterpreted, manipulated like Chinese whispers and liberally extrapolated. The resulting narratives have broad appeal as they are more tangible to the general populous. Storytelling can be effective communication, and there is no reason that it cannot be used by pro-vaxxers without sacrificing scientific soundness and accuracy. Vaccines protect us against a variety of terrible and even fatal diseases, and there is no reason that storytelling cannot be used to make the pro-vax arguments more persuasive and more 'human' than merely clinical trial data. A more liberal use of narrative stories to describe and defend the pro-vax viewpoint should be encouraged.

Artificial Confirmation Bias from Social Media

The sources are varied for misguided perceptions and beliefs. From naïve health gurus to violent anti-vaccination campaigners, right and left wing political agitators and even foreign governments who may wish to sow discord for political gain deliberate misinformation gushes to undermine evidence based medical advice mostly on social media. The total amount of misinformation exceeds anything we've ever seen before according to Van Bavel et al. (2020) who offer ways that behavioural sciences can mitigate the misinformation.

The difference between being *uniformed* and *misinformed* is that the former is a personal choice, while the latter is imposed without choice which is where social media tends to artificially generate confirmation bias by its unilateral presentation of certain viewpoints or so-called trending topics. Confirmation bias in vaccine hesitancy and anti-vax sentiment is often the major process of maintaining error. Such bias may extend beyond user-generated social media to mainstream and other news media outlets. Search engine algorithms and other editing algorithms tend to filter a user's internet experiences on the basis of prior searches and interactions. Thus, a person who has searched for anti-vax topics may in future searches get more or similar anti-vax information, creating a bubble of artificial confirmation bias that limits their exposure to alternative opinions and leaves them living in a fake news silo (Pariser, 2011). In essence, repetition makes the information easier to cognitively process, and this ease is misinterpreted as a signal that the information is actually true (*Truth-by-Repetition (TBR) effect*) creating a massive *group think* propulsion. Fear, confusion and isolation also combine to push our genetic engineering to pay more attention to danger, like *QAnon* material that claims the world is run by devil worshipping, baby killing paedophiles. It is a threat to your existence and scary news spreads 6 times faster than sound news.

It is not only 'crazies' that fall for fantastical misinformation and conspiracy theory. Whatever your opinion about aliens running the world or a flat earth, there is an online group who will validate it and hook you in more decisively. Far-fetched lies spread faster and are easier to digest than boring lengthy complicated truths. Social media has accelerated its impact as a study from Carnegie Mellon University (2020) reported that 5% of 200 million tweets about Covid were managed by bots rather than people. It additionally identified more than 100 false narratives about Covid that are proliferating on Twitter aimed at sowing division by accounts controlled by these bots.

A study of this sort of algorithm-driven social media ecology was offered by Johnson et al. (2020) about a burgeoning anti-vax tendency on Facebook. According to their seminal study, anti-vaxxers are better positioned on Facebook to target clusters of vaccine-neutral users and do so with greater efficiency than pro-vax groups. On the basis of mathematical models of the spread of anti-vax information within the primary network patch, Johnson et al. (op cit) have speculated that anti-vax viewpoints will predominate even to a greater extent in future. This should not be surprising, as evidence suggests that anti-vax information is very attractive to vaccine undecided and hesitant individuals, and this sort of individual can be swayed to make a lasting ideological change against vaccinations in 5 to 10 min (Betsch et al., 2010). Vaccine-sceptic individuals often lack the ability to critically assess online medical information in any case. In a study of 34 vaccine undecided students presented with 40 websites containing varying degrees of factual medical information about vaccinations, 59% of those in the study believed all of the websites contained accurate data when, in reality, only 18 of the 40 were accurate (Kortum et al., 2008).

Conspiracy Theories

Throughout the history of pandemics, conspiracy theories have been propagated alongside them; this combination is nothing new. In Roman times 331 BC, when an unknown plague was killing citizens, purportedly a '*ring of women that were preparing poisons*' was uncovered according to Roman historian Livy.

At the root of any conspiracy theory, psychologists note two themes:

- Firstly, absolute abhorrence and denial of the remote possibility that we are at the mercy of chance or fate, or that sometimes bad things just happen. When bad things do occur, there is a reason usually that someone is responsible. This suggests a level of paranoia present.
- Secondly, this human causation leads conspiracy theories straight into unleashing racist or prejudiced beliefs against those thought responsible, the defence mechanism of projection. The fourteenth-century Black Death led to a strongly supported belief in Europe was that Jews were poisoning wells. It's a pattern of prejudice that repeats itself whenever fear, disease and uncertainty combine, noted in the current pandemic with racism directed towards the Chinese diaspora round the world because of the origin of the virus. In conspiracy terms, the virus is claimed to be a bioweapon purposely created and deployed.

In the 1980s and 90s, an example of a prominent bioweapon conspiracy theory circulated claiming that AIDS was an artificial virus created by the CIA to kill African American people. A 1990 New York Times, CBS poll found that 10 per cent of Black New Yorkers believed that the virus that causes AIDS was deliberately created in a laboratory in order to infect Black people. That's compared to one per cent of white New Yorkers. And according to a survey of young adults in Cape Town, South Africa, 16 per cent of Black respondents agreed that AIDS was invented to kill Black people and created by scientists in America (Nattrass, 2012).

Marques et al (2021) surveyed 1,000 people about their level of belief in various conspiracy theories. About 20% of respondents agreed with the belief that the Australian government was covering up known ill effects of the new 5G technologies, while 10% believed that fluoride was being used in water supplies to dim the minds of ordinary Australians and make them easier to control. To any sensible person, these beliefs sound illogical and ridiculous. Marques suggests that people turn to them as a way to try to make sense of what's happening in society and in their lives. Predictors of increased local and international conspiracy beliefs were considerable disillusionment with government, less trust in others and higher levels of religiosity.

Technological advancements seem prone to conspiracy beliefs whether it's 5G, or 10 years ago 4G, or even 100 years ago AM radio, you can find historical reports where the public is wary of new technologies and potential hazards or dangers of these sorts of things. Socially vulnerable people more likely to be believers. The less control you have, the more you might follow a conspiracy theory, driven by a deep desire to feel more in control of your life circumstances. Anybody who's marginalised whether it's by status, class, gender or race can easily find some scapegoat target for the explanation that would make them feel safer than if they were simply at the mercy of chance.

Current virus conspiracy theories emerged shortly after the first news of Covid and have continued to persist and increase in parallel to the outbreak. Initially, the concern as noted above was about the deliberate origins and encouraged spread of the virus by the Chinese as a biological weapon created to wage war on the US and the West, *or even* vice versa!!. Later, conspiracy theories focussed on prevention and cure, for instance, that conventional medical treatment should not be trusted, with a world conspiracy of scientists promoting dangerous vaccines, and that people should use alternative remedies such as Ivermectin and hydroxychloroquine to ward off the virus (Chap. 11). The conspiracy film 'Plandemic' appeared online in May 2020, attracting millions of viewers worldwide, and soon was one of the most widespread examples of pandemic misinformation (Cook et al., 2020), including such spurious and dangerous health advice, like mask wearing 'activates' the coronavirus.

Delusions of persecution produce other well-disseminated counterproductive messages ranging from absolute denial that the virus exists, that the pandemic is a total hoax devised to enable autocratic rule to be established over sovereign states by their current leaders, to a weird but commonly expressed concern that the virus was spread by the new 5G phone system masts. Even tracking microchips have been surreptitiously implanted with the vaccine by Bill Gates (Sanders, 2020), and that the virus is a scam for big pharmaceuticals to make money, are among other phoney claims. Youths in Australia have expressed the belief that vaccination would render them sterile, while some S. African women refused vaccination because they believed it would render them unable to breast feed their infants!

Covid vaccines have also been accused of causing AIDS. Another claim that mRNA vaccines alter human DNA has been regularly debunked by fact-checkers at Reuters and PolitiFact, but it resurfaced again March 2022 as vaccine sceptics (like influential former TV chef Pete Evans) seized upon a study to suggest that people receiving the mRNA vaccine risked changing or even poisoning their genes (ABC RMIT Corona Check No. 102. 04 03 2022). In a fact sheet issued by the US Centres for Disease Control and Prevention, genetic material contained in mRNA vaccines '*never enters the nucleus [centre] of your cells, which is where your DNA is kept*' (CDC 27 05 2022). Coinciding with vaccines being made available to children aged 5 to 11, in Australia January 2022 a rumour about the apparent vaccine-related death of a seven-year-old boy in NSW spread rapidly online after a Facebook comment was left by a man purporting to be the child's father. This has been debunked by factual information from three sources supposedly involved, the hospital, NSW Health Department and the ambulance service, none of which have any record of the event. This was blatant attempt to convince parents not to vaccinate their children. A world famous Australian cricket player died March 2022, and it only took a few days before fake news claimed he died because of a recent booster shot (totally untrue) again to convince people not to vaccinate.

One could fill a book with similar examples!! Conspiracy theorists and anti-vaxxers try to position themselves as only those who really know the truth and are being punished for letting the cat out of the bag. This leads to worse implications as the messages, behaviour and attitudes of 'conspirators' could result in close relatives, workmates and friends to succumb to a deadly virus.

Douglas (2021) with a sample of 170 in an online study found that labelling an idea as a conspiracy theory doesn't reduce endorsement of it. It is unclear why the conspiracy theory label does little to encourage people to be sceptical about it. The suggestion is that people applying the label are septics, and their evaluation is therefore biased and their influence resisted. Another argument is that people are more likely to endorse conspiracy theories they think are unpopular in order to satisfy their needs to feel different, special and superior. For these individuals, the deliberate labelling of a belief as a conspiracy theory will backfire making it more appealing. Simply calling an idea a conspiracy theory therefore will not help in its demise.

A poll by Ofcom (2020) in the UK found that almost half (46%) of the UK population reported exposure to fake news about the coronavirus. A similar percentage has been reported in the USA (Mitchell & Oliphant, 2020), of which 66% among those exposed were confronted with it on a daily basis. This frequency is dangerous as repeated exposure psychologically reinforces belief in fake news (Pennycook et al., 2018). Moreover, an analysis of the most-viewed coronavirus YouTube videos found that over 25% of the top videos about the virus contained misleading information, reaching over 62 million views worldwide (Li et al., 2020).

Snake Oil Salesmen and Miracle Cures

Fake news about the virus focussing on 'miracle' cures has also been actively promoted by political elites, such as President Trump and Brazilian President Bolsonaro, who both falsely claimed the merits of hydroxychloroquine treatment against the virus (Constine, 2020). Then there were a multitude of claims that drinking methanol could kill the virus, a belief that actually was the reverse of a cure when it killed hundreds in Iran. Another drug Ivermectin has also been promoted at the forefront of alternative drugs advocated by conspiracy theorists to prevent and cure Covid. From Australian Federal MP Craig Kelly to tennis champion Pat Cash, Ivermectin has gained attention around the world as a potential Covid treatment. Ivermectin is actually a vital anti-parasitic (de-worming) medicine used to treat humans and animals, with no valid research evidence to show its value to deal with Covid.

It is not surprising that conspiracy theories have flourished in this novel milieu of a global pandemic. Research suggests that people feel the need to explain large events with proportionally large causes and are more likely to believe in conspiracy theories about events with serious consequences in times of crisis. Thus, conspiracy theories gain increasing traction as more people isolate themselves or are officially isolated and have to rely mainly on some untrust worthy mass media (Graeupner et al., 2017). Coronavirus misinformation has a high disruptive potential and has been linked to mob attacks. In the UK, least 50 phone masts have been set on fire in response to the 5G conspiracy (BBC News, 2020). Social distancing decreased in pro-government areas after Brazil's president inaccurately portrayed the risks of Covid (Ajzenman et al., 2020).

Other harmful consequences accompany belief in conspiracy theories, such as vaccine hesitancy (Freeman et al., 2020), extremist political views and prejudice (Kofta et al., 2020), can all adversely impact the effectiveness of containment strategies as misinformation about Covid fundamentally distorts and generally lowers people's risk perception of the virus (Krause et al., 2020) and increase propensity to reject information from expert authorities (Uscinski et al., 2020) impacting on personal and social wellbeing. This is important as higher risk perception by individuals relates closely to adoption of Covid preventative health behaviours (Dryhurst et al., 2020). Lowering risk beliefs undermines willingness to adopt healthy behaviours.

People who believe that alternative remedies can help them fight off the virus are unlikely to follow health officials' advice and instead opt for less effective (at best) or even lethal (at worst) alternatives. Conspiracy beliefs may also fuel hostility towards groups seen as responsible for the virus. Some evidence suggests that giving people factual information before exposure to conspiracy theories can reduce conspiracy theory beliefs (Jolley et al., 2017), and this strategy might work in efforts to combat conspiracy theories relevant to the current pandemic (see 'Thwarting Fake News and Misinformation' section below for similar findings). However, because believers tend to share misinformation within an 'echo chamber' of like-minded in-group members, combating conspiracy theories remains a significant challenge. WHO have a good myth busters site worth accessing.

Disassembling Symbols and Slogans at Anti-Covid Vaccination Mandate Protests

The heterogeneous anti-vaccine mandate rallies in cities round the world are focussing public attention on a variety of symbols and slogans which represent, in particular group protesters' minds, their emotional feelings and attitudes towards policies and practices put in place by national and state governments to suppress the current Covid surges. The protests have manifested a much more diverse set of individuals and groups than one would have traditionally associated with past anti-vax movements which were more homogeneous in attendance and uniquely focused on infant vaccination. Currently, mandatory Covid policies over vaccination, mask wearing, lockdowns, access to work, travel and entertainment restrictions have galvanised people who may always have had some deep down simmering concerns about government intrusion on a range of their personal and economic freedoms.

So a range of people from many walks of life can be found at these rallies, for a variety of reasons, some illogical and some fairly understandable. The protest movement doesn't manifest a singular thrust. Nurses in scrubs, people in high-vis vests and parents with small children march alongside people in Donald Trump caps and QAnon T-shirts all around the Western world. The symbols and slogans used help decipher the variety of what is driving these protests. Protestors wave a variety of upside-down flags and hold a plethora of signs with messages like '*you cannot stop tyranny by simply saying no*', '*reveal the truth*' *and* '*ban the mandates*', '*mandate freedom of choice*', '*my body my life*', '*you want to destroy my freedom simply to decrease your own insecurities*' *and* '*stop the lock downs*'.

Flags appear ubiquitous in the rallies and have been re-appropriated purposefully. Many flags are being waved upside down which is a sign of extreme distress. It's a way of communicating: '*I am in intense distress, fighting a righteous battle to protect my country. Why can't anybody see how unlawful our governments are?*' Under Australian national flag protocols, the flag should never be flown upside down. But upside-down flags have been used around the world as a protest symbol, including at the Capitol Hill riot in Washington in January 2021. The use of the red ensign is associated with sovereign citizen groups, who dispute that Australian laws apply to them, believing that state governments and their police forces have no legitimate power to enforce coronavirus laws, lockdowns and vaccination mandates. A sovereign citizens group attempted to burn down the Old Parliament House Building in Canberra at the beginning of 2022 with the organisation now identified as a potential terrorism threat by New South Wales Police.

When Australia became a federation, it flew two flags; the blue ensign for Commonwealth government business and the red ensign, which was used for maritime purposes. The red ensign was often adopted as a de facto national flag because it was the only national Australian flag that the general public could use and used extensively by sovereign citizen groups because it was associated with the earlier White Australia policy. The use of the red ensign by the Canadian alternative-right has also appropriated their country's red ensign. The sovereign citizens' movement in the US is also historically white supremacist.

The Australian blue Eureka flag carried by some at these rallies has a long history of being used as a symbol of resistance against government mandates, since it made an appearance in 1854 at one of Australia's first anti-government rebellions. This Eureka flag has sometimes carried statements like '*when injustice becomes law resistance is duty*' *or* '*Freedom is not to be sacrificed to appease the worries of others*' or as graffiti on walls and bridges. The Eureka flag continues to support the protesters' view of themselves as oppressed rebels fighting for freedom against a tyranny of government over-reach.

A number of overseas symbols and slogans have been co-opted and adopted in Australian, UK and EU rallies. For example, the T-shirt of the QAnon conspiracy theory can often be seen, based around a belief that the world is run by a global cabal of Satan-worshipping paedophiles who control American politics and the media. Slogans used by Donald Trump have been widely adopted by the anti-lockdown and anti-vaccine protest movements round the world and popular at rallies with supporters wearing matching red '*Make (relevant nation) Great Again*' caps. Even symbols from Nazi Germany, including the deeply offensive use of the yellow star, which Jews were forced to wear has been used in the US by anti-vaccination protesters to symbolise oppression. The use of this symbol could indicate the involvement of white supremacist groups, or there could also be a genuine feeling in some of the people's minds that they are on the path to some type of socio-economic extermination or genocide. People often used emotional symbols to get their point about excessive government control across.

A different line of attack featured in many street protests worldwide by those who do not support the wild myths of the false information is to claim that compulsory vaccination for employment and social enjoyment, lockdowns, mask wearing and border closures are preventing normal life and are a fundamental attack on personal freedom and an ability to earn a living. So the loss of economic freedoms is a common and observed theme at rallies with '*I want my job back*' cries, and many of these protests are billed as '*freedom rallies*', with some people seeing the vaccine mandate as a restriction on both their ability to work and their afterwork activities as did the truckies who blockaded the Canadian capitol Ottawa for days in Feb 2022.

There's a serious concern with considerable supportive evidence that vaccination mandates could create second-class citizens who don't have access to all of the economic freedoms expected as a member of a democratic state. 'Government' (unqualified) has been labelled 'the virus' with 'medical apartheid' applied to compliance with mandates that provide permission to work, enjoy entertainment in clubs, pubs and sporting events. These mandates produce a serious loss of freedom and a major thrust of the protests with some individual professionals in teaching, nursing/public health, aged care, fire and police losing their income to maintain their right to choose whether to be vaccinated or not. Vaccination mandates present an image of excessive government control with protestors who rally under signs calling for freedom. Some attendees at protest rallies also bear signs/badges claiming '*my body, my choice*', appropriating a key slogan of the pro-choice abortion movement. A lot of this language is common in rallies across the world mostly being transmitted and copied through social and mass media.

So the focus of current street protests tends to be a conglomerate of a range of issues prominent in different social disobedience campaigns and often involves both extreme right and left wing groups ironically allied on the same issues.

Political Beliefs of Protesters

Studies have attempted to discern whether there are particular political beliefs and traits associated with those who live in conspiracy theory la-la-land. Surprisingly, a number of studies have found that extreme right wing political conservatives are largely responsible for the proliferation of conspiracy misinformation rather than the political left (Lawson & Kakkar, 2022). But the studies also reveal that while conservatives are more likely to share fake news, it is only those low in conscientiousness who do so. Those who were high in conscientiousness are more diligent and better at controlling impulses. Highly impulsive low conscientious conservatives are more likely to share false news stories, expressed a general desire for anarchy, to disrupt and destroy the existing political and social institutions. These needs reflect an underlying desire to assert superiority of one's ideas or in-group over others and are especially elevated among conservatives with lower conscientiousness.

High conscientious people are likely to take notice of fact-checker information and not spread fake news. On the downside, Lawson and Kakkar (op cit.) reveal the low conscientious group are less receptive to ways of stopping fake news as they are insensitive to third-party fact-checker warnings and would continue to share fake news that supported their own interests as it didn't matter to them whether it is true or not. In this context, interventions based on the assumption that truth matters may be inadequately invalid.

However, a group of large-scale studies spanning 26 countries with a sample of over 100,000 has found an elongated U-shaped relationship where conspiratorial thinking is common at both ends of the political spectrum with a long low middle section of political moderates who rarely indulge in such behaviour (Imhoff et al., 2022). The conspiracy mentality thus seems associated clearly with both extreme left and extreme right wing beliefs, and that this relation may be due to both feeling deprived of any political control and turn to conspiracy theories, fake news and misinformation as an attempt to fire up self-perceived lack of political influence and power, threatening and demonising the larger remainder of society, which to them is the out group.

The best option is for social media companies to monitor closely fake news that has the potential to hurt others and actively remove such content from their platform.

Thwarting Fake News and Misinformation

Managing the Pandemic

It should be obvious by now that managing the pandemic response will not only require sound pharmaceutical interventions but also the leveraging and adapting of research insights from the behavioural sciences to contain the spread of this misinformation barrage about Covid. The information environment around the pandemic underscores the importance of effective communication of real medical science and the introduction of techniques to defuse science fiction, given that the Covid pandemic has produced a steady rise in conspiracy theories, fake news and misinformation, whereby it becomes difficult for the general public to distinguish the real scientific evidence from information offered by unreliable sources of information.

With so much uncertainty, insecurity and worry around the coronavirus pandemic already, misinformation threatens to undermine and confuse lay people's understanding of the disease and the best ways to protect themselves and their loved ones. Because we're talking about potentially the worst pandemic in 100 years, this misinformation is simply not just of the normal annoyance type offered in the to and fro of political debates. It is a deliberate undermining cyclonic blast to completely upset the road to recovery and induce a recipe for disaster if too many people are taken in. Governments and media will need to create strategies combining psychological research that informs on how to stem the spread of false claims with health campaigns employing the cutting-edge psychology of persuasion as a form of inoculation against misinformation (Chap. 4).

The Role of Debunking

Researchers are starting to use behavioural science to understand and counter the proliferation of fake news given its underlying potentially dangerous consequences. One approach is to '*debunk*' which means to expose or excoriate a claim, assertion, sentiment, as being pretentious, false or exaggerated by using fact-checking and correction. Expertise-level sources, exposing denial and providing corrections that offer causal explanations all tend to increase the effectiveness of countering misinformation (Wittenburg et al., 2020). However, with the internet and social media, increasingly common sources for information, the general public are inundated with large chunks of material in a setting with minimal controls where misinformation easily disseminates, and fact-checking cannot keep up with the vast amount of false information produced in times of crisis like a pandemic. Moreover, there is mixed research regarding whether corrections may actually increase belief in the original misinformation due to the corrections evoking even stronger ego defence mechanisms and denial of real evidence.

Rogan: Podcasts and Fact-Checks

In early January 2021, Prof Van Bavel, a New York academic, was asked to fact-check an unfamiliar scientific concept: '*mass formation psychosis*'. The phrase gained impetus after use on a Joe Rogan podcast. The concept implies millions worldwide who are complying to public health guidelines had been 'hypnotised' to develop their 'willingness' to get vaccinated, wear masks and stay home.

After fact-checking, Van Bavel (2022) found no evidence to support it but in return became the object of a backlash explosion from trolls who continually harassed and threatened him (American Psychological Association, 2022).

This allowed him a rare glimpse into the warped world of conspiracy theorists. Rogan's podcasts have been labelled objectionable and offensive, but also medically and culturally dangerous by thousands of medical and psychological professionals who signed an open letter to Spotify damning among other ignorant statements his support of Ivermectin and labelling vaccine passports as totalitarianism.

While social media giants such as Meta (formerly Facebook), Twitter and YouTube have faced increased public and regulatory pressure over how they manage misinformation, disinformation and extremism on their platforms, podcasting has slipped under the radar, and many have become hotbeds of conspiracy theories and anti-democratic sentiments. Monitoring the spread of podcast falsehoods, let alone slowing it down, is challenging for researchers, particularly given podcasts straddle the space between old and new media. Anybody can start a podcast and be the total focus of their podcast's story as there is no conversation just audience engagement. You listen to a podcaster because you like what they are saying.

It's profitable to be polarising and influential so that if Spotify removed Rogan, it could inadvertently increase his reach, as his content could then be shared across multiple platforms without oversight. After Biden's inauguration, tens of thousands of accounts sharing QAnon-related content and election lies were banned from Facebook, Twitter and other social media platforms in the '*Great De-platforming*'. But many dogged supporters of former president Donald Trump simply shifted their conversations elsewhere. This may be an example of the 'Streisand effect', i.e. when you try to censor something, it becomes more appealing, people are more drawn to it, and in some cases of de-platforming, the exiled influencers and followers actually became more radicalised. Van Bavel's experience showed firsthand how Joe Rogan's seemingly innocuous choice to 'just talk to people' helps legitimise dangerous views not backed by scientific consensus.

Fact-checks also spread slower on social media than misinformation (Vosoughi et al., 2018), making it difficult for fact-checking to be effective on its own. A review by Scott (2020), for example, found that Facebook's fact-checking efforts did little to prevent coronavirus conspiracies from being shared widely in private groups on the platform. Further complications arise from the '*continued influence effect*' of misinformation, which states that people may continue to believe misinformation even after it has been debunked (Ecker et al., 2010; Lewandowsky et al., 2012). In addition, while media literacy initiatives are important, they are often expensive to develop and slow to roll out. Debunking is a strategy that attempts to argue the counter case too late when the misinformation has already been assimilated into the thinking of the recipients. It is apparent that other strategies beyond 'debunking' are needed.

The Inoculation Metaphor—Pre-emptive Debunking

In particular, given the practical challenges of fact-checking and the difficulty of debunking and correcting misinformation after the damage is already done, researchers are now invoking the strengths of ***prebunking*** (i.e. pre-emptive debunking). ***Prebunking*** aims to get valid information into the public arena before it's tarnished with alternative dogma and propaganda. Rather than just debunking after or during the event, a '***prebunking***' approach involving '***psychological inoculation***' prior to reception of fake news, myths and deliberate misinformation seems to have worked on a prior outburst of misinformation on the climate change debate (e.g. Lewandowski et al., 2013). Researchers see it as a strong possibility here. Psychological inoculation follows the biomedical analogy. Triggering protective responses, like antibodies, a strong challenge (e.g. a conspiracy theory) is weakened to the point where it will not change the person's position of being in a healthy cognitive and emotional state and will also trigger protective responses, like enhanced critical thinking.

American social psychologist, William McGuire, developed this approach to fake news inoculation over 55 years ago. The concept originated out of the political tensions of the Cold War between the West and Communism after WW2, when there were serious worries about the potential of foreign propaganda to brainwash citizens in the West, but the approach was forgotten when tensions eased. The analysis by McGuire et al. (1961) concluded that most citizens do possess the knowledge and intelligence to rationally evaluate a false claim but only if they really focus closely on what they hear or read by evaluating, reasoning and thinking. But many people simply don't do that and operate on a superficial level of immediate acceptance that '*someone told me*' or '*I read somewhere…*' without querying or investigating more deeply. This unquestioned acceptance leads to their opinions being massively and rapidly swayed by the propaganda.

To avoid that outcome, McGuire (1962) believed you need to make someone aware of their own vulnerability to the lies; only then would they have sufficient raised awareness to resist persuasion. In his initial studies, he examined participants' susceptibility to dubious health claims. As he'd hoped, initially warning people about the potential threat of misinformation, and then providing them with examples of the fallacious argument, provided the necessary shock to their system so that they were more sceptical of the fallacious material at a later date. Unfortunately, the idea never really took off until around 55 years later, when Van der Linden et al. (2017) unearthed some of McGuire's research and was immediately struck by McGuire's prescience, emphasising the role of networks in the spread of misinformation. Internet now offers that perfect network through which misinformation can disseminate rapidly and widely in a way that is very analogous to how a virus replicates in infected hosts.

Anti-viral Myth-Busting Measures

Many myths are already out there infecting receiver after receiver. But what can be done when the message is already out there? Like a real virus, misinformation relies on its R (reproduction) number; that is how many other people each person will pass it on to. But if we can educate enough people about misinformation, we can make them sceptical enough not to pass it on. In this way, we could generate a state of 'herd immunity' to misinformation.

Initially, that might concern immunity against misinformation on a single topic (like the coronavirus), but the effect might generalise to other issues radically reducing the spread of lies in multiple domains. There is already some evidence that knowledge of misinformation in one domain can inoculate you in another (Cook et al., 2017) and Van der Linden's research programme (Van der Linden et al., 2020) commenced investigating how to maximise the effects, so that the majority of the population start to think more critically about information they are receiving.

Many previous campaigns, such as the widespread attempts to debunk anti-vaxxer myths, may have failed because they struggled to present the information in an effective way. It was too common for myth-busting articles to repeat the false claims, often in bold newspaper or TV headline before trying to debunk. Unfortunately, that follows the precept that first impressions are the strongest, with the reader/viewer remembering the fake headline rather than the subsequent material that debunks the claims (Pluviano et al., 2017). Some campaigns also fail by offering the reader an overload of detail, often statistical, which create more confusion rather than clarity to persuade.

Fortunately, the latest research suggests some principles that should make the central message more apparent and memorable. These tend to centre on the principles of simplicity and fluency in presenting the real facts (Schwarz et al., 2016). Simplicity can lie in a single visual image illustrating the central concept or slick layout with key facts in a bold, easy-to-read font. Fluency can come from vivid storytelling (with the use of colourful anecdotes, say). If possible, *avoid repeating the false claims* as this only reinforces them by repetition but rather home in on the true facts.

Forget trying to list '5 coronavirus myths' and then discussing them one by one. Just focus on the truth about the best ways to reduce coronavirus transmission, which in reverse counters tacitly fake news claims without expressing them. The truth must be the focus not the lie. And, adding the principle of inoculation, there should be an initial warning that a myth is going to be exposed rather than placing a statement of the false claim upfront in a heading and explain how and why they are being misled.

The health domain has actually used inoculation theory-informed public health messages very successfully to increase resistance to unhealthy pressures, like smoking cigarettes (Pfau et al., 1992) or binge drinking (Parker et al., 2010) as well enhancing beneficial health behaviours, like committing to exercise programmes (Dimmock et al., 2016) and stemming the spread of false information about the causes of global warming. For example, Van der Linden's set of experiments (Van der Linden et al., 2020) sought to determine whether an inoculation could stem the spread of misinformation about the causes of climate warming. For around a decade, climate change deniers had been attempting to destroy the scientific consensus on the role of CO^2 on global warming with the so-called *Oregon Petition* a website that claimed to have the signatures of more than 31,000 American scientists who believed '*there is NO scientific evidence that the human release of carbon dioxide will, in the foreseeable future, cause catastrophic heating of the Earth's atmosphere*'. In reality, fewer than 1 per cent of the signatories had a background in climate science, and many of the signatures were clearly false including those of *Charles Darwin* and '*Dr*' *Geri Halliwell* (remember the Spice Girls!). The website looks surprisingly convincing and around 10 per cent of people changed their opinion to become more negative towards the existence of a scientific consensus on the greenhouse effect (fossil fuel emissions warming of the planet) having seen the petition. This was a strong powerful effect for one single piece of misinformation.

To see if an inoculation might prevent them from being swayed, Van der Linden et al. (2020) took a group of participants and offered them one of two warnings before they saw the Oregon Petition. The first was a general message that '*some politically motivated groups use misleading tactics to try to convince the public that there is a lot of disagreement among scientists*', followed by a re-iteration of the actual climate science. Not only did it protect against the misinformation; after seeing the petition, belief in the scientific consensus had risen 6.5% higher than before the intervention.

The second part of the study, Van der Linden (2020) gave other subjects a form of inoculation that involved an even more detailed description of the Oregon Petition itself and its false signatures. This was very effective, boosting the acceptance of the scientific consensus on greenhouse warming by nearly 13%. Both inoculations worked better than a third intervention, which had barely any effect, which involved arming a further group of subjects with the facts about climate change, without a specific warning about potential misinformation on the topic.

Following the controversies over the Trump US presidential election in 2016, Van der Linden next attempted to protect people against political fake news more generally in a study, in which the inoculation was an online game ('*Bad News*') that simulates sites such as Twitter, allowing users to build followers by employing misinformation techniques like impersonating or delegitimising official accounts, create a viral article on a controversial topic like the refugee crisis, appealing to partisan divides or creating a conspiracy theory. After, experiencing the techniques on the board game players was significantly less likely to be persuaded by actual fake news articles on the same issue, compared to a control group who had not played the game (Roozenbeek et al., 2019; Van der Linden 2022).

Bad News Game

The fake news game *Bad News* is a real-world inoculation intervention, and it worked so well that it used by schools and governments to pre-emptively expose people to small doses of misinformation techniques (including scenarios about Covid) which measurably reduces susceptibility to fake news (Basal et al., 2020; Roozenbeek et al., 2019; Roozenbeek et al., 2020a). The game can be embedded directly on social media platforms to provide a simulated social media environment in which people take on the role of a fake news creator and learn about six common misinformation techniques over the course of six levels or 'badges'. It has attracted around a million users to date. The UK Foreign Office quickly noted the game's potential and has now translated the game into other major world languages to help combat misinformation worldwide.

The *Bad News* game now targets the misinformation around Covid, focussing particular attention to the use of 'fake experts' (no real qualifications) to question medical advice, which has become one of the most common strategies being used by conspiracy theorists and fake news perpetrators, in order to pre-emptively warn people about the strategies that may be used to spread misinformation around the pandemic. This will be especially important as we try to maximise vaccination rates in the face of continuing spread and numerous mutations of the Covid virus within a context of an increasing explosion of fake news around safety, effectiveness and mandatory issues. Another new online game can be played for free at www.goviralgame.com. Go Viral! was developed in collaboration with the UK government and the WHO in which players learn to resist three manipulation techniques commonly used to spread misinformation about the coronavirus: fearmongering, the use of fake experts and conspiracy theories.

Although the *Bad News* game is a useful tool, more work is needed to curb the spread of misinformation about Covid. An open question in active inoculation research is the extent to which inoculation can boost truth-discernment skills, that is, not just the ability to spot and resist misinformation attacks but also the other side of the coin, the ability to better identify real or credible news (Guess et al., 2020; Roozenbeek et al., 2020b, 2020c). Covid health messaging should do two things: (a) build resistance to unhealthy influence, like conspiracy theories, and (b) also encourage healthier behaviours, like vaccination, social distancing and mask wearing.

Canadian research (Pennycook et al., 2020) has also focussed on people's tendency to share fake coronavirus news without questioning accuracy before passing it on. But if subtle prompts that '*nudge*' people to consider accuracy were provided and then asking them to rate the reliability of a single headline, the prompt primed people to think more carefully about the messages they were reading and subsequently reduced their willingness to share other fake stories. Pennycook et al. (op cit.) argue there is considerable advantage in prompting users to rate the accuracy of what they are reading, hearing and seeing. Evidence suggests that deliberately forcing recipients to employ analytic reasoning and thinking is associated with and causes reduced belief in false news headlines that circulated on social media (Bago et al., 2020). Platforms could nudge users to think about accuracy by, for example, periodically asking users to rate the accuracy of posts they are reading. The crowd sourced accuracy ratings generated by this process may also be useful for identifying misinformation, as has been found for crowd ratings of source trustworthiness (Penneycook et al., 2019).

Prevention is better than cure. This is true as much for diseases as it is for the spread of misinformation. Thus to effectively counter fake news about Covid around the world, researchers, governments and social media companies must continue to rigorously develop and test interventions. This includes identifying manipulative techniques in posts and providing treatments that effectively reduce belief in misinformation, while not undermining belief in accurate information as some people could become suspicious of everything.

The Health Belief Model

The Health Belief Model (*HBM*), devised by the US Public Health Service, has been found extremely useful in identifying the factors that influence and predict individual health-related behaviours and is widely used for understanding health behaviours, guiding health promotion and disease prevention programmes by focussing on individual and group beliefs about health issues. The 6 key factors that generally influence health behaviours on which the *HBM* is based are:

- An individual's perceived threat of becoming sick or catching a disease (perceived susceptibility),
- Belief of how bad the consequence will be (perceived severity),
- Potential positive benefits of taking appropriate/recommended/mandated action (perceived benefits),
- Perceived barriers to appropriate/recommended/mandated action,
- Exposure to factors that prompt action (cues to action),
- Confidence in personal ability to undertake action successfully (self-efficacy).

A large number of studies across the world have found that cultural differences do not influence responses to the *HBM* in relation to Covid. For example, Karl et al. (2022) reveal that health beliefs showed far stronger relationships with recommended Covid behaviours than demographics in Italy and Rumania and confirmed previously reported relationships from numerous nations that *self-efficacy, perceived severity and perceived benefits* were consistently related to the greater adoption of individual Covid protective behaviours, whereas *greater perceived barriers* were related to lower adoption of health behaviours.

Perceived self-efficacy, the belief of being able to successful protect oneself from being infected, was the most consistent and strongest statistical predictor of health behaviours. This supports general findings in the wider psychological literature that self-efficacy is crucial for understanding most behaviours and behaviour change. The second most consistently associate health belief was perceived benefit. This also is congruent previous studies and implies that individuals are more likely to adopt preventive behaviours that are seen as beneficial for them. In contrast, perceived threat may not be sufficient to motivate behaviour in the absence of a belief in being able to protect oneself through adopting effective measures. This suggest that external locus of control and low sense of self-efficacy are major personal factors that inhibit the adoption of recommended/mandated sound health practice. These two personality factors are closely related and are essentially learned through past experience of not coping or failure at some tasks, particularly in childhood. Psychological programmes exist to facilitate such persons developing stronger self-efficacy beliefs and also move to a more internal locus of control.

In an Iranian study, Karimy et al. (2021) showed that perceived barriers were an essential factor determining the use of preventive behaviours and inhibiting behavioural change. So, focussing (identifying, eliminating) on the barriers which hinder Covid preparedness and response is necessary. Additionally, the study found external cues to action were among the strongest stimulus needed to trigger preventive behaviour. Karimy et al. (op cit.) recommend promoting the adoption of preventive behaviours by mass media, emphasising on the sense of social responsibility and sending notifications via mobiles and social media. All these results align with the findings of Janz and Becker (1984) who researched the effectiveness of health beliefs on the adoption of preventive behaviours in a wide variety of contexts. Chen et al. (2021) in China found it was possible to increase the vaccination rate by reducing perceived barriers to vaccination and by encouraging volunteers to advocate for vaccination to their friends and family members. The central factor for reducing vaccine hesitancy was by enhancing self-efficacy for vaccination, due to its crucial mediating function. Again feelings of self-efficacy appear to be the crucial component in adopting positive Covid health behaviours.

In sum, *HBM* studies indicate that health information campaigns need to (1) emphasise the benefits of preventive behaviours including avoiding the likelihood of getting a chronic disease and complications of the disease, (2) highlight tips and advice to overcome the barriers, (3) provide cues to action by means of showing various reminders in social media, (4) focus on adoption of Covid-related preventive behaviours and (5) perhaps most importantly encourage feelings of self-efficacy in individuals by behaviourist reinforcement techniques and learning coping skills. Overall, the *HBM* has shown considerable utility globally as a basic tool in providing insights into strategies for managing the Covid outbreak.

Some Principles to Guide Our Own Behaviour on Social Media

Firstly, do not repeat false claims and only share material you know to be factually accurate. Even intelligent people can be easily fooled by fake claims because they are time poor or may find material that has some support in their own 'beliefs'.

Secondly, when trying to defuse a false claim, avoid being over emotional and don't be dismissive. Don't publicly shame people for their beliefs. You may be challenging deeply held beliefs that people have, particularly if it relates to a politically sensitive issue. So they're not going to react well to you publicly saying, '*this is a load of nonsense, you shouldn't be saying that*'. As Van Bavel et al. (op cit.) found moderating your language can increase the reach of your message to the people who need to hear it, rather than simply preaching to the converted.

Thirdly, if you want to get another person to be more realistic about some conspiracy theory they're peddling, ask questions rather than simply presenting them with real facts. Try to encourage critical thinking: '*Why do you think that? What the evidence? What are the person's qualifications for saying that?*'. Ask them to explain how this conspiracy works, rather than why they believe it. This shift in focus forces the person to confront the fact that they may not comprehend the details of the issue clearly, which may prompt them to start thinking about the accuracy of what they are sharing.

Useful books elaborating on all this are.

David Robson's *The Intelligence Trap: Revolutionise Your Thinking And Make Wiser Decisions* (Hodder and Stoughton).

Lydia Khahil's on conspiracy theory *The Rise of the Extreme Right*. A Penguin Special.

References

ABC RMIT Corona Check No. 102. (2022). Retrieved 05 March 22 from https://www.abc.net.au/news/2022a-03-04/coronacheck-mrna-vaccines-not-genotoxic-pete-evans/100879220

ABC RMIT Fact Check. (2022). The 'surprising' finding of an online poll about COVID-19 vaccines is not what it seems. Retrieved 28 October22 from https://www.abc.net.au/news/2022b-10-28/fact-check-news-com-au-vaccine-poll-manipulated/101583964

Ajzenman, N., Cavalcanti, T., & Da Mata, D. (2020). More than Words: Leaders' Speech and Risky Behavior during a Pandemic (No. 2034). Retrieved 18 September 21 from https://www.inet.econ.cam.ac.uk/working-paper-pdfs/wp2019.pdf

American Psychological Association. (2022). The anatomy of a misinformation attack. Retrieved 28 January 22 from https://www.apa.org/news/apa/2022/news-anatomy-misinformation

Bago, B., Rand, G., & Pennycook, G. (2020). Fake News, Fast and Slow: Deliberation Reduces Belief in False (but Not True) News Headlines. *Journal of Experimental Psychology: General, 129*, 1608–1613. https://doi.org/10.1037/xge0000729

Bakshy, E., et al. (2015). Political science: Exposure to ideologically diverse news and opinion on facebook. *Science, 348*, 1130–1132. https://doi.org/10.1126/science.aaa1160

Basol, M., Roozenbeek, J., & van der Linden, S. (2020). Good news about bad news: Gamified inoculation boosts confidence and cognitive immunity against fake news. *Journal of Cognition, 3*, 1–9. https://doi.org/10.5334/joc.91

Betsch, C., et al. (2010). The influence of vaccine-critical websites on perceiving vaccination risks. *Journal of Health Psychology, 15*(3), 446–455. https://doi.org/10.1177/1359105309353647

BBC News 24 06 20 Coronavirus: Derby 5G phone mast set on fire. Retrieved 02 February 21 from .https:// www. bbc. com ›uk-england-derbyshire-52790399

Carnegie Mellon University. (2020). 5% of 200 million tweets about Covid were managed by bots. Retrieved 16 July 20 from https://www.cmu.edu/news/stories/archives/2020/may/twitter-bot-campaign.html

Crikey Report. Cam Wilson. (2022). Sick, paranoid, poorer and disorganised: the aftermath of the Convoy to Canberra protests. Retrieved 09 April 22 from https://www.crikey.com.au/2022c/02/18/aftermath-of-the-convoy-to-canberra-protests/

Center for Disease Control and Prevention. (2022). Retrieved 17 October 22 from https://www.cdc.gov/coronavirus/2019-ncov/vaccines/facts.html

CheckMate ABC News investigation. (2022). Retrieved 02 December 22 from https://www.abc.net.au/news/2022-12-02/fact-check-debunking-died-suddenly/101720550

Chen, H., Li, X., et al. (2021). Health belief model perspective on the control of COVID-19 vaccine hesitancy and the promotion of vaccination in China: Web-based cross-sectional study. *Journal of Medical Internet Research, 23*, e29329. https://doi.org/10.2196/29329

Constine, J. (2020). Facebook deletes Brazil president's coronavirus misinfo post. Tech Crunch. Available online at: https://techcrunch.com/2020/03/30/facebook-removes-bolsonaro-video/

Cook, J., Lewandowsky, S. & Ecker, U. K. (2017). Neutralizing misinformation through inoculation. *PloSone 12*(5). https://doi.org/10.1371/journal.pone.0175799

Cook, J., van der Linden, S., Lewandowsky, S., & Ecker, U. (2020). Coronavirus, "Plandemic" and the Seven Traits of Conspiratorial Thinking. The Conversation. Available online at: https://theconversation.com/coronavirus-plandemic-and-the-seven-traits-of-conspiratorial-thinking-138483

Diethelm, P., & McKee, M. (2009). Denialism: What is it and how should scientists respond? *European Journal of Public Health, 19*(1), 2–4. https://doi.org/10.1093/eurpub/ckn139

Dimmock, J. A., Gagné, M., Proud, L., Howle, T. C., et al. (2016). An exercise in resistance: Inoculation messaging as a strategy for protecting motivation during a monotonous and controlling exercise class. *Journal of Sport and Exercise Psychology, 38*, 567–578. https://doi.org/10.1123/jsep.2016-0146

Douglas, K., Sutton, R. M., & Cichocka, A. (2017). The psychology of conspiracy theories. *Current Directions in Psychological Science, 26*, 538–542. https://doi.org/10.1177/0963721417718261

Douglas, K. (2021). COVID-19 conspiracy theories. *Group Processes & Intergroup Relations, 24*(2) 270–275. https://doi.org/10.1177/1368430220982068

Dryhurst, S., Schneider, C. R., Kerr, J., et al. (2020). Risk perceptions of COVID-19 around the world. *Journal of Risk Research*, 1–13.https://doi.org/10.1080/13669877.2020.1758193

Ecker, U. K. H., Lewandowsky, S., & Tang, D. T. W. (2010). Explicit warnings reduce but do not eliminate the continued influence of misinformation. *Memory and Cognition, 38*, 1087–1100. https://doi.org/10.3758/MC.38.8.1087

Franklin, H. (2019). How much does the world trust medical experts and vaccines? Wellcome Trust. Retrieved 03 March 21 from https://wellcome.ac.uk/press-release/how-much-does-world-trust-medical-experts-and-vaccines

Freeman, D., Waite, F., Rosebrock, L., et al. (2020). Coronavirus conspiracy beliefs, mistrust, and compliance with government guidelines in England. *Psychological Medicine, 52*(2), 251–263. https://doi.org/10.1017/S0033291720001890

Graeupner, D., & Coman, A. (2017). The dark side of meaning-making: How social exclusion leads to superstitious thinking. *Journal of Experimental Social Psychology., 69*, 218–222. https://doi.org/10.1016/j.jesp.2016.10.003

Guess, A. M., Lerner, M., et al. (2020). A digital media literacy intervention increases discernment between mainstream and false news in the United States and India. *Proceedings of the National Academy of Sciences of the United States of America, 117*(27), 15536–15545. https://doi.org/10.1073/pnas.1920498117

Imhoff, R., Zimmer, F., Klein, O., et al. (2022). Conspiracy mentality and political orientation across 26 countries. *Nature Human Behaviour, 6*, 392–403. https://doi.org/10.1038/s41562-021-01258-7

Janz, N. K., & Becker, M. H. (1984). The health belief model: A decade later. *Health Education Quarterly, 11*(1), 1–47. https://doi.org/10.1177/109019818401100101

Johnson, N. F., Velásquez, N., Restrepo, N. J., et al. (2020). The online competition between pro- and anti-vaccination views. *Nature, 582*, 230–233. https://doi.org/10.1038/s41586-020-2281-1

Jolley, D., & Douglas, K. M. (2017). Prevention is better than cure: Addressing anti-vaccine conspiracy theories. *Journal of Applied Social Psychology, 47*, 459–469. https://doi.org/10.1111/jasp.12453

Karimy, M., Bastami, F., Sharifat, R., et al. (2021). Factors related to preventive COVID-19 behaviors using health belief model among general population: A cross-sectional study in Iran. *BMC Public Health, 21*, 1934. https://doi.org/10.1186/s12889-021-11983-3

Karl, J., Fischer, R., Druică, E., et al. (2022). Testing the effectiveness of the health belief model in predicting preventive behavior during the COVID-19 pandemic: The case of Romania and Italy. *Frontiers in Psychology, 12*, 627575. https://doi.org/10.3389/fpsyg.2021.627575

Kofta, M., Soral, W., & Bilewicz, M. (2020). What breeds conspiracy antisemitism? The role of political uncontrollability and uncertainty in the belief in Jewish conspiracy. *Journal of Personality and Social Psychology., 118*(5), 900–918. https://doi.org/10.1037/pspa0000183

Kortum, P., Edwards, C., & Richards-Kortum, R. (2008). The impact of inaccurate internet health information in a secondary school learning environment. *Journal of Medical Internet Research, 10*(2). https://doi.org/10.2196/jmir.986

Krause, N. M., Freiling, I., Beets, B., & Brossard, D. (2020). Fact-checking as risk communication: The multi-layered risk of misinformation in times of COVID-19. *Journal of Risk Research, 23*(7–8), 1052–1059. https://doi.org/10.1080/13669877.2020.1756385

Lawson, A., & Kakkar, H. (2022). Of Pandemics, politics, and personality: The role of conscientiousness and political ideology in sharing of fake news. *Journal of Experimental Psychology: General., 151*(5), 1154–1177. https://doi.org/10.1037/xge0001120

Lees, J., & Cikara, M. (2020). Inaccurate group meta-perceptions drive negative out-group attributions. *Nature Human Behaviour, 4*(3), 279–286. https://doi.org/10.1038/s41562-019-0766-4

Lewandowsky, S., Ecker, U. K., Seifert, C. M., et al. (2012). Misinformation and its correction: Continued influence and successful debiasing. *Psychological Science in the Public Interest., 13*(3), 106–131. https://doi.org/10.1177/1529100612451018

Lewandowsky, S., Gignac, G., & Oberauer, K. (2013). The role of conspiracist ideation and worldview in predicting rejection of science. *PLoS ONE, 8*, e75637. https://doi.org/10.1371/journal.pone0075637

Li, H. O.-Y., Bailey, A., Huynh, D., & Chan, J. (2020). YouTube as a source of information on COVID-19: A pandemic of misinformation? *BMJ Global Health, 5*. https://doi.org/10.1136/bmjgh-2020-002604

Marques, M., Ling, M., Williams., M., et al. (2021). Australasian public awareness and conspiracism: Motivational correlates. *Political Psychology, 43*, 177–198. https://doi.org/10.1111/pops.12746

McGuire, W. J., & Papageorgis, D. (1961). The relative efficacy of various types of prior belief-defense in producing immunity against persuasion. *The Journal of Abnormal and Social Psychology, 62*(2), 327–337. https://doi.org/10.1037/h0042026

McGuire, W. J., & Papageorgis, D. (1962). Effectiveness of forewarning in developing resistance to persuasion. *Public Opinion Quarterly, 26*, 24–34. https://doi.org/10.1086/267068

Mitchell, A., & Oliphant, J. B. (2020). Americans Immersed in COVID-19 News; Most Think Media Are Doing Fairly Well Covering It. Pew Research Center. Available online at: https://www.journalism.org/2020/03/18/americans-immersed-in-covid-19-news-most-think-media-are-doing-fairly-well-covering-it/

Nattrass, N. (2012). Understanding the origins and prevalence of AIDS conspiracy beliefs in the United States and South Africa. *Sociology of Health and Illness, 35*(1), 113–129. https://doi.org/10.1111/j.1467-9566.2012.01480.x

Ofcom Report 09 04 2020 Half of UK adults exposed to false claims about coronavirus. Retrieved 20 November 21 from https://www.ofcom.org.uk/about-ofcom/latest/media/media-releases/2020/half-of-uk-adults-exposed-to-false-claims-about-coronavirus

Pariser, E. (2011). Beware of online "filter bubbles". TED Talks. TED 2011 Web site. Retrieved 06 November 21 from https://www.ted.com/talks/eli_pariser_beware_online_filter_bubbles?language=en

Parker, K. A., Ivanov, B., & Compton, J. A. (2010). Inoculation's efficacy with young adults' risky behaviors: Can inoculation confer cross-protection over related but untreated issues? *Health Communication, 27*, 223–233. https://doi.org/10.1080/10410236.2011.575541

Pennycook, G., Cannon, T., & Rand, D. G. (2018). Prior exposure increases perceived accuracy of fake news. *Journal of Experimental Psychology, 147*, 1865–1880. https://doi.org/10.1037/xge0000465

Pennycook, G., & Rand, D. (2019). Fighting misinformation on social media using crowdsourced judgments of news source quality. *Psychological and Cognitive Sciences., 116*(7), 2521–2526. https://doi.org/10.1073/pnas.18067811

Pennycook, G., McPhetres, J., Zhang, Y., & Rand, D. (2020). Fighting COVID-19 misinformation on social media: Experimental evidence for a scalable accuracy-nudge intervention. *Psychological Science, 31*(7), 770–780. https://doi.org/10.1177/0956797620939054

Pfau, M., Van Bockern, S., & Kang, J. G. (1992). Use of inoculation to promote resistance to smoking initiation among adolescents. *Communication Monographs, 59*, 213–230. https://doi.org/10.1080/03637759209376266

Pluviano, S., Watt, C., & Della Sala, S. (2017). Misinformation lingers in memory: Failure of three pro-vaccination strategies. *Cognitive Processing., 21*(3), 321–330. https://doi.org/10.1007/s10339-020-00974-8

Romer, D., Winneg, K., Jamieson, P., et al. (2022). Misinformation about vaccine safety and uptake of COVID-19 vaccines among adults and 5–11-year-olds in the United States. *Vaccine, 40*, 6463–6470. https://doi.org/10.1016/j.vaccine.2022.09.046

Roozenbeek, J., & van der Linden, S. (2019). The fake news game: Actively inoculating against the risk of misinformation. *Journal of Risk Research, 22*, 570–580. https://doi.org/10.1080/13669877.2018.1443491

Roozenbeek, J., Maertens, R., McClanahan, W., & van der Linden, S. (2020a). Differentiating item and testing effects in inoculation research on online misinformation. *Educational and Psychological Measurement, 81*(2), 1–23. https://doi.org/10.1177/0013164420940378

Roozenbeek, J., Schneider, C. R., Dryhurst, S., et al. (2020b). Susceptibility to misinformation about COVID-19 around the world. *Royal Society Open Science,7*.https://doi.org/10.1098/rsos.201199

Roozenbeek, J., van der Linden, S., & Nygren, T. (2020c). Prebunking interventions based on "inoculation" theory can reduce susceptibility to misinformation across cultures. *Harvard Kennedy School (HKS) Misinform Review, 1,* 1–15. https://doi.org/10.37016//mr-2020-008

Sanders, L. (2020). The difference between what republicans and democrats believe to be true about COVID-19. YouGov. Available online at: https://today.yougov.com/topics/politics/articles-reports/2020/05/26/republicans-democrats-misinformation

Schwarz, N., Newman, E., & Leach, W. (2016). Making the truth stick and the myths fade: Lessons from cognitive psychology. *Behavioral Science and Policy., 2*, 85–95. https://doi.org/10.1353/bsp.2016.0009

Scott, N., Palmer, A., Delport, D., & Hellard, M. (2020). Modelling the impact of reducing control measures on the COVID-19 pandemic in a low transmission setting. Medical Journal of Australia. Pre-print published online: 2 September 2020. Final version retrieved 26 February 22 from https://www.mja.com.au/journal/2021/214/2/modelling-impact-relaxing-covid-19-control-measures-during-period-low-viraltransmission

Stock, S. J., Carruthers, J., Calvert, C., et al. (2022). SARS-CoV-2 infection and COVID-19 vaccination rates in pregnant women in Scotland. *Nature Medicine, 28*, 504–512. https://doi.org/10.1038/s41591-021-01666-2

Uscinski, J. E., Enders, A. M., et al. (2020). Why do people believe COVID-19 conspiracy theories? *Harvard Kennedy School (HKS) Misinform Review, 1*, 1–12. https://doi.org/10.37016/mr-2020-015

Van Bavel, J. J., & Pereira A. (2018). The Partisan Brain: An identity-based model of political belief. *Trends in Cognitive Sciences, Mar, 22*(3), 213–224. https://doi.org/10.1016/j.tics.2018.01.004.

van Bavel, J .J. V., Baicker, K., & Boggio, P. S. et al. (2020). Using social and behavioural science to support COVID-19 pandemic response. *Nature Human Behaviour, 4* 460–471. https://doi.org/10.1038/s41562-020-0884-z

Van Bavel. (2022). Report by Adams, Z. American Psychological Association. 25 01 2022. The anatomy of a misinformation attack. Retrieved 10 February 22 from .https: // www. apa. org›news›apa›2022›news-anatomy-of-a-misinformation-attack/

Van der Linden, S., Leiserowitz, A., Rosenthal, S., & Maibach, E. (2017). Inoculating the public against misinformation about climate change. *Global Challenge, 1.* https://doi.org/10.1002/gch2.201600008

Van der Linden, S., Roozenbeek, J., & Compton, J. (2020). Inoculating against fake news about COVID-19. *Frontiers of Psychology., 11*, 566–790. https://doi.org/10.3389/fpsyg.2020.566790

Van der Linden, S. (2022). Sander van der Linden on how psychological inoculation protects against false news. European Science Media Hub. Retrieved 23 November 22 from https://sciencemediahub.eu/2022/09/07/sander-van-der-linden-how-psychological-inoculation-protects-news-consumers-against-false-news/

Vosoughi, S., Roy, D., & Aral, S. (2018). The spread of true and false news online. *Science, 359*, 1146–1151. https://doi.org/10.1126/science.aap9559

Waszkiewicz, P., Lewulis, P., Górski, M., et al. (2022). Public vaccination reluctance: What makes us change our minds? Results of a longitudinal cohort survey. *Vaccines, 10*(7), 1081. https://doi.org/10.3390/vaccines10071081

WHO Mythbusters Site. Online at https://www.who.int/emergencies/diseases/novel-coronavirus-2019/advice-for-public/myth-busters

Wittenberg, C, & Berinsky, A. (2020). Misinformation and its correction. In N. Persily & J. A. Tucker (Eds.), *Social media and democracy. The state of the field, prospects for reform* (pp. 163–198). Cambridge University Press. https://doi.org/10.1017/9781108890960

CHAPTER 4

Following Doctors' Orders: Persuasive Communication Delivery

Abstract This chapter explores the problems of ensuring compliance with public health orders/medical advice and how best to persuade people to follow instructions. Psychological studies of persuasive communication suggest that a variety of interacting factors are at play. The credibility of the communicator is important, and community opinion leaders are vital. The structure of the message itself is important in terms of sequence of the argument (e.g. which comes first pros or cons; positives or negatives). The use of fear is counter-productive, but encouraging public commitment in a group context is valuable for ensuring compliance. Handouts, posters, etc. should be tested for readability so that they are written at appropriate language level for recipients. Psychological reactance can be evoked with an unproductive boomerang effect if a too forceful imposition or one imposed unreasonably occurs. Personality characteristics can mediate persuasion and compliance with for example high IQ and high internal locus of control are harder to persuade, while those with low self-esteem are easily influenced.

Keywords Compliance · Opinion leaders · Argument presentation · Group commitment · Readability · Psychological reactance

Following Doctors' Orders

In this chapter, strategies for engaging in effective communication and persuasion around health issues will be presented. Although much of the psychological research on this is pre-Covid, it can clearly inform and show relevance to health officials who currently and urgently need to persuade

© The Author(s), under exclusive license to Springer Nature Singapore Pte Ltd. 2023

R. B. Burns, *The Human Impact of the COVID-19 Pandemic*,
https://doi.org/10.1007/978-981-99-1710-5_4

swathes of the population to make and sustain a number of drastic behaviour changes and follow health policies willingly, such as isolating, mask wearing or reporting voluntarily for medical testing. Humans enjoy their individuality, and in multiethnic populations now common worldwide where cultural and religious factors additionally come into play, it can prove difficult to gain high levels of commitment. Perhaps, we will only know a long way down the track with enquiries finding exactly what did transpire in communities' responses to the demands of the Covid context. But in the political and medical circles, it does seem like there was debate over human nature in terms of '*people must do this*' and consequently '*how do we get people to do this*', with the subsequent highly restrictive mandates and sanctions seemingly on quite a pessimistic view of human nature, sceptical that people would step up and respond in the way that was needed.

The importance of a community perspective to accept restrictions was exemplified by the UK's Dominic Cummings affair when Boris Johnson's advisor broke the non-essential travel ban, and the Downing Street drink parties at a time such gatherings were disallowed. Appeals by politicians for people to '*come together*' in emergencies need to be backed up with real practical attempts to engender and maintain such collective unity; otherwise, it risks becoming empty rhetoric that will simply fall on deaf ears if the top ranks of government may not feel obliged to follow national mandates.

Politicians generally do not realise some of the levers that government pull are in essence psychological in that they affect the way people feel, think and behave. Some people will understand and conform, some people will be obstinately negative, and then there will be everything in between. Psychologists are willing to accept uncertainty and communicate that people are complex and explain why they're complex. Governments usually want a straightforward simple formula to apply uniform response and given human complexity that is out of the question. Behavioural scientists are comfortable accepting that behaviour is on a continuum recognising '*everyone is different*', including the same individual from one day to the next. Will I panic buy toilet rolls? Probably not, but if the whole family goes down with a severe tummy bug, perhaps I would.

Virologists and epidemiologists have outlined the various things people need to do to minimise transmission and reduce risk with vaccination, physical distancing, handwashing, mask wearing as the most straightforward examples, then covertly it is the mission of the behavioural scientists to get everyone to do those things. Psychology has ways of understanding and explaining that people are human, emotional and complex in a way that epidemiologists, economists or health bureaucrats perhaps can't. Covid is affecting everything we think, feel and do and that is the field of psychology.

Compliance Versus Adherence and Internalisation

Communication is the major social process in the exchange of information between sender and receiver, in this case between government and its agencies and the general public. One of the major problems in the field of medicine and health promotion is to find ways of persuading clients and general public to follow instructions which will hopefully ameliorate or prevent deficiencies in health status. A lot of previous psychological research use the term '*compliance*' in this context. Compliance is where a person may agree with another person or group of people, but privately may disagree with that advice, viewpoint or behaviour. The individual then only changes their behaviour, in a temporary manner to maintain a good relationship or group membership, but not necessarily their opinions. For example, a person may laugh at a salacious joke because their group find it amusing but deep down the person finds the joke distasteful and would never repeat it. Another example is where a person may feel pressurised to smoke because the rest of their friends do. Social influence leads to compliance because the person now smokes just for show and maintain group acceptance but deep down they wish not to smoke. This sort of change may be quite temporary as the person changes in-group allegiances. Some people who join in anti-mandate rallies may simply be complying to retain friendships and particular group memberships and be seen as '*one of us*'.

Many health researchers now tend to use the term '*adherence*' rather than '*compliance*' because as examples show above compliance provides an image of the message receiver as passive, submissive and unable to hold onto their own positions or decisions and the message sender (s) as all-knowing, all powerful, who knows what is best or what is the '*truth*'. If doctor's clients got ill, therefore it was their own fault for not complying. *Adherence* provides greater focus on what people do and why, leading to their understanding of what should be done. This focus on creating this understanding leads to the concept of *internalisation* which occurs when people begin to accept other's ideas and take on the attitudes, values and beliefs of these others as their own, so they are not just complying at a surface level but acting almost unconsciously *to behave in the way they have chosen*. Sound adherence is achieved when internalisation has occurred. We make the behaviour and beliefs our own because we're happy with it being part of us.

An example of internalisation is any time that we accept influence as the result of rational persuasion. Someone makes arguments, gives evidence and produces facts/statistics, and we critically consider that evidence and come to the conclusion with a number of some of the following thoughts: '*Yes, you seem to be right*'; '*I accept these arguments*'; '*They are consistent with my beliefs*'; '*I accept the evidence as valid*'; '*I accept the speaker or the persuader as someone with credibility who has expertise and who's telling me the truth, and therefore I'm going to change my attitude or my behaviour as a result*'. This is what those seeking to obtain adherence by others to public health messages and mandates are trying to achieve. Unfortunately, internalisation also works for the anti-vaxxer and conspiracy groups if individuals feel their message is most persuasive creating a strong bonding, making it difficult to reverse.

In the domain of health science communication, scholars have explored, through decades of research since the 1960s, a host of messaging approaches, to aid public and patient decision making through increased understanding, action and internalisation (Trevena, et al., 2013). Failure to adhere to medical advice compromises the full benefits of the treatment/advice and suggested behaviour changes and is likely to increase disease transmission, hospitalisation rates, rehabilitation needs, on occasion's death rates and decrease the possibility of an informed decision being made involving a future healthy lifestyle option. Ley (1972) reports that over 50% of people forget to take the full number of their antibiotic tablets for the full period of time prescribed. Masur (1981) discovered that between one-third and one half of patients fail to adhere to their treatment. Failure is even greater when it involves a change in lifestyle like stop smoking/drinking or the essential current needs in designated circumstances to social distance, mask wear and use QR check-in tracing systems.

In general failure of an individual or the public at large to adhere to instructions and advice that are not simply requested but mandated in pandemic situations can be due to a variety of factors, involving inter alia one or more of:

- Poor ability to understand the message intellectually, or what have I got to do?
- An insufficient ability among second language persons to use the presentation language for reading and hearing,
- Unwillingness to comply, often due to prior indoctrination with misinformation and fake news,
- Personality issues, like low self-efficacy or competence to carry out the behaviour as well as external locus of control beliefs mentioned in the Health Behaviour Model discussion,
- Unwillingness/inability to do so through cultural beliefs, political beliefs or economic constraints.

The problem is that health officials and governments must always remember they are not just trying to manage a health issues like a disease but also '*manage persons*'. While the treatment and public health advice can rarely be varied, the nature of the relationship between the professional and the individual or public must frequently be massaged to suit the recipient(s) and appear more down to earth, humane and individualised, using a calm, manner to deliver material translated if necessary at a level most people can understand, void of medical and technical jargon (see readability below). The bedside manner needs to be displayed even when conveying public health advice and instruction on TV and other mass media. Alarmist messages, with emphasis on negative aspects of the pandemic (number of seriously ill people or deaths) rather than on positive ones (number of recovered), use of alarmist expressions (*'even young people are dying'*), and stories rich with elaborated focus on victims' personal details are as counter-productive as hyperbolic positivity and optimism, which produces a paradoxical effect that the unrealistic positive messages may lead to greater mistrust (*'what are they are hiding'*).

Psychological Studies in Persuasive Communication

Psychological studies into persuasive communication through half a century of research have generally discerned four major factors that influence adherence levels:

- The source of the message,
- The message itself,
- The context in which the message is transmitted,
- The recipient characteristics.

The interaction of all these variables can be quite complex, and as Laswell (1948) summarised succinctly very early on, we need to know, *'who said what to whom with what effect'*. We will consider the four elements one by one although recognising they mingle intricately. The research studies reported below were not always within the health ambit, but the general principles still apply whatever the context.

The Source of the Message

Credibility

It obviously matters a great deal who is communicating with us. If the communicator, organisation, institution or other group is perceived as trustworthy, then we are more likely to pay attention to the position being advocated. A well-informed professional such as a health professional, community leader or politician who is seen as motivated by a genuine concern for our welfare and not by self-interest is more likely to have their public health advice followed. A credible effective communication involves having a clear objective, knowing exactly what the message is that must be communicated to the receiver and choosing the most effective communication channel, e.g. personal presentation, video, written material, for the particular situation.

Hovland and Weiss (1951) tested the source credibility effect by giving subjects an initial questionnaire which included questions on why illegal drug abuse is wrong. A week later, four newspaper articles were presented to the subjects. Two provided arguments in favour of the issue, while the other two argued against. In addition, one article in each pair was attributed to a prestigious medical journal, while the other was a less credible source, a mass circulation newspaper. A second questionnaire was then given and attitude change measured. High credibility source positive change of + 22% was obtained towards the issue, while the low credibility positive change was + 8%. This difference is the result of source. If there is a time lag say a month or more, the differences decrease greatly. This presumably is due to the credibility of the source becoming less important and detached from the communication through passage of time. So if compliance is required immediately, the source must be perceived as credible. This was found in a recent mask wearing effectiveness study in Bangladesh (Abaluck et al., 2021) involving 342,183 adults in 572 villages. In villages receiving mask interventions from credible local health leaders, symptomatic prevalence of the virus was reduced by approximately 9% relative to comparison villages. Moreover, cloth mask distribution, role-modelling and active mask promotion tripled mask use to 42.3% in intervention villages compared to 13.3% in comparison with villages.

Attractiveness

Tannenbaum (1956) found that the amount of positive attitude change is directly proportional to the degree of rated attractiveness of the communicator rated on a range of bipolar dimensions. It is almost a replica of the interviewing mantra of '*first impressions count*'. Power to persuade is greatly increased if presenter credibility and trust is linked to being presentable, neat and pleasant in tone and manner, offering some charm and a sensitive appropriate humour. Politicians and senior medical officers need these qualities to gain acceptance and follow through for the content of their health messages.

Opinion Leaders

Information and advice that is acted upon has been conceptualised by psychologists as a stepped flow of information from opinion leaders to followers, then on to contacts, colleagues, etc. Opinion leaders must also have qualities raised in the two aspects above, such as being perceived as credible, trusted, respected, presentable, popular and 'in the know'. This leads to willingness to follow the 'advice' and behave in certain ways and hold particular opinions. An opinion leader need not hold an official or high position, but they are often well known and respected within their particular circle. Various internet platforms often use another name for these people; they can be called *influencers*. These opinion leaders can often be invaluable in persuading others to follow medical advice and government health instructions especially among immigrant groups with limited English skills and among First Nation groups and communities. These cultural/ethnic groups have particular cultural and religious beliefs and customs which can prevent some health messages from being accepted and may even be considered an attack on their culture.

Therefore, a trusted senior member of a community is often the best person to transfer the message in their cultural terms and even demonstrate adherence themselves, e.g. being vaccinated in public at the local clinic or using a mask.

While a popstar might be a good influencer for younger mainstream people, a respected elder or a sports star from that community would be a far more effective messenger than a person with no connection or understanding of the group's culture. Outgroup (i.e. government or predominant culture) imposition of a vaccine mandate or mask wearing, for example, may be viewed as a deliberate imposition or a threat and rejected by the in-group. But if the new behaviour is modelled, explained and demonstrated by a trusted in-group leader considerable fear, doubt and threat are removed to be replaced by more willing acceptance and imitative behaviour. There is often a step-like flow in the transmission of information as it passes down the line to lower level influencers such as a senior family member or local religious leader taking over the next stage to explain the message onto family members or congregation and encourage them to comply.

Research from the deadly West Africa Ebola crisis of 2014–2015 strongly supports the policy of enlisting local voices to help build engagement and trust in health officials and increase the success of such public health measures. For instance, specialised Ebola treatment facilities that employed community liaison officers and social mobilisers to raise awareness and resolve misconceptions were associated with increases in reporting Ebola cases (Christensen et al., 2020). Correlational evidence from Liberia also suggests that explicit government efforts to reach out to the population and create trust in institutions, and governments also may play an important role, like door-to-door canvassing, and are associated with compliance with crisis management policies like bans on gatherings (Tsai 2020) or to abide by mandated social distancing policies and using clinics for care during the Ebola outbreak (Blair et al., 2017).

Opinion leader trust was also related to decisions to adopt preventive measures such as Ebola vaccinations in the Democratic Republic of Congo (Vinck et al., 2019). Trusted voices of religious leaders have been shown to make public health messages more effective in changing behaviour during the West African Ebola crisis, for example, in Sierra Leone where religious leaders across faiths advocated for practices such as handwashing and safe burials. The engagement of the faith-based sector was considered a turning point in the epidemic response (Greyling et al., 2016). Therefore, finding the correct credible sources for different audiences is an effective strategy. Conversely, a lack of trust in public health officials may lead to negative effects on utilisation of health services. Reliable information and public health messages are certainly needed from national leaders and central health officials, but local voices can amplify these messages and help build the trust that is needed to spur behavioural change.

Of course credibility and trust can work for both facilitating health work and the opposite, of obstructing it, because such personal skills and qualities can also be hallmarks of demagogic leaders who rile against vaccination and other mandated behaviour and that constitutes very dangerous power. A good example of a persuasive Australian politician whose words are accepted like

Table 4.1 Death rate per 100,000 within 60 days of testing positive over 3 weeks to 21 November 2021

Age group	*Double vaccinated*	*Unvaccinated*
Under 18	0.0	0.1
18–29	0.0	0.3
30–39	0.3	1.1
40–49	1.0	3.6
50–59	2.2	13.0
60–69	7.8	32.8
70–79	21.1	69.3
80 +	66.6	161.0

Data adapted by author from UK Health Security Agency Report. Dec 13, 2021

a Papal Bull by followers occurred when one national party leader misused statistical evidence in her campaign against mandated vaccination speaking at a so-called freedom rally mid-December 2021 in Queensland. She claimed it was a fact that in England, more people are dying with COVID-19 who are double-vaxxed than unvaxxed, using data from UK Health Security Agency (13 12 2021) which shows that of 3726 Covid deaths over a three-week period to November 2021, 2903 were fully vaccinated, compared to 708 unvaccinated people. However, those figures were used in a deliberate misleading fashion and do not mean that vaccinated people are at a higher risk of death from Covid. Using the same data, the correct index from which to judge effectiveness is the death rate per 100,000.

Table 4.1 reveals that the death rate among unvaccinated people across the UK was higher for every age bracket when compared to those who were double-dosed in terms of the death rate per 100,000. Fully vaccinated people were around 90% less likely to die than those who weren't vaccinated.

Presenting the Message

The communication must be presented at a level that the particular recipients can understand. This may not necessarily be a second language problem but also can occur with first language recipients if their reading skills are poor and also when the material is spoken or written in a complex manner with many long tortuous sentences and technical terms unlikely to be understood. The measurement of readability levels is introduced below.

Communications can also be improved by visual material on hand outs, internet, YouTube, etc. For example how to use a mobile phone to operate the apps needed to successfully use QR codes to log in at shops, cafes, etc. for potential contact tracing purposes or copy vaccination records from government sites on to a mobile or computer. Memory too is very pertinent to failure in following health advice. From the work of Ebbinghaus, Iate in the nineteenth century, it has been known in repeated experiments that considerable forgetting of information can occur soon after presentation with 66% loss after two hours when using artificial verbal material termed nonsense syllables, i.e. meaningless material. When normal meaningful verbal material is employed, the forgetting is less severe. The differential rate of forgetting between meaningful and meaningless material occurs because some of the meaningful material can be related to and integrated with previous knowledge and experience. Meaningless material has nothing to lock onto. Since many members of the public can find communication from health professionals difficult to comprehend, it actually functions like meaningless material, cannot be related to anything they really know or have experienced and is therefore rapidly forgotten. To support this contention, Ley (1973) showed from a wide range of studies that between 37 and 50% of health advice and instructions is forgotten within an hour. The imperative here is to ensure the meaningfulness of the message match the language skills, experiences and understandings of the recipient(s).

One-Sided or Two-Sided Presentation

One-sided messages only present the advantages of taking action and fail to mention any possible disadvantages, for example educating mothers only about the benefits of the oral contraceptive pill, but not explaining the side effects or risks associated with the pill. The same issue arises with the Covid messages; do we simply provide information about the benefits of each particular restriction but also provide information on the downsides of not complying. This issue is concerned with whether the communication gives both sides of the argument or just one. Hovland et al. (1949) revealed that the effects of one or two-sided presentations depended on the initial opinions of the recipients towards the topic.

- In obtaining behaviour change/acceptance of the communicator's message, a two-sided presentation is more effective than only giving the communicator's arguments for those initially hold opposing beliefs and attitudes.
- The one-sided approach was better in generating higher levels of acceptance of the message in those initially in favour.
- Better educated persons were less influenced by one-sided than two-sided, while conversely poorly educated persons were more influenced by a one-sided presentation and confused by the pros and cons of a two-sided argument.

Overall, there are several good reasons for presenting a one-sided argument. The first reason is focus; it's hard enough to maintain attention for very long, so you want to make your point quickly and then offer only the information you need to bring the point home. The second related reason is that you really don't want to confuse matters by bringing in contradictory information/ argument. It might encourage some recipients to pause and say to themselves '*I never realised that*' and perhaps change their opinion in the wrong direction to the one you are proposing. In this way, you have the best chance to maintain clarity and conciseness, which are both important factors in credibility.

While these are powerful arguments for leaving out contradictory information, they all have weaknesses. Showcasing alternatives can actually clarify your case and shorten your argument, because our facts and evidence make stronger sense when seen in comparison with contradictory information. Besides, while clarity and conciseness are important to credibility, confidence tends to trump both, and confidence is strongly demonstrated by presenting arguments against alternatives rather than being afraid to shine a light on alternatives. Thus, in attempts to convince people to comply with advice or health instructions consider the recipients' present opinions, their level of education and their ability to weight up the benefits and drawbacks of various alternatives.

The best reason to use a two-sided argument is that many studies show it to be the most effective for an educated and involved audience. After analysing the results of 26 studies that compared the effects on attitude change of three different approaches, viz.: one-sided arguments, two-sided arguments, in which counter-arguments were listed, and two-sided arguments, in which counter-arguments were listed and refuted, Allen (1991) found:

- The least persuasive messages were two-sided with no refutations.
- Second were one-sided arguments.
- The most persuasive were those in which the speaker offered their desired arguments then listed counter-arguments and refuted these.

This implies that when you're trying the hardest to get your message across by focussing only on the strengths of your own arguments, when you're most passionate and enthusiastic about your own position, you are actually not as persuasive as when you devote some air time to refuting the other side. This is because from the audience's perspective, their brain starts searching for counter-arguments if none are given. Second, one-sided, 'no-brainer' arguments subtly imply that there is no decision to be made, which robs the audience of their power to choose.

So, generally good practice is to include and refute contradictory information/arguments in your communication. Finally, give a short summary reverting back to your message to bring your point home with strong positive arguments in favour of your position, delivered with enthusiasm, conviction and even passion about what you see as the way forward.

Order of Presentation
This variable is concerned with how should we order the arguments or facts to maximise adherence to the message? Many presenters when trying to convince the audience to follow a particular behaviour are not sure whether to articulate the positive argument first or the negative first.

- Research (McGuire, 1957) strongly suggests that the positive message/argument should come first with the negative second. The reason for this seems to be that when negative features are presented first, the subject is likely to accept the truthfulness of it, finds it unpleasant and tunes out, not paying sufficient attention to the later positive message.
- Starting with the pleasant matters keeps the audience focussed on the benefits before the negative elements lower attentiveness and interest.

So health professionals should focus on positive advantages accruing from adopting whatever is suggested or required with information about the consequences of not complying coming later.

Discrepancy Effects
Messages congruent with a person's or group's values and attitudes will be more acceptable and acted on than those that are incongruent as the contradictory information and required new behaviour will often create tension and stimulate an attempt to find ways to reduce it like denial of the credibility of the communication or refusing the accept the credibility of the communicator or downright suspicion and rejection of the communicator's agenda.

The greatest change in an audience occurs when a credible communicator advocates a position not too far removed from that of the receivers. People seem able to accept a position within a small range of latitude from their own. An extreme difference creates automatic rejection.

Acceptance is most likely to occur when neither communicator nor audience holds extreme views and the behaviours, requirements are clearly expounded and within the capabilities of the recipient to undertake.

Effect of Emotional Factors of Fear and Threat
One of the central emotional responses during a pandemic is fear. Humans, like other animals, possess a set of defensive systems for combating ecological threats (Mobbs et al., 2015). Negative emotions resulting from threat can be contagious and spread through a community like a virus (Kramer et al., 2014), making threats appear more imminent (Cole et al., 2013) (also *cf* climate warming deliberate panic creation). Witte et al. (2000) in a meta-analysis found that targeting fears can be useful in some situations, but not others since inducing fear leads people to change their behaviour if they feel

capable of dealing with the threat, but leads to defensive reactions like denial when they feel helpless to act. The results suggest that:

- Strong fear appeals produce the greatest behaviour change only when people feel a sense of efficacy that they can carry out the requirements. They are likely to respond with positive comments like '*that's interesting, I will try it out*' or '*it sounds difficult but I think I can re-organise my life around it*'.
- Strong fear appeals where recipients believe they are unable to change their behaviour appropriately produce the greatest levels of defensive responses such as *'I don't think I can manage to do that'* or *'I really don't understand what you want me to do' or 'I don't believe it is that serious' or 'I think there is a hidden agenda behind what you say'* (Remember the self-efficacy and external locus of control factors in the Health Behaviour Model, Chap. 3).

Appeals that arouse strong fear or offer threats do not generally increase motivation to follow the advice or accept the communicator's message. A '*boomerang effect*' can occur where fear creates defensive reactions such as inattentiveness, denial, repression (deliberate forgetting as ignorance is bliss and knowledge is stressful), resulting in shutting one's eyes and closing one's ears to it all. Reaction formation, where the recipient takes up the opposite behaviour, is another Freudian defence mechanism that powers up the process of denial, distortion and the disguising events which preclude realistic action and proactive problem solving.

As an example, Janis and Fechbach (1963) showed that varying the amount of fear in 3 messages on dental care affected level of action taken. The group receiving the most fear condition showed on self-report the greatest level of anxiety and worry, but this did not turn into action but actually decreased willingness to act on the advice. Fear, as a tactic to gain attention and agreement, has limited usefulness. In excess, it is counter-productive. Action to a fear communication seems to work better when the communication is followed immediately with specific advice and instructions. Leventhal (1976) found that after a fear talk about the dangers of tetanus infection, only 1 in 30 went for their shot. When instructions were also given in the talk about where and when to get a shot and its benefits 1 in 3 did so. It is therefore necessary to focus on the benefits of vaccination, mask wearing, social distance, etc. to gain optimal responsible behaviour in the current situation.

It is also believed that the relationship between fear and attitude is an inverted U-shaped graph. At low levels of fear content, the audience may simply tune out with disinterest. As fear content increases, more attention is paid with increased action followed. But at high fear content level, the reception of the message decreases again as an '*I do not want to know or hear this*' response inhibits attention.

Factors such as likely prior knowledge and attitudes to the message content, self-esteem level, personality issues and message complexity as well as audience ability to carry out behaviour they are being asked to do, all need to be taken into account in working out the degree of fear to be generated. More knowledgeable and intelligent persons are less likely to respond to a fear tactic. Those who generally display a high anxiety level (neurotic persons) will block out even minimal fear-inducing messages. Extroverts on the other hand will tend to require high levels of fear messages before they are likely to take any notice.

Emotion and Risk Perception

Some people function on the belief that bad things are less likely to befall them than other people. This is called the '***optimism bias***', and while optimism bias may be useful for avoiding negative emotions and facilitating more positive thinking about their ability to control their lives, it can lead to an underestimation of their likelihood of contracting a disease, an '*I'll be alright Jack*' sentiment and subsequent ignoring of public health warnings about mask wearing, social distancing, etc. (Wise et al., 2020). Social distancing and hand hygiene were most strongly predicted for those who perceived a high probability of personally being infected. Communication strategies must strike a balance between breaking through optimism bias without inducing excessive feelings of anxiety and dread.

Sound health decisions depend on accurate perceptions of the costs and benefits of certain choices for oneself and for society rather than optimism. Emotions often drive risk perceptions, sometimes more so than factual information (Loewenstein et al., 2001). An emotional response to a risky situation can influence thinking in two stages according to (Peters et al., 2006). First, the emotion's quality (e.g. positive vs. negative) focusses people on congruent information (e.g. negative information is picked on when feeling negative). That information, rather than the feeling itself, is then used to guide judgement at the second stage. For example, Noar et al. (2016) found that smokers exposed to more explicit pictorial negative emotional health warnings experienced more negative emotion towards warnings and smoking, spent more time examining warnings and recalled more risks, with subsequent positive effects on risk perception and quitting intentions. As negative emotions increase, people may rely on negative information about Covid more than other information to make decisions.

In the case of strong emotional reactions, people may also ignore important numeric information such as probabilities, which unfortunately are rarely given and have to be calculated personally. For example in the current pandemic, most TV news reports and newspapers tend to report negative facts such as total number of infections, hospitalised persons, deaths, ICU and ventilator cases on daily and periodic bases. These bland figures look horrendous, as we solemnly note another 40 deaths and 15 more on ventilators, creating a sense of despair and doom. However, a bit of quick maths by the presenters could allay a lot of fear if people were told the death to infection rate only represents (say) 1 death in every 10,000 hospitalised case (0.0001%). Negative framing captures too much unwanted attention, especially for people who are less mathematically skilled, and a focus on more positive data would be beneficial to many worried people, for example, by reporting the huge numbers of people infected who recover or experience only mild symptoms. While the negative information may increase negative emotion and sensitise people to otherwise neglected risks for themselves or others, we noted above that fear is generally not a good motivator for positive proactive behaviour and may lead to despair and a '*why bother I am going to get it anyway*' sentiments. Research is needed to determine whether a more positive frame could relieve negative emotions and lead the public to adopt increasingly public health behaviours as they see their destiny is in their hands.

Context of Presentation

Group Decision Making

Information and advice offered to groups is likely to be acted upon more than advice to individuals particularly if the presenter allows discussion to occur where '*public*' commitment by some members can convince waverers, leading to a consensus. This has been found in health and safety issues over the use of safety gear like PPE, safety helmets and evacuation procedures. For example, Lewis (1952) talked to groups of mothers to encourage them to give their infants cod liver oil and orange juice, then asked each participant to state openly whether they would follow the advice. Making a commitment with group members present was far more effective than having an individual talk. This technique has also been a very effective strategy to keep alcoholics and weight watchers moving forward. Always remember that communication is a two-way process and turns the group situation into a conversation where all have a chance to comment, ask questions, seek clarification, etc. all of which will facilitate improved understanding and increased adherence. In a group situation, the best way of increasing person-to-person communication is to seat people including yourself in a circle, then you look seem less of a teacher or a person in authority. Remove physical barriers, and no more sitting behind the desk making pronouncements like an autocrat.

In-Group Pressure

Very similar to group commitments by members who were not already convinced is the issue of in-group or peer-group influence on a person who may wish to be accepted as a member because relatives, friends and other significant others already are members which can be used both for encouraging socially positive compliance with public health directions but also with negative rejection behaviours. A very interesting and early demonstration of group pressure to induce compliance was a study by Asch (1951) involving a

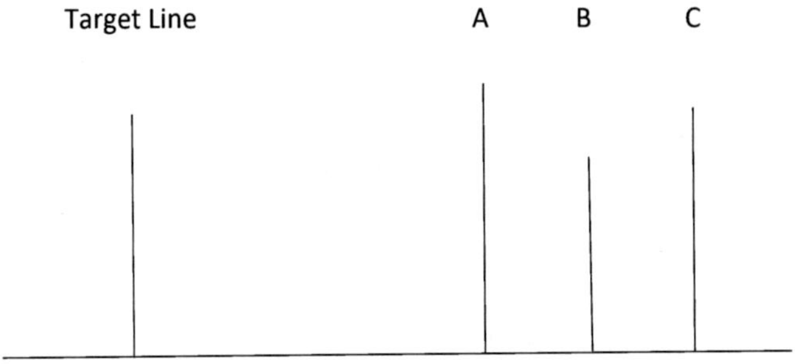

Fig. 4.1 Artificial example of the sort of layout of Asch's experimental design with target line and three comparison lines

series of experiments to demonstrate how people conform in groups. Participants were shown three lines of different lengths, then asked to select which line matched a fourth 'standard' line. When others in the group (who were planted) selected the wrong line, many participants would conform to group pressure and also select the wrong line length when the answer was fairly obvious. The confederates had agreed in advance what their responses would be when presented with the line task. The real participant did not know this and was led to believe that the other seven confederates/stooges were also real participants like themselves (Fig. 4.1).

Each person in the room had to state aloud which comparison line (A, B or C) was most like the target line which changed on every trial in a random fashion. The answer was always very obvious. The real participant sat at the end of the row and gave their answer last. There were 18 trials in total, and the confederates gave the wrong answer on 12 trials (called the critical trials). Asch was interested to see if the real participant would conform to the majority view. Asch's experiment also had a control condition where there were no confederates, only another real participant.

Asch measured the number of times each participant conformed to the majority view. On average, about one-third (32%) of the participants who were placed in this situation went along and conformed with the clearly incorrect majority on the critical trials. Over the 12 critical trials, about 75% of participants conformed at least once, and 25% of participants never conformed. In the control group, with no pressure to conform to confederates, less than 1% of participants gave the wrong answer.

The important factors that influence conformity appear to be:

- Being in the immediate presence of a group makes conformity more likely. Nowadays, this would include an online group.
- People are more likely to conform when they believe that they want to be part of the group and share something in common with the person or group such as attitudes, beliefs and/or values.

- A person is more likely to conform when all members of the group agree and hold the same views.
- The likelihood of conformity increases with the number of people present. If only one or two people are present, a person might argue against the group opinion and hold to their own position. With larger numbers or a few who are important significant others, then compliance is more than likely.

The important message from Asch (op cit) is when group affiliation is important to people, they are more likely to conform with social pressure, even though it may seem wrong. Real judgement is clouded by desire for acceptance, being seen as one of the group and supporting group values, beliefs and attitudes. A negative context examples are possibly a bikie group or a reclusive religious sect and a positive one the Boy Scouts, a mainstream church, a surf club or the Rotary club. In the context of Covid, this in-group compliance process leads to increasing extension to others of the main thrust of being *anti* any restrictions imposed for sound public health reasons, and because of the ubiquity of online groups hatching, nurturing and disseminating misinformation, there is facilitation of the easy entrapment of others without any significant personal contact.

Social Norms

Asch's experiment and many others pointedly show that people's behaviour is influenced by social norms: what they perceive that others are doing or what they think that others approve or disapprove of. A large literature has distinguished different motives for conformity to norms, including the desire to learn from other people and to gain affiliation or social approval (Cialdini & Goldstein, 2004; Wood, 2000). Although people are influenced by norms, their perceptions are often inaccurate. For example, people can underestimate the benefits of health-promoting behaviours (e.g. handwashing) and overestimate the minimum effects of unhealthy behaviours (Berkowitz, 2005).

Changing behaviours by correcting such misperceptions can be achieved by public messages reinforcing positive (e.g. health-promoting) norms. Providing accurate information about what most people are doing is likely to be helpful if what most people are doing is desirable (health-promoting). But if what most people are doing is not desirable, providing purely descriptive normative information can backfire by reducing positive behaviours among people who already engage in them, unless it is accompanied by information signalling that most people approve of these actions (prescriptive as opposed to descriptive norms) (Schultz et al., 2007).

Perceived norms are also most influential when specific to others with whom common identities are shared, including for the spread of health behaviours. Therefore, messages that provide in-group models for norms (e.g. members of your community) may therefore be most effective (Christakis et al., 2013).

The virus itself spreads from person to person, and since people centrally located in networks come into contact with more people, they are often among the first to be infected (Christakis et al., 2013). But these very same central people may be instrumental in slowing the disease because they can spread positive interventions like handwashing and physical distancing by demonstrating them to a wide range of people (Kim et al., 2015). Some research suggests that a larger proportion of interventions can come not from direct effects on people who receive the intervention, but from indirect effects on their social contacts who copied the behaviour (Bond et al., 2012). We may therefore leverage the impact of any behaviour change effort by targeting well-connected individuals and making their behaviour change visible and salient to others.

Another way to leverage the impact of norms falls under the general category of '*nudges*' (Halpern, 2015). Because people are highly reactive to the choices made by others, especially trusted others, an understanding of social norms that are seen as new or emerging can have a positive impact on behaviour. For instance, a message 'nudge' with compelling social norms might say, '*the overwhelming majority of people in your community believe that everyone should get vaccinated*'. Nudges and normative information can be an alternative to more coercive mandated means of behaviour change or used to complement regulatory, legal and other imposed policies when widespread changes must occur rapidly.

The Medium

There is virtually universal agreement that personal influence is more effective in persuasion than any other source. Documents, emails, notices pinned on notice boards, video presentations and the like can be ignored and forgotten. The presence of an effective communicator in a face-to-face situation with a group creates an opinion leader effect, offers increased attention and acceptance. This context also enables further explanation and answering questions which add to comprehension of the message and perceptions of credibility, knowledge, honesty and appeal in a communicator who can support the message by showing they are at ease, can generate a positive pleasant milieu, display empathy and present as genuine.

In a face-to-face context, the communicator can, like a good teacher, be aware of who is following and who is not, realise where interest is declining and provide immediate repair to the situation in a sensitive manner. Mass media presentations unfortunately tend to be one-way systems with little opportunity to correct misinterpretations or obtain immediate feedback. Even newer systems of the Zoom type may seem too user-unfriendly for many people who can have difficulty in negotiating the logging in, camera angles, etc. These electronic systems have shown that there is a divide between the computer/mobile savvy and the non-savvy, mainly less well educated and also older members of society, as the population tries to manage contact QR systems and amalgamate various documents of vaccination history onto the QR page. This is not to downplay the role of mass media in contemporary society where they have enormous influence in the continuing flow of information in a step-like process via opinion leaders to groups and then to individuals. Thus, the term mass media does not imply a substantial direct effect on the masses but a thrust to start a drip down effect.

Using tracking and tracing apps to persuade people to self-isolate has only had limited success. Arguably, the most important behaviour, in terms of reducing infection rates, after vaccination is self-isolating. The vast majority of people (86%) say they are willing to self-isolate if requested. But only 50% with a cough or fever actually reported adhering to guidance to self-isolate during the early phase of the pandemic, according to the Department of Health and Social Care tracker data (Smith, 2021). Similarly, in a pilot scheme of a manual track and trace system, only one-third of people fully cooperated. People do question the credibility of the app message to self-isolate because they can react defensively to messages that make them fearful. They may need persuading that contact with an infected person really happened, and an app message may not be able to do this.

Contact tracing is likely to be more effective if done by someone who is trusted, and linking from the app to a trusted member of the community could provide valuable reassurance and advice about self-isolating, thereby reducing anxiety. The valuable role of a respected opinion/community leader was raised earlier. Another factor affecting credibility is that some people will probably be asked to self-isolate multiple times, as they repeatedly come into close contact with people with Covid. This is especially likely for people with job roles that mean they are in contact with large numbers of people, those living in areas with higher population densities, those who use public transport and those who choose to mingle in entertainment venues where physical distancing is difficult to maintain. But requests to self-isolate, especially on more than one occasion, are likely to be influenced by a person's perception that what they are doing is making a difference. If during a period of self-isolation they do not go on to develop symptoms or test positive for Covid, then their response may seem pointless and increase the likelihood of ignoring any further requests to self-isolate subsequently. It is a bit like crying 'wolf' although there is still the probability that they will get infected on some future occasion.

To combat this, the app could feed back positive personalised messages that emphasise how self-isolation reduces the need for other lockdown measures. And motivational messages could also be sent such as messages that ask people to reflect on the regret they might feel if they didn't self-isolate and were responsible for infecting someone.

Many health campaigns using posters do not necessarily get over the message that was intended. The UK Health Education Council produced a poster aimed at discouraging pregnant women from smoking which displayed a nude heavily pregnant lady smoking with a written message in the poster about the effects the behaviour could have. Evaluation of the poster showed that the photograph was so novel it distracted viewers from the underlying primary message to do with smoking during pregnancy. Many found the woman ugly and ungainly with responses like '*it would put women off having babies, not off smoking*'. A younger mother only 4 months pregnant was horrified and found the picture frightening, '*am I going to be that big; the photo is surely out of proportion*' (Noar et al., 2016).

Readability: Use Appropriate Language
When communicating (verbal statement, email; notice; letter) to a wide audience, e.g. all employees, all clients or the general public, ensure the written or spoken material is presented at a level the poorest reader will understand. Don't pretend to be erudite using technical language, rare Latin derived words and/or long involved sentences.

> Given the contemporary trends in our operational and human resource downsizing, henceforth you will interface inter alia with an AI robotics configuration

After blank stares from the production team, the manager recovered the situation by stating:

> In future with fewer employees much of our work will be computerised

There exist several reading ease assessment techniques. The most popular is the *Flesch Reading Ease Formula* (Flesch, 1974) which can be applied to randomly selected 100 word length samples of writing (or speech) to assess their 'readability'. The formula derived from using a statistical process known as regression analysis is:

$$\text{Reading Ease} = 206.835 - 1.015\,\text{S} - 0.846\,\text{W}$$

where

S average length of sentences in words,
W average number of syllables per 100 words.

Readability scores range from 0 (practicably unreadable) to 100 (very easy for anyone).

It is very salutary to check out the readability of some of the email/ document/presentations you write using the Flesch Reading Ease Formula scale. The relationship of scores to age is very rough as there are very good young readers and very poor adult readers. You need to aim for a score within the range of 65–80 to ensure most readers will understand your email/ document/poster as this is around the level achieved by school leavers who are not proceeding to university (Table 4.2). Obviously if your 'audience' are generally graduates, then a lower score is acceptable but avoid the clever jargon.

Flesch also made one of the few attempts to quantify a measurement of human interest the message material will have for the reader. This involves counting the number of personal words and personal sentences. Personal words are essentially first, second and third person pronouns both singular and plural like '*you*' and '*we*' (which refer to persons rather than things) as well as all the words that have a gender connotation. Personal sentences include those with questions, commands, praise and requests that address the reader. .

Again a regression equation technique was employed using 100 word length randomly selected samples. His score formula is:

$$\text{Human Interest} = 3.635\ \text{pw} + 0.314\ \text{ps}$$

where

pw the number of personal words per 100 words,
ps the number of personal sentences per 100 sentences.

The total is the human interest score which places the material in a range from 0 (no human interest) to 100 (full of human interest) (Table 4.3).

Research with school texts (Burns & Charleston, 1997) and with health advice (Ley et al., 1977) show that readability is an important factor in determining successful comprehension and consequent behavioural action, and that much material is often too difficult for the populations they were designed for. Ley (1976) found that many leaflets, such as dental care and X-ray leaflets, as measured by the Flesch scale were too difficult to understand as they were written at a level at which only 25% of the population could understand them. By rewriting at a lower Flesch scale level, Ley (1976) found that a leaflet explaining the effects of anti-depression and anxiety drugs reduced significantly the errors made by patients who had the normal leaflet.

Serry et al. (2022) using readability tests (including Flesch) found Covid public health information on 367 individual web pages from the Victorian government's Department of Health and Human Services (DHHS) and the Department of Education and Training (DET) websites during the first year of the pandemic often too difficult to understand by the general public. The researchers discovered a senior secondary reading level of year 10 or above, which was required for effective engagement with the government website, Covid information and mandated requirements. About half of the Australian population reads at an education level of year 10 or below. The Australian Federal Government has endorsed accessibility guidelines that require communications should be written to suit a lower secondary level of education. This equates to students at around Year 7 to cater to differences in English ability, migrant persons, education level, disability status and access needs and is critical in reaching high levels of population coverage during a pandemic or epidemic, with key content such as when and where to wear masks, social distancing, vaccinations, when children can and can't go to school and valid reasons for going outside the home. This research also found older migrants relied quite heavily on their communities than official channels of information.

In response, a government spokesperson indicated public health communication throughout the pandemic had not been limited to information on websites, but included inter alia social media, newspaper and on train stations. None of them were assessed but may equally have been as unsuitable.

Numerous other studies have investigated the readability level of Covid health advice and regulations in other countries and repeatedly found it generally too difficult for the average person, e.g. Basch et al. (2020); Berg et al. (2021); Ferguson et al. (2021); Halboub et al. (2021); Mac et al. (2021); Mishra et al. (2020); Szmuda et al. (2020); Worrall et al. (2020); Wrigley et al. (2021).

However, a number of criticisms of readability ease scores do exist. The predictor variables appear to be simplistic, with formulae implying that word and sentence lengths are the only criteria of understandability, as it is obviously possible to write short sentences with short words that are hard to understand particularly in medical and health advice. Other variables that may impact on readability include the use of the passive voice, negatives, introduction of new concepts/jargon and abstract sentences. Textual variables like layout, and font size, are known to impact readability, as do reader characteristics such as motivation, actual reading ability and second language issues. An additional issue with reading interest involves the fact that much official material distributed by government, health practices and advertisements in newspapers providing impersonal command information on current advice, mandates and procedures to follow and employ a general unspecified '***you***' with whom the reader may not identify.

As a little experiment, you might like to try and check out the readability of some of the written Covid advice about social distancing and washing hands, of mandated issues of what can and cannot be done, about where and how long to quarantine, how to transfer your vaccination record to your mobile, of who to contact concerning adverse reactions or where to sign up for a vaccination. Table 4.2 shows that you really need to try to achieve a score of around the high 70's to ensure most people understand what they have been presented with. Anything less than the high 50's will prove difficult for around half the population to fully comprehend and act on what they have read or heard.

Using Visual Materials

The literature shows that non-text communication formats can improve attention, increase understanding and help with information recall, when compared to text alone. Houts et al. (2006) have reviewed the literature to understand

Table 4.2 Interpretation of reading ease scores

Reading ease	*Score*	*% adults able to understand material*	*Level of reading—approx. age range*	*Average sentence length in words*	*Average no. of syllables per 100 words*
Very easy	90–100	93	4 to age 9	8 or less	123 or less
Easy	80–89	91	5 to age 10	11	124 -131
Fairly easy	70–79	88	6 to age 11	14	132 -139
Standard	60–69	83	Age 12 -16 and average adult	17	140–147
Somewhat difficult	50–59	54	Age 17–18. Final year school	21	148–155
Difficult	30–49	33	University	25	156–167
Very difficult	Below 30	5	Post-grad	29+	168 plus

Collated by author from data in the manual

Table 4.3 Interpretation of the human interest score

Human interest score	*Description*	*Typical material*	*% personal words*	*% personal sentences*
60–100	Dramatic	Fiction	17	58
40–59	Highly interesting	Family emails	10	43
20–39	Interesting	Newspapers/magazines	7	15
10–19	Mildly interesting	Unsolicited mail/flyers/ meeting agendas, etc.	4	5
0–10	Dull	Scientific/professional	2	0

Constructed by author from material in the manual

the role of pictorial material in improving health communication, and based on this review, they suggest several design principles:

- Pictures closely linked to written or spoken text can, when compared to text alone, markedly increase attention to and recall of health education information. In particular, people with limited literacy or language skills can benefit from illustrations which can be quite simple stick people drawings with verbal bubbles or simple captions explaining the sequence with simple words to take home as reminders.
- Visuals enable people take in information faster and more accurately and remember it better, improving attention to, comprehension of and, most importantly, recall of technical and health information (Houts et al., 2006; Osborne, 2012).

- Pictures can also improve comprehension when they show relationships among ideas or when they show spatial relationships.
- Incorporating visual messages alongside text has been shown to be more persuasive and more stimulating, in turn generating an emotional response in the reader and triggering memory systems within the brain to provide a rapid response
- Pictures can change adherence to health instructions, improve behavioural intentions but emotional response to pictures affects whether they increase or decrease target behaviours and can reduce anxiety and minimise emotional stress associated with risk communication and getting negative prognostic information (Kim et al., 2020).

Visual narratives or infographics are promising tools for science and health communication, especially for broad audiences in times of public health crisis according to Brown et al. (2021) who produced an app with an illustrated 'flashcard' course platform to deliver visual narratives about Covid and then assessed their impact on behavioural intentions with 1775 health app participants. After viewing, each participant answered questions about their understanding of the course, how much they learned and their perceptions and behavioural intentions towards Covid. Participants generally evaluated 'flashcard' courses as easy to understand and were associated with improved self-efficacy and behavioural intentions towards the Covid disease. Findings supported the use of visual narratives to improve health literacy and provide individuals with the capacity to act on health information that they may know of but find difficult to process or apply to their daily lives.

Other researchers using infographics have also found significant improvement in individuals' understanding of information described in numeric or scientific terms with this enhanced comprehension resulting from infographic exposure subsequently increasing self-efficacy (Reddy, 2020) and/or lead to positive behavioural change (Cokely & Garcia-Retamero, 2013; Houts et al., 2006). Results of a large longitudinal survey with young adults showed that the effects of simple and memorable visual aids can be as effective as extensive educational interventions when being used to promote condom use among this population (Garcia-Retamero et al., 2015).

Even those who possess higher health literacy skills prefer shorter, simpler text. A scientific infographic needs to present adequate verbal and visual simplicity to render itself accessible and convincing to the audience (Ancker et al., 2006). Infographics of modest complexity are commonly used to convey knowledge to non-experts. Li et al. (2021) examined how Americans' awareness of 'flatten the curve' charts relates to their perceived effectiveness of social distancing measures, perceived controllability of the pandemic and behavioural intentions towards social distancing measures. Individuals exposed to the explanations of the 'curve' and the role of social distancing in altering the curve were more likely to see social distancing as an effective way to slow the spread of Covid. Thus, they were more willing to adopt social distancing behaviours.

In summary, when using pictorial and graphical material, presenters should:

- Consider 'how best can I use pictures to support key points?',
- Minimise and if possible remove distracting details in pictures,
- Use simple language in conjunction with pictures,
- Closely link pictures to text and/or captions,
- Be sensitive to the culture of the intended audience (using familiar objects and symbols) in creating or selecting pictures for use in health education materials and include people from the intended audience/culture in designing pictures,
- Have health professionals involved in planning the pictures, not artists,
- Evaluate pictures' effects by comparing response to materials with and without pictures in pilot runs.

The Recipient/Audience Characteristics in Susceptibility to Persuasion

Considerable research has been conducted to discover if there are individual differences between people in their susceptibility to persuasion. Various personality traits appear to be implicated as major factors in levels of impressionability.

- Those with low esteem appear to be more easily impressed by others.
- High intelligence is associated with low persuasibility.
- Persons of high internal locus of control tend to be less influenced by persuasion as they feel more in control of their own decision making (Richardson, 1963).

Facts about health dangers by themselves seem to evoke little change in behaviour and attitude. Those we need to convince and persuade to take appropriate health actions whether in relation to pandemics, drug abuse, alcoholism, etc. need also to be provided with the personal skills to:

- Learn to say '*no*' to others who would try to compete with fake information,
- Learn how to be assertive,
- How to make decisions,
- How to build up personal self-esteem to be confident in their own beliefs and decisions.

We need a more detailed analysis of motives, personality and interests that sensitise a person to their response to source and content of health messages and of ego defence processes like repression and reaction formation that distort, reframe and filter aspects of the perceived message. In terms of personal issues, Richardson's study (1963) of health advice on fluoridisation of water supplies found that those opposed to the introduction of the 'treatment' had a sense of powerlessness and felt controlled by external events rather than being in control of their own lives. Their negative attitude was their only strategy of showing power by ignoring or saying 'no' to the faceless 'them'.

There are also ethical considerations involved in attempting to persuade others to adopt some behaviour or attitude. Always consider whether we are trying to impose our personal view and behaviour on others in the disguise of a supposed requirement if we do not make it seem as being soundly based on evidence. Without giving the audience means or opportunity to evaluate whatever evidence there is and the sources of that evidence, we also may be bordering on the edge of misinformation, propaganda and manipulation.

Psychological Reactance

Remember when you were young (and even now!) and read a sign saying 'KEEP OFF THE LAWN' you probably felt compelled to walk deliberately on the lawn. Disobeying this forceful curt sign occurred for several reasons. These could include: it annoyed you; secondly, you saw no reason for it; thirdly you object to control and conformity thus refusing to obey; and finally, you enjoy the thrill and risk of getting away with behaviour that has been banned. I was a bit of a rebel at a UK grammar school as a boy where wearing the school cap to and from school was mandatory. I often removed it enroute and occasionally ended up in detention. This psychological reversal of behaviour or what is aptly named the '*boomerang effect*' means that health messages, advice and mandates can backfire, make things worse and need to be carefully managed.

Communicative messages transmitted in the public health field are often constructed strategically by the creators usually striving to curtail specific anti-social or unhealthy attitudes and behaviours manifested by the target audience. However, these messages are not always successful in achieving the intended effect. Messages with a specific intent can backfire and cause the opposite to the intention and can actually firm up the unhealthy or anti-social attitude or behaviour targeted for change and even increase the numbers holding such beliefs. A message can be either more or less consistent with one's initial belief or attitude on an issue, i.e. pro-attitudinal, or discrepant from one's belief or attitude, i.e. counter-attitudinal. It is in the latter situation where the strategy for change can backfire enormously.

An analysis of theoretical mechanisms for the effect suggests two distinct paths to the boomerang (Byrne & Hart, 2009). One path predicts that message receivers will process harmful elements in a message at the expense of those that were intended; that is their focus precludes understanding of the intent of the message. The other path predicts that receivers will understand the message as intended, but then resist complying with it as their views are more strongly held.

Note that a boomerang is distinct from a failure to persuade which suggests non-movement of a message receiver's belief, given a persuasion attempt. In other words, a boomerang is not merely ineffective, and it is quite counter-productive. That is, a belief boomerang occurs when a message receiver's belief position moves in a direction opposite to the advocated position in a message when compared with a baseline (Byrne & Hart, 2009). The baseline can be one's initial position or a control group's position.

The negative outcome when persuading may stem from:

- The target's desire to conform to and maintain membership of some valued in-group
- When the communicator's position is too far from the recipient's position and thus produces a 'contrast' effect and thus enhances their original attitudes,
- An attempted attitude change is considered as an impediment to a person's freedom; the more the implication of threatened freedom, the more inclination towards the regaining of that freedom (Brehm & Brehm, 1981),
- The target's misinterpretation of the message,
- When the persuasion triggers aggression or unalleviated emotional arousal,
- The target's aversion for emotionally confronting information such as something that causes cognitive dissonance (see below) or induces a high fear level,
- The target's resentment at feeling manipulated or challenged,
- When new information presented as part of an argument against a position actually reinforces the target's faith in their current position.

On the other hand, due to the human need to preserve a positive self-image, it is likely that directing attention to people about biases they hold also may cause a boomerang effect in order to save face in cases where being associated with a specific bias implies negative social connotations.

Cognitive dissonance (Festinger, 1962) has been applied to explain the boomerang effect and describes the mental discomfort experienced while dealing with two conflicting attitudes, beliefs or values. People in a state of cognitive dissonance prefer to take action that enables them reduce the extent of their dissonance. One of the common examples can be a situation when an individual smokes (behaviours) and at the same time knows that smoking is the prime reason behind cancer (cognition); they will be in the state of cognitive dissonance. They often resolve the clash by claiming that since the percentage of smokers getting cancer is small, they won't be affected and therefore continue smoking—a false self-justification or rationalisation.

Work done in the field of commitment and post hoc justification has found that negative consequences of behaviour can actually increase the likelihood that a person will justify it and resist change like the smoker above. Of course, the same sorts of arguments are used by those who resist vaccination, avoid mask wearing, social distancing, etc. in the mistaken belief that they will not catch the virus or that these actions are ineffective. All this involves a complex of denial, rationalisation, reaction formation, repression and a mistaken belief that freedom of choice is sacred. In cognitive dissonance theory when an individual is faced with information that does not coincide with their world view or positive self-concept (which contains the complete picture of themselves including beliefs and attitudes), they are likely to find a way to discredit the new information in the attempt resolve the dissonance that is created by the information and maintain their concept of themselves rather than allow it to be destroyed. '*I am not stupid; I know I am right*'.

If we return to the KEEP OFF THE LAWN sign, there would be more acceptance and compliance if it had been more gently explained with a sign devoid of capital letters and reading '*please stay off the lawn because new seed has just been spread*'. An order thus turns into an explanatory request. Similarly with a verbal health advice, the delivery should be explanatory, calm and clear, offering opportunity to question and discuss. The decision to change behaviour/attitude should come from the recipient(s) themselves rather than imposed, locking them into a corner from where they fight to get out. Of course in a public health emergency as we have now, time is of the essence and mandates are necessary, but as discussed in Chap. 10 on the ethics of mandates where the arguments for justification are given, these are still only value judgements and some leniency needs to be applied where windows of personal responsibility can be opened and managed adroitly minimising the boomerang effect.

This chapter provides some insights from the past work on related issues in the social and behavioural sciences that may help public health officials, politicians and the media mitigate the impact of the current pandemic. Some social scientific insights for Covid pandemic responses for public health experts, policymakers and community leaders to be a persuasive communicator could include some of these:

- Demonstrate expertise and knowledge to make yourself credible and trustworthy to provide an opinion leader style.
- Be aware when to provide one-sided or two-sided arguments as appropriate.
- Plan a logical step-by-step explanation and argument, simple, concrete and clear using a language or readability level for lay persons generally, and add clear simple pictorial/graphical illustrations that are memorable.
- Be empathic and aware of signs of audience confusion or difficulty in understanding as well as listening attentively to their questions.

- Don't instil fear or advocate extreme views unless there is imminent severe danger.
- Never suggest changes in behaviour or attitude without clear explanation why, showing the audience clearly what is the benefit for them and offer the changes in a step-like sequence.
- Try to get a public commitment from as many in a group as possible.
- As was noted in combatting fake news, nudging recipients to think more critically and carefully about material aided their acceptance of alternative more sound advice and behaviour.
- Create a shared sense of identity or purpose by addressing the public in collective terms and by urging '**us**' to act for the common good as a big in-group '*in it altogether*' that will protect loved ones, neighbours and the community in general.
- Identifying special opinion leaders, for example, religious, community, sports leaders that are credible to their specific audiences to share public health messages can be effective.
- Norms of prosocial behaviour are more effective when coupled with the expectation of social approval and modelled by in-group members who are central in social networks.
- Leaders and members of the media should highlight bipartisan political support for Covid-related measures, to reduce polarisation and lead to less-biased reasoning.

References

Abaluck, J., et al. (2021). Impact of community masking on COVID-19: A cluster-randomized trial in Bangladesh. *Science, 375*(6577). https://doi.org/10.1126/science.abi9069

Allen, M. (1991). The effectiveness of one-sided and two sided appeals as a function of familiarization and context. *Western Journal of Speech Communication., 55*(4), 390–404. https://doi.org/10.1080/10570319109374395

Ancker, J. S., et al. (2006). Design features of graphs in health risk communication: A systematic review. *Journal of the American Medical Informatics Association., 13*(6), 608–618. https://doi.org/10.1197/jamia.M2115

Asch, S. E. (1951). Effects of group pressure upon the modification and distortion of judgment. In H. Guetzkow (ed.) *Groups, leadership and men*. Carnegie Press: Pittsburgh, PA

Basch, C. H., Mohlman, J., Hillyer, G. C., & Garcia, P. (2020). Public health communication in time of crisis: Readability of on-line COVID-19 information. *Disaster Medicine and Public Health Preparedness, 14*(5), 635–637. https://doi.org/10.1017/dmp.2020.151.14(5):635-7

Berg, S. H., O'Hara, J. K., Shortt, M. T., et al. (2021). Health authorities' health risk communication with the public during pandemics: A rapid scoping review. *BMC Public Health, 21*(1), 1–23. https://doi.org/10.1186/s12889-021-11468-3

Berkowitz, A. (2005). An overview of the social norms approach. In L. Stewart & L. Lederman (Eds.), *Changing the culture of college drinking* (pp. 193–214). Hampton Press.

Blair, R., et al. (2017). Public health and public trust : survey evidence from the Ebola virus epidemic in Liberia. *Social Science Medicine, 172*, 89–97. https://doi.org/10.1016/j.socscimed.2016.11.016

Bond, R., et al. (2012). A 61 million person experiment in social influence and political mobilisation. *Nature, 489*, 295–298. https://doi.org/10.1038/nature11421

Brehm, J. W., & Brehm, S. S. (1981). *Psychological reactance—a theory of freedom and control*. Academic Press.

Brown, P., et al. (2021). COVID ISSUE: visual narratives about COVID-19 improve message accessibility, self-efficacy, and health precautions. *Frontiers in Communication., 6*, 712658. https://doi.org/10.3389/fcomm.2021.712658

Burns, R., & Charleston, R. (1997). The Readability of English medium texts in Brunei primary schools. *Australian Journal of Language and Literature., 20*, 290–302.

Byrne, S., & Hart, P. S. (2009). The boomerang effect a synthesis of findings and a preliminary theoretical framework. *Annals of the International Communication Association., 33*(1), 3–37. https://doi.org/10.1080/23808985.2009.11679083

Christakis, N., et al. (2013). Social contagion theory. *Statistics in Medicine, 32*(4), 556–577. https://doi.org/10.1002/sim.5408

Christensen, D., et al. (2020). Community based crisis response from Sierra Leone Ebola outbreak. *American Economic Review, 110*, 260–264. https://doi.org/10.1257/pandp.20201510.26085/C34K58

Cialdini, R., & Goldstein, N. (2004). Social influence, compliance and conformity. *Annual Review of Psychology, 55*(1), 591–621. https://doi.org/10.1146/annurev.psych.55.090902.142015

Cokely, E., & Garcia-Retamero, R. (2013). Communicating health risks with visual aids. *Current Directions in Psychological Science, 22*, 392–399. https://doi.org/10.1177/0963721413491570

Cole, S., Balcetis, E., & Dunning, D. (2013). Affective signals of threat increase perceived proximity. *Psychological Science, 24*(1), 34–40. https://doi.org/10.1177/0956797612446953

Ferguson, C., Merga, M., & Winn, S. (2021). Communications in the time of a pandemic: The readability of documents for public consumption. *Australian and New Zealand Journal of Public Health, 45*(2), 116–121. https://doi.org/10.1111/1753-6405.13066

Festinger, L. (1962). *A theory of cognitive dissonance*. Stanford University Press.

Flesch, R. (1974). *The art of readable writing*. Harper Row.

Greyling, C., Maulit, J. A., Parry, S., et al. (2016). Lessons from the faith driven responses to the W. African Ebola epidemic. *The Review of Faith & International Affairs, 14*, 118–123. https://doi.org/10.1080/15570274.2016.1215829

Halboub, E., Al-Ak'hali, M. S., Al-Mekhlafi, H. M., & Alhajj, M. N. (2021). Quality and readability of web-based Arabic health information on COVID-19: An infodemiological study. *BMC Public Health, 21*(1), 1–7. https://doi.org/10.1186/s12889-021-10218-9

Halpern, D. (2015). *Inside the Nudge Unit*. Random House.

Houts, P. S., Doak, C. C., Doak, L. G., & Loscalzo, M. J. (2006). The role of pictures in improving health communication: A review of research on attention, comprehension, recall, and adherence. *Patient Education and Counseling, 61*(2), 73–90. https://doi.org/10.1016/j.pec.2005.05.004

Hovland, C., & Weiss, W. (1951). The influence of source credibility on communication effectiveness. *Public Opinion Quarterly, 15*(4), 635–650. https://doi.org/10.1086/266350

Hovland, C., et al. (1949). *Experiments in mass communication.* Princetown University Press.

Janis, I., & Feshbach, S. (1963). Effects of fear arousing communication. *The Journal of Abnormal and Social Psychology, 48*(1), 78–89. https://doi.org/10.1037/h0060732

Kim, D. A., Hwong, A. R., Stafford, D., et al. (2015). Social network targeting to maximise possible behaviour change. *Lancet, 386*, 145–153. https://doi.org/10.1016/S0140-6736(15)60095-2

Kim, M. T., Kim, K. B., Ko, J., et al. (2020). Health literacy and outcomes of a community-based self-help intervention. *Nursing Research, 69*, 210–218. https://doi.org/10.1097/NNR.0000000000000409

Kramer, A., Guillory, J. E., & Hancock, J. T. (2014). Experimental evidence of massive scale emotional contagion through social networks. *Proceedings of the National Academy of Sciences of the United States of America, 111*(24), 8788–8790. https://doi.org/10.1073/pnas.1320040111

Laswell, H. (1948).The structure and function of communication in society. In L.Bryson (ed) *The Communication of Ideas.* Harper: New York.

Levanthal, H., (1976). Findings and theory in the study of fear communication. In L. Berkowitz (ed) *Advances in Experimental Social Psychology.* Academic Press: New York.

Lewis, K. (1952). Group decision and social change. In Swanson, G. et al. (eds) *Readings in Social Psychology.* Holt: New York.

Ley, P. (1972). Comprehension, memory and the process of communications with the patient. *Journal of International Health Promotion Education, 10*, 23–36.

Ley, P. (1973). The measurement of comprehensibility. *Journal of International Health Promotion Education, 11*, 17–26. https://doi.org/10.1080/03073289.1973.10805309

Ley, P. (1976). Towards better doctor-patient relationships. In Bennet, A. (ed) *Communication in Medicine.* London: OUP.

Ley, P., Jain, V., & Skilbeck, C. (1977). A method for decreasing patients' medication errors. *Psychological Medicine, 6*, 599–601. https://doi.org/10.1017/S0033291700018237

Li, M. et al. (2021). Can scientists use simple infographics to convince? *Public Understanding of Science, 30*, 898–912. https://doi.org/10.1177/0963662521103 8719

Loewenstein, G. F., Weber, E. U., Hsee, C. K., & Welch, N. (2001). Risk as feelings. *Psychological Bulletin, 127*(2), 267–286. https://doi.org/10.1037/0033-2909.127.2.267

Mac, O. A., Muscat, D. M., & Ayre, J. (2021). The readability of official public health information on COVID-19. *Medical Journal of Australia, 215*(8), 373–375. https://www.mja.com.au/journal/2021/coronavirus-covid-19-vaccination-information-must-pay-attention-health-literacy

Masur, F. (1981). Adherence to health care regimes. In C. Prokop & L. Bradley (eds.), *Medical Psychology*. New York: Academic Press.

McGuire , W. J., (1957). Order of presentation as a factor in conditioning persuasiveness. In C. I. Hovland et al (eds). *The Order of Presentation*. New Haven: Yale

Mishra, V., & Dexter, J. P. (2020). Comparison of readability of official public health information about COVID-19 on websites of international agencies and the governments of 15 countries. *JAMA Network Open, 3*(8), e2018033.

Mobbs, D., Hagan, C. C., Dalgleish, T., et al. (2015). The ecology of human fear. *Frontiers in Neuroscience, 9*, 55–66. https://doi.org/10.3389/fnins.2015.00055

Noar, S. M., Hall, M.G., Francis, D. B., et al. (2016). Pictorial cigarette pack warnings: A meta analysis of experimental studies. *Tobacco Control, 25*, 341–354. 10.1016.

Osbourne, H. (2012). *Health Literacy from A–Z*. Jones and Bartlett.

Peters, E., Västfjäll, D., Gärling, T., & Slovic, P. (2006). Affect and decision making: A hot topic. *Journal of Behavioral Decision Making, 19*, 79–85.

Richardson, A. (1963). Attitudes to Flouridation in W. Australia. *Australian Dental Journal, 8*, 513–524.https://doi.org/10.1111/j.1834-7819.1963.tb03289.x

Schultz , W., Nolan, J., Cialdini , R., et al. (2007). The constructive, destructive, and reconstructive power of social norms. *Psychological Science, 18*(5). https://doi.org/10.1111/j/1467-9280.2007.01917.x

Serry, T., Stebbins, T., & Martchenko, A., et al. (2022). Improving access to COVID-19 information by ensuring the readability of government websites. *Health Promotion Journal*. https://doi.org/10.1002/hpja.610

Smith, L. E., (2021). Adherence to the test, trace, and isolate system in the UK: results from 37 nationally representative surveys. *BMJ*. 372. https://doi.org/10.1136/bmj.n608

Szmuda, T., Özdemir, C., Ali, S., et al. (2020). Readability of online patient education material for the novel coronavirus disease (COVID-19): A cross-sectional health literacy study. *Public Health, 185*, 21–25. https://doi.org/10.1016/j.puhe.2020.05.041

Tannenbaum, P. (1956). Initial attitude towards source and concepts as factors in attitude change in communication. *Public Opinion Quarterly, 20*, 413–425. https://doi.org/10.1086/266638

Trevena, L. J., Zikmund-Fisher, B. J., Edwards, A. et al. (2013). Presenting quantitative information about decision outcomes: A risk communication primer for patient decision aid developers. *BMC Medical Informatics and Decision Making, 13* Suppl 2(Suppl 2), S7. https://doi.org/10.1186/1472-6947-13-S2-S7.

Tsai, l., Morse, B., & Blair, R. (2020). Building credibility and cooperation in low trust settings in Liberia during the 2014–15 Ebola crisis. *Comparative Political Studies, 53*, 1582–1618. https://doi.org/10.1177/0010414019897698

UK Health Security Agency. (2021, Nov 23). Retrieved 14 December 21 from https://twitter.com/ukhsa/status/1470038788198080520

Vinck, P., Pham, P., Bindu, K., et al. (2019). Institutional trust and misinformation in response to the 2018-19 Ebola outbreak in the Congo. *The Lancet Infectious Diseases, 19*, 529–536. https://doi.org/10.1016/s1473-3099(19)30063-5

Wise, T., Zbozinek, T., & Michelini, G., et al. (2020). Changes in risk perception and self-reported protective behaviour during the first week of the COVID-19 pandemic in the United States. *Royal Society Publishing* open science. 7200742200742. https://doi.org/10.1098/rsos.200742

Witte, K., & Allen, M. (2000). A meta analysis of fear appeals: Implications for public health campaigns. *Health Education Behavior, 27*, 591–615. https://doi.org/10.1177/109019810002700506

Wood, W. (2000). Attitude change persuasion and social influence. *Annual Review of Psychology, 51*(1), 539–570. https://doi.org/10.1146/annurev.psych.51.1.539

Worrall, A. P., Connolly, M. J., O'Neill, A., et al. (2020). Online readability of COVID-19 health information: A comparison between four English speaking countries. *BMC Public Health, 20*(1), 1635. https://doi.org/10.1186/s12889-020-09710-5

Wrigley, K., Murray, K., McCarthy, C., et al. (2021). An objective analysis of quality and readability of online information on COVID-19. *Health Technology, 11*(5), 1093–1099. https://doi.org/10.1007/s12553-021-00574-2

CHAPTER 5

Impacts on the World of Work

The only way to do great work is to love what you do. If you haven't found it yet, keep looking. Don't settle. Steve Jobs
Clients do not come first. Employees come first. If you take care of your employees, they will take care of the clients. Richard Branson

Abstract The crucial issues of this chapter focus on the way Covid has affected unemployment levels, where work is conducted, and what personal benefits employees seek from work now. Restrictions imposed by national governments in developed countries involving quarantine periods, drastically reduced travel limitations, social distancing, mask wearing, limitations on numbers gathering together, all conspired to limit work opportunities and consumer ability to seek purchases, leading to economic slowdown with minimal activity for, and even closure of, many businesses. Hence, unemployment surged and many employees, where feasible, worked from home. The pros and cons of work from home (WFH), including the employee preference for continuation in the hybrid form, are reviewed along with discussion of the 'Zoom' effect. Employees are showing increasing propensity to move from their preCovid employment and seeking either more WFH, or to be entrepreneurial or joining more caring companies that have employee well-being more central in their philosophy. The pandemic has changed the priory rankings of reasons why people work with money less salient while intrinsic motivations like achievement, self-esteem, personal satisfaction and better life-work balance in a flexible system will contribute more significantly in the future.

Keywords Unemployment · Work from home · Hybrid work · Zoom · Return to office reluctance · Employee work preferences

© The Author(s), under exclusive license to Springer Nature Singapore Pte Ltd. 2023

R. B. Burns, *The Human Impact of the COVID-19 Pandemic*,
https://doi.org/10.1007/978-981-99-1710-5_5

Why Do People Work?

This seems a rather simple question, but the answer has many facets. This is reflected to some extent in the aphorism, *do we work to live or live to work?* The exploration of this issue as it was before Covid and what changed due to Covid impacts can shed light on the effects of the pandemic on the ways people now approach work and the socio-psychological effects of the changes.

PreCovid the major motivator was income because it provided the finance to fund basic needs like food, housing, clothing, etc., and if possible, a good life with a car (or two) and holidays (maybe overseas), and also for many an eventual retirement fund, even though some may not have enjoyed what they did. Wages/salary/bonuses are extrinsic motivations or external rewards. It motivated promotion and career development to facilitate a keeping up with the Jones'. But earning money is a limited view of the value of work for the individual. Given the drastic upheavals of Covid involving for some mental deterioration from stress and even early death from infection, many employees are realising that there is more to life than money. In fact, psychologists such as Maslow (1943) had argued that once basic biological needs like food, shelter and security are met, then humans are motivated to seek more personal and social needs such as feelings of achievement, self-esteem, affiliation with others, personal identity and improved life-work balance, and these are becoming increasingly embraced as Covid recedes, and income becomes less salient. Why were these other personal factors important preCovid and more so than income in the future:

- The sense of achievement and self-fulfilment provides intrinsic motivation (internal reward). Job title, occupation and/or promotion are useful measures of personal standing particularly when asked *what do you do?* The job bestows a role, purpose and identity on you and recognition from others (compare an ICU nurse with a used car sales person). Your sense of identity of who you are, what you can do, is closely tied to your job. It is also a crucial part of you as an essential factor that shapes your definition of who you are as an individual.
- Humans are social animals, and work provides social connection through the workplace peer group, often people with similar skills, interests and views. It helps provide acceptance and companionship like Friday post-work drinks, and picking you up to go to work when the car breaks down. The social benefits also include being able to gain some relief from personal home problems as other topics can be a different focus among close friends and colleagues. For many people, their closest friends are the ones whom they have met at work, and these friendships can often last during retirement. In a way, your work friends often feel like your tribe. When this link is broken through becoming unemployed or retirement you can feel very alone and depressed missing your friends.

- Work induces routine into life with its daily requirement to be at a particular place at a particular time. It is then easier to plan other activities doing what provide you with genuine enjoyment and satisfaction in other parts of your day to create a good work-life balance. Losing a job removes the structured life and creates a disrupted time as you may stay in bed longer, watch TV/play computer games for long hours, lack energy, developing feelings of loneliness, depression and social exclusion.
- Employment is generally good for your mental health for the reasons above as it allows you to meet people, boosts your self-esteem, feels supported and gives you a sense of purpose and identity. The thought of contributing to something bigger than yourself can make you feel more fulfilled with your life.

However, preCovid, in big corporations, the personal intrinsic reasons noted above were often subjugated to more economic core drivers prior to Covid such as the influence of Harvard Business School-style management theory and HR, the MBA syllabus/qualification, the decline of allegiance to unions, career advancement, the 24/7 'workaholic' drive, and the co-option of employees' hearts and minds into profit-driven projects. The late 1990s and two decades of the twenty-first century represented to many the peak capitalism of the dot.com era, with an invincible future where employment was the only source of meaning, rubbing out the Woodstock search for meaning brand. Values were still important but limited to those of the company, the over-riding one being to align employee values to growing the business.

The impact of Covid on the world of work changed the meaning of work for many. It is easy to see why changes to work practices such as having to move your desk on to the kitchen table at home or becoming unemployed because of Covid lockdowns might lead to demoralisation, loss of self-esteem, loss of identity and loss of social/peer support and alienation from society. But paradoxically, as employers are realising now, as they try to get workers back to the workplace, many employees actually gained more satisfactions from home working, setting their own routines with less big brother watching closely over them, more contact with their children and obtaining social support by meeting colleagues or other friends at a café, maintaining limited but psychologically important time in company of their choosing at times that fitted their schedule, part of which might be in some cases working in the evening when the children were in bed. The priority of income declined and other more personal issues gained impetus and importance.

Covid Changes to the World of Work

Covid is certainly not responsible for the total change to the way work is organised although it has accelerated some changes. Gradual movements in the world of work have been noted by many researchers in the area for the last three decades. The major changes have involved the casualisation of service jobs, the increase in female participation, job hopping, the growing importance of transferable skills and lifelong learning, changing consumer buying habits and working from home which were highlighted by Burns (1993). These changes and others have been greatly amplified by the pandemic as the workplace and even work itself became disrupted as lockdowns, quarantine, contact isolation, social distancing, restrictions on cross-border and international movements of skilled professionals and student travel, plus vaccine mandates for certain workplaces took hold of economic and social life. Living through the coronavirus pandemic has brought about a fair amount of soul searching for both employers and employees.

Two major impacts of the Covid infection were (1) an insidiously sudden *increase in unemployment* as very restrictive rules and extreme safety measures were introduced around the world since no one really could envisage what the impact of Covid would be in the early days and (2) an increase in *working from home (WFH)*. For employees and employers, it was all new territory for both parties and of course for governments which had to manage it.

Unemployment

Unemployment mainly hit part-time employees in hospitality, tourism, retail and small business like hairdressing and owners of such businesses all over the world. Much unemployment stemmed from lockdowns, quarantine orders, and social distancing (numbers allowed on premises) which caused forced closure, and later as things started to look up, vaccination mandates and personal isolation for close contacts took effect, disabling small businesses with loss of employees particularly in cafes/restaurants where applied density numbers and 'takeaways' would not provide sufficient income to carry on from Los Angeles, the Costa Brava, the Greek islands, Fiji, London, and Melbourne. Businesses in national border areas suffered drastic loss of income as travel between neighbouring countries were banned for a time.

The toll that the COVID-19 pandemic has exacted on the global economy has been significant, with the International Monetary Fund (IMF) estimating that median global GDP dropped by 3.9% from 2019 to 2020, making it the worst economic downturn since the Great Depression. As a result, similar scenarios were evident in most developed and undeveloped countries.

In the UK, the number of people in work fell by 825,000 people between January–March 2020 and October–December 2020, while unemployment rose by almost 400,000, and the number of people who were economically inactive rose by 327,000. Redundancies reached record highs while UK working hours dropped to the lowest since 1994 (House of Commons Library Research Briefing, 2022). Two years after the start of the pandemic, employment levels in the UK were still around 350,000 lower than they had been before it began. The youngest and oldest workers were most likely to lose their jobs or be furloughed at the beginning of the pandemic. Low paid workers were more likely to work in sectors most affected by the pandemic, particularly hospitality and non-essential retail, so were most likely to be put on furlough or experience falls in income at the beginning of the pandemic. Over 11.7 million jobs were furloughed in total on the UK's government's support Coronavirus Job Retention Scheme. Youth employment recovered quickly from spring 2021 and had nearly returned to prepandemic levels by January–March 2022, but many older workers opted to retire early. However, the rise in vacancies in 2022 was driven by low paying jobs, and by February 2022, unemployment rates in low occupation had almost completely recovered (House of Commons Library Research Briefing, 2022).

A similar rapid and sudden hit on employment occurred in the USA. Of the 16.9 million people unemployed in July, 2020, 9.6 million (57%) were unable to work because their employer closed or lost business due to the pandemic. The recession induced by the pandemic resulted in steep job losses, pushed the unemployment rate to a high of 13.0% in the second quarter of 2021. Total US civilian employment fell by 8.8 million over the whole year, as the brought economic expansion to a sudden halt (U.S. Bureau Of Labor Statistics Monthly Report, 2021) Service occupations, food preparation and serving-related occupations such as personal care were the most affected, with jobless rates that were nearly 4 times higher than they were in 2019.

Poorer countries were not exempt. A study of smaller countries in Asia Region and some in the West Africa Region who were all involved in the *US President's Emergency Plan for AIDS Relief (PEPFAR)* revealed that in the majority of these *PEPFAR* countries, GDP fell in 2020, the year the pandemic emerged, compared to 2019. In 11 of the countries, there was a contraction of GDP greater than 10% with *PEPFAR* countries coming off worse than other regional nations. Moreover, while the global economy was estimated to have recovered in 2021, this did not happen in *PEPFAR* countries. While almost all *PEPFAR* countries were experienced some GDP growth in 2021, the projected growth, at least through 2023 remains below prepandemic projections (10–13% below). By contrast, the current projections of global GDP exceed the prepandemic projections (Oum et al., 2021). This leads to significant uncertainty facing economic recovery in PEPFAR countries, which will be highly dependent on the future course of the pandemic variants, international economic relief efforts, and access to sufficient vaccine. By 2021 less than a third of the population has received at least one vaccine dose in 30 of the 53 *PEPFAR* countries.

Australia did not escape the employment mayhem. The immediate impact on employment in early and mid-2020 was sizeable; 870,000 people had lost their jobs already by mid-2020 reported in a report from the Australian Institute of Health and Welfare (2021). The seasonally adjusted unemployment rate for the population aged 15 and over rose steeply from 5.3% in March 2020 to 7.4% in June and July 2020 (highest level in 22 years), before gradually declining by Nov 2022 to around 3.5% as economic business picked up.

Unemployment rates in the UK and Australia have each reached an incredibly low 3.5% late 2022, and many service employers are desperate in 2023 in their search for staff. Unemployment rate remains at 3.5%, (Australian Bureau of Statistics Labour Force Report, 2022). These low figures appear to result from many unemployed not returning to their old jobs leaving hospitality and caring services short but setting up as small-scale self-employed such as gardeners and Uber drivers. Other apparently dropped out of the labour force statistics as they give up the search for work.

In most nations, younger employees and casuals bore the brunt of the lowering employment rate at the onset of the pandemic. In Australia for example, the 15–24 age group recorded the largest drop in employment rates (proportion of the age group who are employed), falling from 60 to 50% between March and May 2020, the lowest rate since the Labour Force data series began in 1978. This was followed by that for the 25–34 age group (from 81 to 76%). Casual workers also bore the brunt, due to their over-representation in hospitality, retail, and other service sectors adversely affected by lockdowns or severely restricted during lockdown. Casually employed workers accounted for nearly two-thirds (63%) of the job losses in the initial Covid attack between February and May 2020 with the fall resulting in around 540,600 fewer casual employees (Australian Institute of Health and Welfare Report September 2021).

A differential effect of the pandemic was revealed as the movement of those who could transfer to working from home contrast led to the number of people earning $1000 or more per week ($52,000 + pa) increasing by 8% in Australia between August 2019 and 2021. These could maintain income although also still being impacted with other non-monetary causes of distress. Thus, one group was insulated to some extent while another group of casuals and service workers suffered economic and social privation. Financial impacts also were borne by business during 2020, with 72% of businesses having less income as a result of Covid, 22% having revenue remain the same and 7% reporting a revenue increase.

In early 2020, Governments in Australia, New Zealand, UK, USA and Japan were quick to provide an array of economic stimulus packages early and throughout the pandemic to keep as many people in employment as possible and support those who had lost their jobs. These actions significantly helped to offset the adverse impacts on the labour market ensuring they could pay rent/ mortgage and buy essentials as other epidemiological measures slowed the spread of the virus. It was these packages that mitigated the immediate financial problems for many people and combined with gradual relaxation of restrictions facilitated a return to near normal with employment levels recovering into 2022. But during two years of being without a job and partial hours was stressful and traumatic, and the social distress of this period will be discussed later in Chap. 8.

Carpe Diem. Changes to Work Contexts

Covid has changed many things in our lives, not least where some of us work. The restrictions imposed to control Covid enabled millions to experience a different and for many a better experience in the way of working. Companies and employees are now both finding it hard to return to the old normal. Several decades ago, the world of work was glossed up by a book '*Better Than Sex: How a Whole Generation Got Hooked on Work*' (Trinka & Fox, 2004) with inanimate computers, spread sheets and emails presented as the focus of engagement and intimacy which had immense appeal especially for those who were less adept in personal relationships and group dynamics. In this way, they could live many years of personal satisfaction in their 'love' affair with work. Now that Covid has provided other opportunities to experience and gain increased satisfaction from different forms of working, many are looking to seize the moment to disengage from the world of work as organised previously.

Some employees were lucky being employed in businesses that did not necessarily require them to be present physically, undertaking activities that only required a desk and computer. This facilitated an increase in working from home (*WFH*). This venture was not novel as many entrepreneurs and small business have functioned in this way in the past, and of course school teachers and university lecturers would argue they have been undertaking a lot of required work at home, even over weekends, such as marking, planning the next day's lesson/lecture and completing administrative tasks, for many generations in a hybrid form of work, a format more seek to embrace now.

Working from Home (*WFH*)

WFH became a natural uncontrolled 'experiment' imposed across the developed world. In the UK, the proportion working exclusively at home rose from 5.7% in January/February 2020 to 43.1% in April 2020 according to the HomeOfficeLife blog which also contains a mass of other WFH data for the UK. The USA census data reveals a similar increase with the number primarily working from home tripling from 5.7% (roughly 9 million people) to 17.9% (27.6 million people) between 2019 and 2021. (U.S. Census Bureau Release, 2022). In the USA, WFH is often renamed 'remote work'. Even though the immediate pandemic problems have eased, the level of *WFH* in the developed world is likely to remain much higher than it was before the pandemic as it provided a revelation to many employees that they could do their jobs at home just as well as in the workplace.

It is said that there is no place like home; but home ain't what it used to be for many! Residential has morphed into '*resimercial*' as private homes combine sometimes unwillingly with the commercial world. In Australia, prior to the pandemic, approximately, 24% of employees were engaged in some degree of *WFH*. These were mainly entrepreneurs or single business owners who regularly did their job from home for most of the time. The percentage of employed people working from home on a regular basis had been steadily increasing by around a percentage point every two years.

In developed countries approximately 35% of workers had jobs prior to Covid that were amenable to working from home but few actually did so. This low level of *WFH* was likely due to management practices and companies reluctant to invest in necessary technology given uncertainty about its benefits (Productivity Commission Report, 2021).

The *WFH* figure jumped in Australia to 41% during the pandemic in Australia with higher rates in those states with severe lockdowns (New South Wales, Victoria and the Australian Capital Territory) in late 2021 as the Delta impacts were deepening. *WFH* continued to be more common in some occupations. The potential to engage in *WFH* is associated with higher levels of education, higher incomes, and full-time jobs. Close to two-thirds (64%) of managers and professionals were doing it regularly in August 2021, compared with around a quarter (25%) of people across other occupations. While the pandemic has seen a large shift in people working from home, there haven't been similarly large changes in other working arrangements such as working Monday to Thursday only (Australian Bureau of Statistics (ABS) media release, 2021).

There has been a power transfer towards employees facilitated by the pandemic particularly in the way people don't want to be seen simply as an asset to be exploited. During two years of Covid disruption, lockdowns, work from home, the accelerated adoption of digital technology, Zoom type interfaces and an increasing shortage of skilled labour meant more options have become available around how to integrate work in our lives. All this has changed the meaning of work for many. There is no general rejection of work, but employees are realising the past lack of humanisation in work. *WFH* for two years has been a real-life experiment of some other alternative non-standard work environment that they are finding more pleasant, with a more self-managed style of earning a living.

Will WFH Affect Our Wellbeing?

Working from home can affect various aspects of wellbeing, including physical and mental health, work-life balance and family functioning. It may also open up work opportunities for people who face barriers to labour force participation or full-time employment, such as people with disabilities or caring responsibilities. Min et al. (2021) gathered real-time data off Twitter to discern how employees across the English-speaking world were responding to *WFH*. As expected benefits emphasised were increased productivity, no commute, and the ability to structure workdays as desired. But while they enjoyed not having to sit in a cubicle all day, numerous parents reported that working from home was stressful because of blurred boundaries and competing demands from family. Similar results were obtained in a series of studies by Oakman et al. (2020) conducted over the 2020/21 period using focus groups of managers and non-managers from a range of sectors. Most participants' experiences were more negative than positive, due in part to extreme lockdowns including curfews and loneliness/isolation, with childcare and school closures for some compounding their work from home experiences.

Working from home can improve physical and mental health by giving people more time and control over their day to sleep, exercise and cook nutritious food, for example. But it can also worsen physical and mental health due to decreased incidental exercise, increased isolation and the elimination of the boundaries between home and work life.

Evidence shows that working from home reduces physical activity levels. For example, the average UK public transport commuter misses out on 21 min of incidental exercise for each day that they work from home. One in five (19%) of those working from home more frequently is exercising less often, while nearly a third (31%) are eating more (YahooLife UK, 2022).

Avoiding the commute reduces the 'cost' of working, and this is expected to induce an increase in labour supply, with more work opportunities for people who face barriers to labour force participation. This includes carers, parents of young children, some people with disabilities, as well as people living in remote or regional areas of larger nations where there are often fewer job opportunities in close physical proximity. Working from home policies can also promote a more gender-balanced workforce (Australian Productivity Commission Report, 2021).

Some Identified Issues with WFH

Rules for *WFH* are not always clear and vary from employer to employer, who are struggling with how to operate it, leading to demand for at least a continuing hybrid model by many employees. The general direction of specific negative aspects of *WFH* discerned by Min et al. (2021), Oakman et al. (2020), and many other studies during the pandemic are identified as these:

- There are blurred boundaries involving working longer hours and weekends, invasion of privacy (using Webcam and private phone for work) and work impinging on carer responsibilities. Health impacts of WFH were different for men and women. Women, for example, were less likely to report any positive health changes compared to men (Oakman et al., 2020). Fathers who WFH reported increased stress and mothers working from home experienced decreased happiness. Women were more likely to report higher levels of work exhaustion than their colleagues who continued to work in the office.
- Both managers and non-managers reported exhaustion associated with increased working hours and long periods of work without taking leave
- Negative physical outcomes such as increased musculoskeletal pain and weight gain from sitting long hours at home in non-ergonomic chairs

and decreased incidental exercise were commonly reported as working from home reduces physical activity levels. For example, the average UK public transport commuter misses out on 21 min of incidental exercise for each day that they work from home.

- Negative outcomes on mental health arose due to increased feelings of isolation and disconnect from work, particularly for those living alone in isolated lockdown who could not socialise. There was continual potential for conflict between household members over use of facilities and time spent on work matter. In a UK study, 81% of younger workers say that they would feel more isolated without time in the office, 48% reported that they are pressured to communicate more to demonstrate their value, 60% reported that they feel less connected to colleagues while 30% have found it difficult separating their home lives from their work lives with the biggest struggle being not able to 'unplug' (The Homeofficelife blog, 2022).
- A noted negative financial impact for employees was increased utility bills and purchase of additional equipment.
- Companies are concerned with perceived productivity and costs of working from home, which may increase co-ordination costs, reduce effectiveness of collaborative processes of knowledge-sharing and creativity. There is also the worry that separation from managers may enable workers opportunity to slack off.

Some the answers to these issues lie with managers equipping workers with proper home office setups, helping employees maintain structure by setting aside times for work, meetings and family time/relaxation. However, there were a number of quite positive aspects emphasised in the studies including:

- Improved work-life interaction, particularly for employees not in mandatory lockdown situations, including flexibility to fit in parenting, household chores, dog walking and exercise. *WFH* can improve physical and mental health by giving people more time and control over their day to sleep, exercise and cook nutritious food, for example.
- However, the main benefit claimed by workers was avoidance of the dreaded daily commute. In 2019, full-time workers in Australian major cities spent an average of around 67 min per day commuting, which in terms of forgone earnings amounted to $49, not including vehicle costs. For those taking public transport, the average time value and transport cost totalled $57 per day.
- The increased operation of online communication platforms such as Microsoft Teams and Zoom resulted in improved communication and bonding within teams and between departments, as well as cross-business collaboration.

- Productivity increases due to working longer days and not being distracted in the office, contributed to the positive financial impact for employer organisations. In Australia, about three-quarters of workers surveyed considered that they were at least as productive working from home as from the office because they had better control over their time and enjoyed better work-life balance. A similar view was held by many employers too.
- Firms believe they will be able to tap into a larger pool of labour.
- Some firms may also be able to realise office rent savings.

The overall messages from studies of *WFH* during the pandemic is that to optimise *WFH* employers should:

- Support workers to set boundaries between work and home management, and support of flexible work hours.
- Ensure clarity about employees' roles, including workload and performance indicators.
- Provide appropriate technical support, equipment and software for home use.
- Provide regular online communication and performance management adjustments where necessary.
- Encourage networking by training and supporting managers to supervise remote teams.

Of course, the majority of workers haven't and can't enjoy the luxury of working from home; many jobs simply can't be performed remotely. Only around a maximum 35% of the total workforce in Western countries was working remotely during the pandemic. Garbage collectors, maintenance and repair persons, police/fire, long distance delivery drivers and public transport workers are examples of those who cannot take advantage of staying at home to work. Those who have been at their physical workplaces since the pandemic's beginning, especially health care professionals are suffering both high infection rates and burnout. Ingoglia (2022) notes that a 2021 KFF/Washington Post poll, for example, found that 3 in 10 health care professionals in the USA have considered leaving the field.

Is WFH a Goer?

When lockdowns began in 2020, companies were concerned about workers skiving off and working less. The indication is that this has not happened. Home workers report spending longer, unpaid hours on the job when they work from home, resulting in a higher output for the same paid hours. Organisations initially believed *WFH* working from home would be a temporary expedient, but now employers are experiencing challenges to return employees back to the office desk after experiencing their suburban scenes and family at weekday lunchtimes.

It is difficult to assess whether working from home is as productive as in the office. It all depends on each employee's risk factors, the context and many family/home variables that are differentiated individually and often subjective. Some women with young children may struggle, as may new starts and people who live alone. Some employees claim that they are more productive at home to relieve boredom and some may work harder and longer to justify *WFH* to the boss, while others wish to be perceived as trusted and have earned the right to work at home. However for workaholics, the downside may come later with work-life balance out of kilter. This has led to the call for a '*right to disconnect*'. In other words, there needs to be legal and reasonable limits on working time, able to disconnect from work emails, telephone calls and other forms of contact outside of agreed scheduled work hours.

Physical and mental health are psychological issues especially social isolation, which may be helped by arranging small co-working hubs where people can meet in person or online to be more creative and network. There needs to be clever planning in place so people do not overcommit, yet meet organisational demands, and also enjoy a chosen personal life. In addition, some employees have concerns about invasion of privacy when Zoom or similar video features are used, peering into one's home and belongings.

WFH and Its Implications in the Home

Employee wellbeing is important, whether they're in the office or at home. People are generally happier working from home because it allows for more flexibility, but there are psycho-social problems in attempting to replicate the office in a small duplex or two bed with one big open plan room where everyone lives, plays, eats and watches TV.

Disturbance is inevitable, and bedrooms are usually unable to accommodate a table. House routines and ways you share various duties may have to be renegotiated. There is a need to develop psycho-social plans down to the individual level. For example, many organisations rightly are concerned with the home physical working environment and ensuring ergonomic safe desks and chairs but it must extend beyond this to consider how to build in a daily walk or cycle, hit some balls at the driving range or visit a local cafe or other preferred activity, and having strategies to switch off mentally and physically. Therefore, managers must support staff at home, and it is not just a matter of productivity and managers need training for this so they can 'train' their people. Governments keep making comments about getting people back to the workplace but fail to understand that for some there are difficult issues to surmount to return to the old way, it isn't simply a matter of having an early breakfast and jumping on the train.

The pandemic has shown that modern white-collar workers do not really have to sit alongside their colleagues to be productive. That's not to claim that employees are better off psychologically or healthily interacting solely with their laptops in their kitchen or local coffee shop, rather than with others in the office, but evidence suggests that productivity of remote or hybrid workers increases due to the improved pleasant, self-managed and flexible environments. On the other hand as employers note that working at home alone is often more efficient, there is the danger they are likely to ignore possibilities of work stress and mental health deterioration in isolated workers and simply calculate the financial benefits of decreasing office space and support for distributed workforce.

The Abandoning of the Central Business District (CBD)

The restrictions due to Covid such as lockdowns, movement controls and person numbers in any space had an immediate and drastic effect on *CBDs*. The 'knowledge' jobs amenable to working from home were concentrated in the *CBDs* of the world's biggest cities but the employees generally lived in the inner and middle suburbs. As *WFH* was strongly injected into the work context, lowered commuting reduced *CBD* economic activity such as in retail, hospitality and personal services. With increasing *WFH,* many city and town retailers were being abandoned by former customers. Some of these businesses have gradually moved to the suburbs.

The shift is having consequences, as major employers weigh up the need to keep paying for half-empty city skyscrapers, with the added demand for suburban and regional hub offices that can accommodate teams and individuals sometimes only for several days per week. This desire not to attend office is also exacerbated by the lengthy lockdowns and negatively affects small café and newsagents as well as transport in big conurbations. As a percentage of the preCovid rate, the Property Council of Australia February 2022 Report noted occupancy compared to 2019 in Melbourne was just 15%, Sydney was just 18%. Even cities that avoided the brunt of lockdowns such as Brisbane (41%), Adelaide (47%) and Perth (55%) are seeing far more empty desks than in 2019. This decline in demand for *CBD* office space arose from some firms downsizing or relinquishing their offices and a few shutting up for good.

Sydney is only gradually making a recovery from a record 80% slump in retail activity during the lockdown. Data collected by Google since the beginning of the pandemic shows movement around the centres of Parramatta, and Sydney is unlikely to recover to prepandemic levels. April 2022 in Parramatta, there were 34% fewer people heading into the office compared to early 2020 (ABC News, 2022). Fewer workers travelling to work means fewer café customers with around 23% less using public transport. Some *CBDs* will survive as many firms are experimenting with hybrid or work from anywhere models and will maintain their *CBD* offices because of their central location and accessibility. The hybrid model will also maintain workers' link to cities as the benefits of close proximity sharing and learning are strongest in high density companies.

Some well-known restaurants in London are still having to close due to staff shortages despite increasing customer and tourist demand following the easing of coronavirus restrictions in 2021. The pressure on fewer staff working in the hospitality industry is increasing their mental health deficits worse than at height of the pandemic, according to a survey reported by BBC News 23 April 21 with almost a third of the 200 respondents saying their mental health was worse than in 2020 as 45% of the UK respondents are having to ask staff to work longer hours. A key reason for this is the high number of vacancies within the industry, with a massive staff shortage as hospitality closures during lockdown caused workers to rethink their career choices. This is exacerbating employee ability to cope. A survey by hospitality mental health organisation The Burnt Chef Survey (2022) showed that one in five hospitality workers was planning on leaving. Worldwide the hospitality industry is struggling with a severe shortages as locals and tourist visitor numbers rise with mandates removed, yet staffing numbers continue to drop. Work-life balance ranks highest as to why people do not want to return to what once was the third largest sector in the world.

The Hybrid WFH Arrangement

Many employees would prefer have the flexibility of spending some time working in both the office or from home. It's been dubbed *'hybrid working'*, operating with two desks; one in a quiet (perhaps not always quiet) spot at home and the other in a more chatty position in the office. The hybrid model appears intuitively appealing, balancing the benefits of home working for focussed work such as analysis, research, writing or interacting in detail with clients via technology with workplace for group discussion and socialising where more creative and innovative activity can occur, providing a break to the occasional dramas or interruptions of family life. Evidence is mixed on how any particular combination of office and home work location period affects productivity for individuals in practice. But, over time, as firms and workers negotiate outcomes, learn and adapt and become more effective at working from home, this issues should gain more clarity. In reality, as part of the negotiation to mutually agreeable outcomes, many firms are likely to try out the hybrid model, where workers spend two to three days a week in the office and two to three days working from home. In practice, the hybrid model may be more difficult to execute well, due to increased management and co-ordination costs.

Return to Office Reluctance

Many companies are facing a dilemma about whether or not to require employees return to the workplace. 47% of American workers prefer to work in a hybrid model, and 32% don't want to return to the office again (Bloom, 2021). In the UK, 59% of workers prefer to work in a hybrid model as the average UK office workers attended the workplace 3.8 days per week prepandemic, but post-Covid, this has reduced to an average of 1.4 days per week with only 13% of workers attending the office on a Friday (BBC News, 2022). Other UK data shows the proportion of people hybrid working as risen in 2022. 14% worked from home exclusively between 27 April and 8 May 2022, while 24% both worked from home and travelled to work, with high earners more likely to be hybrid workers as 38% of workers earning £40,000 or more hybrid worked between 27 April and 8 May 2022, while only 8% of those earning up to £15,000 reported hybrid working (UK Office for National Statistics, 2022).

Over half of employees in Australia (55%) would prefer to be remote at least three days a week once pandemic concerns recede. In contrast, 68% employers want at least three days a week of employee attendance to maintain a distinct company culture. Least experienced workers (0–5 years) felt the need to be in the office the most, and 30% of them prefer being remote no more than one day a week. The least experienced workers are also more likely to feel less productive while working remotely. They're more likely to value meeting with managers or company training programmes than their more experienced colleagues. A recent Australian Bureau of Statistics Job Mobility report (2022) reveals that a job churn has come true in Australia with 1.3 million (about 10% of the workforce) changing jobs in 2021 to find jobs that better suit their needs adding to the complexity of hybrid work and who will allow me that freedom. The hybrid model promises negotiating difficulties as it currently lacks any legal basis in most developed nations.

Not surprisingly, workers may be willing to accept lower wages to continue *WFH*. Survey data from the US suggests that the ability to work from home two or three days per week may be equivalent to a 7% pay rise to workers reflected in *Owl Labs and Global Workplace Analytics' 'State of Remote Work' Report (2022)* where 46% of workers said they would be willing to take a 5% pay cut to work remotely at least part of the time. 37% offered a pay cut of over 10%. Meanwhile, a survey from *GoodHire* (2022) found that 61% of respondents would be willing to take a pay cut to maintain remote working status. Some workers even suggested that they would take a 50% pay cut to avoid returning to the office. The same survey found that 70% would forfeit benefits like health insurance, paid time off and retirement accounts to continue remote work. In reverse, one international law company has offered its employees the option to work from home permanently but only if they take a 20% pay cut. In the USA, Bloomberg News (2022) notes the popularity of hybrid work with only 33% returning to the office in the first week of February 2022.

Job switching and negotiation on wages provide firms with information about what attracts workers. In this way, firms will try different arrangements, note outcomes, and retain only those that yield desirable results. The pandemic has accelerated trends towards more flexible work arrangements and encouraged workers to seek new jobs that better suit their needs and preferences ('*the great resignation*'). Workers and employers are now diverging in their desires. In a tight labour market, employers need to factor in a potential loss of staff if they push too hard to get people back in behind their 'desks'.

A variation of the hybrid model is the '*work from anywhere*' approach, where workers have considerable control over where they work each day, but with an expectation of some minimal office time. Flexibility was once seen as a benefit; now, it is becoming an expectation but must be managed adroitly. W*ork from anywhere policies*' have been observed among high-tech firms where use of collaborative technologies is commonplace and access to a global talent pool is important. For example, KMPG and Atlassian have this policy for their global work force. This has afforded them the ability to recruit some outstanding people who would have been lost to them under preCovid demands to work in a centralised office. The only rule for the latter company is that staff must be prepared to attend for face-to-face meetings four times each year. This approach certainly doesn't mean sacrificing productivity or lowering those KPIs. Low-skill jobs, such as call centres where monitoring is easier and collaboration is less important, have also adopted the work from anywhere policy.

Women Not Benefitting from the Hybrid Model

The lockdown periods have prompted a disruption in gender relations, but not for the better, with women typically picking up their usual more than fair share of home school duties and domestic chores, all while trying to keep their own professional lives on track. So *WFH* in a hybrid model has not proved to be an answer to the prayers of many women as latest research of over 5000 women in 10 countries (Deloitte Women @ Work, 2022) reveals unintended consequences of hybrid models exacerbating existing bias with women less likely to receive recognition and rewards than male peers. Women also miss out on face-to-face support and not being seen as serious workers. Online meetings have intensified the struggle for some women to be heard or even included. Over 90% of women feared asking for a more flexible work schedule would scupper their chance of promotion; 64% in hybrid roles had been given no set formal expectations on about how they worked, and around 50% complained of a lack of contact with team leaders. The hybrid model has the potential to intensify the gender gap and create power differences between those in and those out of office. However, many women felt they worked better remotely than in person.

Some Major Surveys of WFH and Its Variants

Several important reports and surveys offer an insight into the issues and problems of where and when work is done. These include the

Bendelta Survey, 2022 (https://www.bendelta.com) A Feb 2022 survey across 16 countries.

PricewaterhouseCoopers (PWC) Survey USA 2021. Involving 133 executives and 1200 office workers in November and December 2020 https://www.pwc.com/us/en/services/consulting/business-transformation/library/covid-19-us-remote-work-survey.html.

Global Workplace Analytics. (2020) *Work From Home Experience Survey.* Global survey of 3000 employees. https://globalworkplaceanalytics.com/global-work-from-home-experience-survey

LinkedIn (2022). *Workplace Culture Shifts Report.* (https://www.socialmediatoday.com/news/linkedin-publishes-new-report-into-workplace-culture-shifts-and-what-they/617801/

Mainstreet Insights Australian Report (2022) *Workplace and the Future.* (https://mainstreetinsights.com.au/).

Australian Productivity Commission Report Working From Home (2021) (https://www.pc.gov.au/research/completed/working-from-home.)

Medallia's Return to Work Report (2021) based on very large US sample https://info.sense360.com/hubfs/210824_Sense360_Return%20to%20Work%20Insights_v2.pdf.

These surveys have identified major trends across the globe.

Strong Support for the Hybrid Model

Unanimously, the surveys demonstrate that while the demands are quite vocal for more hybrid work, the workplace office will stay with a change in its role. Less than one in five managers want to return the office to what it was prepandemic and are grappling with how widely to extend hybrid/remote work options, with 13% of executives prepared to let go of the office totally. Meanwhile, 87% of employees say the office is important for their top-rated need of collaborating with team members and building relationships, a fairly common theme. Employees generally want to return to the office rather more slowly than employers expect and most prefer an arrangement, with 3 days of 'home' work per week as the sweet spot. For employers the best post-Covid sweet spot compromise appears to be three days in the office because they genuinely believe some time together is better for mental health, ideas and customer attention, and are keen to keep tabs on workers on at least some days. About half of workers said they would be very or somewhat likely to seek employment elsewhere if their preferred setup was not available. 61% of US employees are expecting to spend half their time in the office in 2022 (PWC Survey, 2021). Market research firm Medallia (2022) revealed fewer than 1 in 5 US employees currently working remotely want to return to an exclusively in-person workplace.

Employees in the USA (PWC survey, 2021) also want the flexibility to work remotely part or all of the week as they juggle their work, home lives, caregiving responsibilities, and mental health. Almost a fifth (19%) of all respondents would like to be fully remote, even if Covid were no longer a concern. An almost equal number (22%) would like to be mostly in the office, and 21% indicate the nature of their work does not allow them to work remotely at all. The remainder prefer a hybrid work setup, with some days in the office and others remote. Similar to the USA, the Australian Productivity Commission (2021) and Mainstreet (2022) reports claim that working from home is expected to remain a feature of working life continuing at higher levels than before the pandemic.

But few workers prefer fully remote work, and most want to spend some time working from the office. The Mainstreet report (2022) for example notes like the other reports that most do not want to work from home all the time with 60% of respondents preferring a hybrid model of work, with only 15% opting for permanently working from home, and 18% preferring the workplace most of the time. The PWC (2020) reveals US executives and employees are converging around a post-pandemic future with a lot more flexibility, and by design or default, most companies worldwide appear to be heading towards a hybrid workplace where a large number of office employees rotate in and out of offices configured for shared spaces. Yet few are prepared to completely abandon the office space. This model embraces the flexibility that most employees (and some employers) crave after working from home for months. It's also a complicated way to organise the work week and is likely to transform a company's culture, employee engagement, the way the work gets done and how office space is used. The Mainstreet report (2022) notes remote work is an overwhelming success for both employees and employers, with a shift in positive attitudes towards remote work evident: 83% of employers now say the shift to remote work has been successful for their company, compared to 73% in 2020.

Benefits of Working from Home

The Productivity Report (op cit) found evidence some people might even take a pay cut to negotiate life in the home office or around the kitchen table, when taking into account numerous advantages of at-home work, such as saving time and money on daily commutes. This replicates findings from the US surveys. In 2019, full-time workers in Australia's major cities spent an average of 67 min each day commuting, and for those taking public transport, the average time value and transport cost totalled $57 a day. Thus the commute for many employees is a meaningful cost in terms of the time and money spent and it's large enough that it might make a difference to the choice of work location and even to a job change. This commute issue was emphasised in the HILDA (Household, Income and Labour Dynamics in Australia 2021) survey, an epic research project from the University of Melbourne that examines how we live our lives, which also found that a long commute to work is a negative hit on people's satisfaction with their jobs. Other reasons why workers preferred to be at home included the ability to have more time and control over their day, to sleep, exercise or cook the food they preferred rather than quick takeaways, to work while the house was empty and be free to enjoy the children after school (attendance at after school sport, etc.).

What Are Downsides of Working from Home?

A number of the reports found *WFH* can worsen physical and mental health due to less incidental exercise, increased isolation and having no boundaries between home and work life. That has led to the call for a '*right to disconnect*', arguing there need to be legal and reasonable limits on working time, including allowing people to log off from telephone calls, work emails and other work-related contacts. The Productivity Commission (op cit) urged governments to monitor the labour market and regulatory settings to make sure they were fair and continued to protect workers.

Impact on Future Career

Hybrid working brings concerns for future career prospects for many employees. The disadvantage for staff not wishing to return to the workplace is that they can easily miss out on professional development, promotion, attachment to the most exciting projects and working with the most talented colleagues. This perception occurs because *WFH* and its variants reduce opportunities for collaboration and networking, reduce face-to-face interaction with managers, all of which may confer long-rm career consequences and prospects. Nonetheless, many employees worldwide are willing to change jobs or accept lower wages in order to continue *WFH*.

Complementary Use of Work Location

Hybrid working is here to stay but the argument that home and work space should be used for different activities. Is a common one. Employees consistently preferred the office for spontaneous meetings, collaboration and problem solving, while preferring home or other remote place for focussed work, independent problem solving and participating in training. There was a definite desire by over two-thirds of responders to all surveys to work no more than two days per week in the office. Even though the employee believes that they are very productive at home, and they felt the need to pose questions to themselves like, how well are you contributing to team cohesion; how well are you contributing to the social fabric of what makes your organisation what it is; how are you doing mentoring your junior people? The work context cannot be just about them. When employees work at home their connections with other workers are less spontaneous, limited to a quick chat in messages, so the quality of the relationships may become a bit more eroded. In the office, on the other hand, they can have more dynamic interactions. Pop in on people and say 'hi' and have spontaneous conversations over coffee; seek quick advice. Employees can develop much more meaning and relational aspects with colleagues (rather than only managers) when in the office which offsets any sense of loneliness, from quite limited contacts at home often only a more formal one-way call from the manager or supervisor when you're working from home.

Provision of or Access to Technology

Virtually, all employees claim to have access to the technology that they need to be productive but less than third in each survey were resentful or are disturbed by any hint of being monitored by digital surveillance.

Management Support

Most employees felt supported by leaders (average 85%), or felt leaders were skilled at managing a dispersed team (average 80%), but many did not believe they were given equal opportunities to those working in the office (average 37%). And while supported by leaders, some still felt challenged by remote working. All surveys note the need to consider what extra support people are going to need, what skills are needed and how to help employees develop competence and motivation and fortitude to work alone at home. Covid has made employers realise that working from home is a viable option some employers are also placing controls round working at home policies and not creating a sense of trust in their employees which is required for this system to work. Productivity gains and worker wellbeing must both be forefront. Benefits and risks will need a flexible framework as employees are not all the same and one size will not suit all.

Increased Awareness of Sense of Community and Connectivity

The major downside of *WFH* noted by the studies was the loss of connections to other colleagues which had been a lifeline for many workers, despite all the complaints and comedies about office politics and getting along with co-workers. While home working has been a boon to most not only in the flexibility it offered and the cut in petrol costs or fares, it seems many surveyed did actually miss the social aspect of the workplace during Covid lockdowns according to the surveys.

For example, Mainstreet Insights (2022) surveyed employees aged 18–65 to see how they were faring during 2021 found that 70% of these Australians reported that their most meaningful and regular social connections were still at work, outranking both their homes and community. The desire to return to a group workplace is strongest among Gen-Z workers (aged 18–26), who are perhaps the most social group and possibly still living at home and don't want elderly parents to be their only social connection. This group also reports the most impact on their mental health was Covid-related isolation as their lifestyle prior to isolation was going out enjoying mingling with peers. Australian workers in particular are more appreciative of their workplace and the connections they experienced there than they were two years ago as a result of Covid disconnect experiences. Compared to 2019, Australian workers are more likely to consider their colleagues as trusted friends (78% cf. 72% 2019) and experience meaningful interactions with their colleagues (88% cf. 80% 2019). Gen Zs not only believe that a weekly check-in is optimal, more than one in two (58%) want check-ins to be entirely in person. (Mainstreet 2022) It is an unexpected finding that despite comfort and familiarity with using technology. After the experiences of social isolation and household upsets for those in long lockdowns. 70% Australian workers now appreciate that they are more likely to experience meaningful and regular social connection in their workplace. To some, work is still simply a job, but to many it's a lifeline to social interaction, purpose, identity and a place of belonging and this explains why hybrid work is highly desired combining the beat of both worlds.

Employees Seek More Than Money. Prioritising Wellbeing in the Workplace

Workers in all developed countries are beginning to express a strong desire to be looked after, i.e. the importance of work wellbeing, flexibility and social connection have become more important than before for employers to consider in retaining old and attracting new staff whether working at home or at the workplace (Productivity Commission op cit). 0ne in two Australian workers would like their leaders to be proactive in making them feel well taken care of (54%) and prioritise their mental health and wellbeing (51%). The various surveys reveal that employers have started to realise that employees worldwide want jobs that provide personal achievement, opportunity for advancement and develop new skillsets, not just money, and corporate rhetoric is beginning to resound with enough integrity for employees, pushed by shareholder meetings, to feel their efforts are worthwhile and will be able to attract talent. More and more employees also want to work for organisations that don't harm others or the environment. Glassdoor (https://www.glassdoor.com.au) is a Website where current and former employees review and rate their companies. It identifies companies that do not satisfy criteria that loom large for many workers such as climate change, ethical supply chains for clothing and other manufactured goods, anti-slavery measures, non-military products, gender equity and animal rights. The previous criteria like office design, parking spaces or good superschemes have declined down the list that signifies an employer of choice.

The focus has now changed to how a company positions itself in the broader society in terms of external behaviour that can make the difference in recruitment. In sum, people seek work that keeps them engaged in a good job that uses their skills, and expertise, with a dedicated supportive manager, in an organisation they can be proud of, where they have a future. Companies that haven't changed will become less popular employers. But the impending worldwide economic downturn may cause to focus back to job and income security and away from any luxury and freedom to try and match work to personal, moral, social and purpose values.

Management Response

The Productivity Commission (2021) expects workers and firms will negotiate mutually beneficial hybrid arrangements, and that governments should facilitate a smooth transition to post-Covid different models of work. Most surveys do accept that more than 60% of jobs can't be done from home, so for millions of frontline workers who need to be physically present to undertake their work, little will change for such as bus drivers, refuse collectors, hospitality workers, airline pilots and tradespersons.

Employers' plans also vary widely, with some expecting all employees to work in person (19%), some aiming for remote or hybrid arrangements (22%), and most anticipating a mix of different policies for different staff (33%). Some entrenched organisations want to drag their employees back even if they are kicking and screaming (Productivity Commission op cit). The PWC Survey found that 65% of employees are looking for a new job with 88% of businesses seeing higher turnover than normal. Several U.S. technology companies, such as Square, Twitter, and Coinbase Global, have embraced remote work and declared themselves fully remote. As in Australia, many employees are voting with their feet if they are not permitted the work patterns they prefer and are likely to leave even if this involved a pay cut. Some are prepared to sacrifice a lot for the flexibility to work in the way that best suits their needs and preferences.

The majority of employees in all surveys wanted management to support them to continue working in a hybrid format but while they highly valued the ability to work from home found that they were working longer hours and instead of working a fixed 9–5, preferred flexible hours that change daily to accommodate other commitments. These trends reveal a historic shift in the way employees want to balance work and family life. The sooner employers understand and adjust to their employees' desire for more flexibility and recognise that Covid was a catalyst in this regard the faster society will arrive at the 'new normal'. Working from home is here to stay long after the Covid pandemic. A survey of 5000 Australian federal public servants (Williamson et al., 2020) highlighted a mismatch between needs and preferences of managers and those of employees. More than a third of federal public servants in Australia would like to work from home all the time or at least 4 days per week and certainly not return to the office for a 5 day week. 40% of them indicated that they would consider leaving the organisation if they were not permitted to work at home.

Managing the New System

Surveys emphasise that managers will have to devise new forms of sensitively negotiated but carefully planned working arrangements suitable to the organisations activity to keep staff not only motivated but also on the payroll, with some staff in the office and others elsewhere. Two days in the office must involve meaningful meetings with colleagues and clients, not more Zooming or Microsoft Teams to others in the team. Under hybrid conditions, the organisation must ensure all required members are in on the same days too. Flexibility may not go as far as being able to dictate which days you work where. Co-ordination of activities must still be an important criterion. Flexible work has to be proactively managed as work post-Covid must work both for the employee and employer. Workers have proved that they can remain highly productive under flexible, changeable conditions. From the management side, the ease of collaboration remains a major issue but can be helped if managers ensure that all team members are present in the office on the required day for face-to-face group meetings and planning and not for more Zoom. Managers should also evaluate employees not on the amount of time they spend at work but on the impact they're making with their work.

The only people pushing back on working from home and hybrid approaches are executives, who are struggling to adapt to it. One common reason discovered is that most senior leaders have the lowest levels of digital understanding and are the ones who don't know how to set up Zoom calls to multiple staff and set the camera right. Of course, some people like the structure and organisation of the office environment, along with the social benefits, and so there are strong arguments to be made for employers designing flexible approaches related to job requirements and employee wishes.

Managing the Future of Hybrid Work. Flexibility Versus Performance

The future needs to ensure that hybrid models don't normalise discriminatory practices and balance the trade-off between full autonomy and team commitments by bridging the expectation gap of employees understanding why the employer might want them back in the office and the employer understanding why the employee might want to work from home for some period of the week. There's no possibility of a general rule on the optimal balance of work days at home vs. in the office as it depends on the type of work, the home context and the personal characteristics of the individual employee. But failing to strike the right balance between working in these two locations can leave some people feeling lonely and disconnected. The side effects of loneliness can have varying impacts on an employee's wellbeing and can be as devastating as triggering depression (ABC News, 2022).

People with an extroverted personality can find it harder to work from home alone than do introverts, when missing chunks of actual face-to-face interaction. While people need autonomy, and competence for psychological growth, relatedness which is to feel connected or have a sense of belonging or connection to other people is vitally important. We lose relatedness working from home for many leading to melancholic, anxious, lonely and isolated feelings. A lot of people like coming into the workplace cause it is a busy and active place, offering dynamic interactions as you stop in on people and have spontaneous conversations or a coffee break with learning and development opportunities, a sense of community, plus a sense of connection that brings meaning and purpose. At home, it is difficult to replicate this in the home office as connections with other workers are less spontaneous with only a quick chat in messages, which erodes the quality of relationships. It's also important to have interactions with colleagues rather than managers both when in the office and even when working from home. Managers should be promoting socialisation, both in the office and online. Researchers have been looking into the ideal number of days spent working from home versus in the office to reduce the onset of loneliness, the so-called *'magic ratio'*. Research on this actually does show that it's around two to two and a half, so any more than two and a half days at home is probably a bit too much (ABC News, 2022).

It's a misconception to think a worker's loneliness is their problem alone, rather than an organisational matter. This has to be fixed by the organisation or their employee will not be producing to their best when the environment doesn't give each employee what they need. It is noted in Chap. 6 that loneliness can led to mental and physical distress which can trigger depression and over 50% of respondents to several national surveys from the Australian Institute of Health and Welfare (e.g. Annual Report October, 2021) had felt lonelier since the onset of the pandemic.

Attracting New Talent. Flexibility Is the Criterion

There's no doubt from the various reports that flexibility is now a critical factor when it comes to attracting new talent and keeping current employees happy. It's the fastest-growing priority for candidates considering new jobs; and employees who are satisfied with their flexibility on work schedules or location are 2.6 times more likely to be happy working for their employer and 2.1 times more likely to recommend working for the company. On LinkedIn (2022), of the searches in the United States that use remote, hybrid, and onsite job filters, job seekers are craving remote work with 84% of searches for hybrid and remote jobs. On average, those remote jobs also receive 4 times the applications that onsite jobs do. Being able to hire people, through a *WFH* option has also given employers a bigger pool to select from, and has given employers and employees a chance to focus on what works best for them. What didn't exist before the pandemic forced bosses to change was trust that employees working remotely would put in the effort required.

Sick Leave Becoming Redundant in WFH

Another interesting development is that *WFH* has killed sick leave. There is no soldiering on anymore, but encouragement in the Omicron variant surge from government and management to actually go home, stay home and work from there if there is a hint of a sniffle, as businesses recognise their duty of care to other employees, customers and communities. No need for sick leave or reporting unplanned absence. Even if an employee falls sick at home there is ample opportunity after taking a couple of tablets to shuffle the work load around to permit an extensive period of rest each day with a bit of work here and there. This saves sick leave for when it is really needed. All that had to be done such as a visit to doctor, chemist and dentist which could not be done at weekends is very possible in normal opening hours when working at home. The central workplace will remain the dominant for the foreseeable future. But the increase in working from home is potentially of great benefit to a substantial portion of nation's workforce.

Legal Complexities

In many countries, there is reluctance to return to the workplace full time. Advice from workplace lawyers is for employers to consult and communicate with employees, even though employers have the upper hand legally. The employer is also on firm grounds to require the employee back to the workplace if they can cite operational reasons, such as collaboration, training supervision and mentoring. Australian contract law, for example, provides no right in law for an employee to be able to choose their workplace and clearly states that employees have an obligation to obey a lawful command of their employer, except where it is over-ridden by health and safety laws.

Another legal minefield relates to workers' compensation rules. If an employer wants to be covered for a claim arising from employee injury sustained while working at home, the employer needs to have verified that the home is safe and keep records of work at home hours. This detail has been ignored in the Covid turmoil. A more complex issue not yet addressed is that of employee health due to their work activities which when work is performed in the workplace is still the responsibility of employers. For example, workplaces need to have Covid contingency measures in place, such as separating a toilet just for anyone who is deemed to be a close contact and regular resting of all employees. Then, there is the issue of who should supply the exposed workers with hard-to-find *RATs*. Workplace health and safety laws already stipulate that workplaces have to provide their staff with any gear they needed to keep them safe which would include *RATs*, masks and ventilation during a pandemic. The Unions argue no employee under any circumstance should be forced to pay for the items needed to keep them safe at work.

Lawyers have raised the sticky issue of when other workers did not want to work alongside unvaccinated essential staff. The issue here is not just the people being asked to come into work, they're not necessarily the ones at risk. It's the people that are already in the workplace that are now going to be exposed to a returnee who has not been vaccinated. What if you don't want to work near an exposed person? Its gets a bit tricky as each employee has a right to a safe workplace. That's a fundamental right under workplace health and safety legislation.

If the employer does not provide a safe workplace it may be judged negligent, in which case the employee could sue. For some company owners, all of these risks and considerations are not worth it, and some small businesses are not opening or simply working with minimum staff. To sum up, the employer imposing a return to workplaces while Covid is still around must provide a work environment that, depending on type of business, inter alia:

- Monitors and maintains any required social distancing guidelines between employees and visitors.
- Safely manage the flow of people in and out of the workplace/business premises.
- Plan for collaboration spaces, meeting rooms and hot desking and the technology to support.
- The requirement for an unvaccinated person to wear a mask if the employer claims it is necessary to ensure health and safety of other employees and the general public. The Australian Fair Work Commission has accepted this argument.
- Ensure employee safety, mental and physical wellbeing.
- Establish stringent cleaning and sanitation protocols for desks, meeting rooms, bathrooms, end-of-trip facilities and shared kitchen spaces.
- Ensure the provision of personal protective equipment (PPE) appropriate to the business such as face masks, gloves, alcohol wipes, handwashing stations and hand sanitisers if necessary, with notices and demonstration posters around the workplace.
- Have a risk management process that involves, if relevant, travel policy reviews and tracking of employee compliance with health regulations.
- Have a contingency plan ready should there be another spike in Covid cases.
- Determine which employees are essential in the workplace by role, location and demand and which can continue to work effectively from home with ways to further support remote working for those who need it.
- Understands the new situations employees face as a result of the Covid pandemic which should be taken just as seriously as business-related considerations. These include stress and anxiety for people who may not yet feel comfortable or safe returning to work, alternative transport methods for staff who rely on public transport. Reviewing operation of meal/washroom breaks and other safety protocols.

The Zoom Effect

A major focus of the *WFH* experience interesting psychologists is the phenomenon of Zoom fatigue. The onset of the pandemic thrust many employees into remote work arrangements, and face-to-face meetings were quickly replaced with virtual meetings as lockdowns and social distancing were imposed. A considerable number of individual comments led to increasing popular press discussion of what they termed virtual meeting or videoconferencing fatigue (i.e. now generally termed 'Zoom fatigue'). This was painted as a feeling of being drained and lacking energy following a day of virtual meetings staring at and self-attempting to present a good impression on screen.

Shockley et al. (2021) conducted an experiment in the USA which 103 employees were randomly assigned to have cameras either on or off for 2 weeks and then switch conditions for 2 additional weeks, involving 1408 daily. Everyday after work the participants completed measures assessing how fatigued they felt during the day, how engaged they had felt in the meetings and whether or not they felt they had a voice in the meeting. Shockley (op cit.) found that the relationship between having the camera on and fatigue level was stronger for women than men and also for those who were new to the organisation rather than the old hands. These two groups also reported being less engaged in meetings, and less like they had a voice in meetings. These losses seemed to be due to issues of self-presentation that goes with having the camera on. It becomes cognitively taxing looking at yourself and being hypervigilant about how people are reacting to you. Feeling watched increased the need to manage others' impression of one and directs focus inwards causing the fatigue.

Women and new hires may be particularly prone to anxious self-presentation because of heightened need to be regarded as competent and effective. It may be that having the participants' camera feeds hidden from them would help to mitigate the negative effects. So there is a situation arising where many people having to work from home feel drowned, tired and miserable after several hours on Zoom or Microsoft Teams and often also report eye ache and head ache form focussing intently for period of time. However, some positive effects were noted in comments that with camera on, participants felt more related to their colleagues. Supplemental analyses of the Shockley data (2021) suggest that fatigue affects same-day and even next-day meeting performance. Such is the pressure that some companies are instituting a Zoom free Friday. Given the anticipated prevalence of remote work even after the pandemic subsides, this study offers insights for ongoing organisational best practices surrounding virtual meetings. In the future research, Shockley plans to investigate whether using avatars or side-view cameras that simulate a typical meeting space would help.

In another study of examining the nature of Zoom fatigue, Bennett et al. (2021) in Australia investigated when it happened and what Zoom characteristics were associated with it. From both qualitative and quantitative data of 279 meetings, they found that fatigue is real and as expected occurs close to the end of each conferencing session. This Zoom fatigue is different from general work fatigue which generally is an end of work. Zoom fatigue is related to time of day with lower fatigue developing after middle of the day meetings likely due to the impact of increasing energy levels after a lunch break. Turning the microphone to mute and building greater group cohesion ameliorated the fatigue somewhat, with the latter being the most effective protective factor. Paralleling Shockley's findings, Bennett et al. (op cit.) also determined that the more cameras were on, the less voice participants felt they had and this increased fatigue as well as decreasing group cohesion, and this was stronger for women and new employees. Again, these were ascribed to issues of self-presentation and managing others' impressions.

While there is no one size fits all some suggested recommendation from Bennett et al. (op cit) for reducing zoom fatigue include,

- Hold meetings early in the day or just after lunch when it is least fatiguing.
- Increase group bonding and cohesion by encouraging some part of a session for chit chat and having a happy hour at the end where again they can chat and eat/drink. This facilitates more connection with each other and more interest in participation.
- Mute the microphone if not speaking. Fatigue can result from mental effort of continual attention. Muting enables background noise to be eliminated and reduces the amount of time spent worrying about maintaining a quiet atmosphere (child or dog interruptions, etc.).
- Switch off the Webcam from time to time. Consider 'hide self' view. This reduces the stimuli onscreen and reduces the time spent worrying about self-presentation or even how tidy the house looks, otherwise the pressure is always there to smile, look pleasant and seem interested. However, keeping Webcam on may help you feel more engaged with the group.
- Take breaks during the zoom conference. This gives opportunity to detach mentally and take a little exercise like walk round the room. Such built in breaks could also be used for chit chat building relationships.
- Establish group norms, e.g. use of mute and Webcam, when to speak, etc. The agreements remove ambiguity of what is acceptable behaviour. This should reduce worry and fatigue. Group norms are also a reflection of high group cohesion and productivity.

In summary, communicating with others visually online can easily become too much for several reasons.

Firstly, there's the presence of gaze from others online, which can be overwhelming. The same goes for not showcasing the whole body, and leaving the body out physically. Nonetheless, having the feeling of constantly being watched but not knowing if people are looking, and where, can be anxiety-inducing. Contributing to this is the fact that that we are now oftentimes included in the view on the screen, in a way seeing what others are seeing. This takes the position of '*being on the outside looking in*', constituting the ideal place from which to judge oneself, which can easily become weary in relation to the ongoing multitasking. The presence of the image and idea of ourselves are thus ever so close, with the boundaries between the internal and external, work and the personal, increasingly blurred, reinforcing the constant, ongoing evaluation part of contemporary society, where our private lives are now also up for scrutiny and affects our professional lives (as evidenced for example by the not uncommon process whereby one's professional career is 'cancelled' due to something that went on in private).

Secondly, there is no possibility of sharing food or beverages online, actions which normally mediate and make more bearable the presence and proximity of others in face-to-face meetings. Adding to this, the inability to spontaneously form one-on-one interactions means one is stuck in group conversations whether one likes them or not. All of the above-mentioned contribute to the collapse between work and leisure time, with not enough difference between the two and the inescapability of 'work'; work never ends and leisure becomes work. All of this places further demand on the individual to actively create their own boundaries to mediate the presence of others and obligations, boundaries which were previously spontaneous, external, such as the office closing in the evening and travelling in personal transport to and from work.

Changes to Perceived Reasons for Working Induced by Covid

This chapter opened with a review of reasons why people worked in the preCovid era, however, the pandemic has raised a twenty-first century's developing focus on flexible work practices and challenged the perception that only work done in '*facetime*' has any use. The global pandemic has enabled displaced and existing employees from a range of industries with a range of talents, encouraging employers, HR and occupational psychologists to appreciate the growing flexibility of what work is, what it represents, who carries it out, when, where and how. This thinking has commenced to mature over the last two years as the worth of skilled, competent and experienced workers became more fully recognised, especially when they could transition easily to a new role to better support society and the economy in novel working conditions.

Consequently, the reasons for working are little different from before Covid and changed their level of importance. In general, income has lost some drawing power with more focus and importance placed on intrinsic motives like personal development, self-esteem, self-satisfaction and social connection coming to the fore.

Prognosticating the Post-Covid Landscape

What employees want out of work is changing from those listed for the preCovid context in the opening paragraphs of this chapter. With talent in high demand, employees are in a stronger position to create the world of work they want, where managers trust them, work policies embrace flexibility, and the career growth path is clear. The rising generation of employees recognises that the skills they build and experiences they acquire today shape their career opportunities of tomorrow and will be quick to move between employers if they feel that their growth is limited. To compound this trend, remote work is giving many, particularly those outside of major metropolitan areas, more job options to consider without disrupting where they want to live.

Some trends expected from 2022 onwards according to the LinkedIn Workplace Culture Shifts Report (2022) and from the Microsoft Report Work Trend Report (2021) a study of more than 30,000 people in 31 countries and an analysis of trillions of productivity and labour signals as the post-pandemic world of work continues to evolve in the future will include:

1. *People are re-evaluating what work means to them and a tightening labour market will generate a rise in job mobility*. This implies that the power will be in the job seeker's hands to ask for what they want from a job, whether that be better benefits, flexibility or remote working, and for some to be picky resigning from one job to take another, or threatening to do so unless they get the sort of work system they want. This employee power will ensure employers embrace flexibility, internal mobility and skills-based hiring if they hope to stay competitive in attracting and retaining talent. LinkedIn's report (op cit.) into workplace cultural shifts shows the number of times 'flexibility' was mentioned in company posts on LinkedIn since 2019 has increased more than 362% and prognosticates that this will continue. It also reveals three in five Australians and more than half (59%) of working Americans are thinking about switching jobs in 2022/23.
2. *Various forms of hybrid working will continue to increase* well into the future as the pandemic has shown that many companies can, in fact, operate remotely, and many employees have found that the freedom that can bring affords them many lifestyle benefits, which they're not so willing to give up by returning to the office full time, even willing to drop in income. It's not about dropping out of work, but doing it differently in a way that satisfies the individual.

3. *Office space will be redesigned.* 66% of business decision makers are considering redesigning physical spaces for the future to better accommodate flexible seating, communal work spaces and meeting spaces with virtual reality enabling individuals to effectively collaborate when necessary, regardless of location (Microsoft report op cit.). There's no one size fits all formula for hybrid work so success in this will employ developing multiple strategies, embracing employee feedback and iterate constantly.
4. *Entrepreneurship is becoming a popular career path* having offered some offering opportunities and flexibility experienced during Covid. This wave of new businesses will include a surge of female founders, with new passion project businesses launched in 2022 onwards.
5. *Employers are starting to put increased focus on employee skilling and training*, a vital support where in the emerging hybrid world, there are fewer opportunities to ask the colleague next to you for help. Talent retention will increase in importance in the future with more internal mobility programmes. The LinkedIn report (op cit.) finds that employees at companies with high internal mobility are projected to stay almost 2 times longer than those who don't, and those who have found new roles internally are 3.5 times more likely to be still engaged in the future than those who haven't. For those looking to transition to a new role need to be helped to see how their skills could be repurposed. A lifelong learning mind-set will have to be incorporated in an organisation's future policy commitments as it is crucial to facilitate for adaptation of the organisation and its employee into the future. This will require the HR role to collaborate with other departments to foster learning and development programmes.
6. *Employee/employer contracts won't be just about work*, they will start to focus more on employee wellbeing in the future as a key part of contractual arrangements particularly with women. LinkedIn (op cit.) reveals that employees who feel cared about at work are 3.2 times more likely to report being happy to work for their current company (this likelihood has increased by 35% since the onset of the pandemic and is expected to continue), and 3.7 times more likely to recommend working for their company. This likelihood has increased by 49% since the onset of the pandemic and is also expected to continue. 'Happier' companies outperform their competitors by 20% and will continue to do so. Employers are recognising these changes with the mention of 'wellbeing' increasing by 147% since 2019 to early 2022 and a 41% increase in women engaging with 'wellbeing' posts (LinkedIn op cit.) all a direction sign to the future of recruitment advertising. This means that managers will need to continue to adapt their styles and build soft skills to attract and retain talent in the future of work. Feeling cared for buffers against stress, increases positive emotions, promotes resilience and enables employees to perceive they are viewed as people, not just workers.

7. *Employees are beginning to seek stronger company culture* as a top priority for accepting a job, for example, 50% in the Netherlands, 47% Australia and New Zealand, France 46%, 45% in Spain, UK 45%, 42% in Canada and USA 41% (Linkedin Report op cit.). Many employees are deciding that what they want is a job that they feel proud of and that aligns with their personal and ethical values; showcasing a company's authentic commitment to equity matters more than ever. More than three-fourths (78%) of job seekers on LinkedIn expect to find diversity, equity and inclusion (*DEI*) information on a company's LinkedIn Page as well as wellbeing matters. From reducing bias when screening candidates, building *DEI* into company culture isn't a 'nice-to-have' or virtue signal, it is becoming both a moral and business imperative post-pandemic ethos.
8. *Hiring will become less interested in degrees and diplomas* with more focus on transferable skills enabling employers to broaden talent pools, as well as levelling the playing field for job seekers from non-traditional backgrounds. 46% of remote workers surveyed are planning to move to a new location this year because they can now work remotely. Talent is everywhere in a hybrid world. It's good for democratising access to opportunity as companies in major cities can hire talent from underrepresented groups that may not have the means or desire to move to a big city. Remote opportunities will be more attractive to minority group applicants (Microsoft Report op cit.).
9. *Authenticity will spur productivity and wellbeing* as employees navigate unprecedented impacts, balancing childcare and home schooling, work from living rooms, quieten barking dogs and push away curious cats; work has become more human. One in five claim to have met their colleagues' pets or families virtually, and one in six (17%) have cried with a colleague (Microsoft report op cit.). The shared vulnerability will provide a huge opportunity to bring real authenticity to company culture and transform work relationships for the better in the future and where people feel more comfortable to be themselves. People who interacted with their co-workers more closely than before not only experienced stronger work relationships but also reported higher productivity and better overall wellbeing (Microsoft report op cit.).

Conclusions

Clearly, the above are significant issues and signs to the future prosperity of businesses in the post-Covid era. Employers who wish both to 'catch' the best new hires and retain staff they want, must pay attention to these post-pandemic trends as they evolve post-Covid workplace models and present the messages in both internal and external advancement/recruitment policy. Taken together, the effect of Covid shows that we are no longer bound to traditional notions of space and time to work together and that physical attendance does not imply performance. Business needs to set aside long-held assumptions and alter course to embrace considerable flexibility. Employees everywhere are re-evaluating their professional goals in the context of the life they wish to lead, not just the career track they are on. This includes questioning when, where, how and for whom they want to work.

In a market of insufficient employees with requisite skills, trying to force employees back into a straightjacket of 9–5 five days per week against their will is not going to be acceptable to many. Covid has wrought changes we are not yet able to fully understand. But the lockdowns liberated some workers to find more satisfaction in work by allowing for a different approach to how we might think about paid work and have accelerated changes that were already bubbling away about why, where and how we work in the future. It is almost impossible to incentivise an employee to put their child in before school care at 7am, drive and try to park somewhere close to their train station, jam in to the carriage of a train probably running late, commute for an hour, take the lift up to their work space and do it all in reverse at the end of the day. In short, Covid taught employers and employees that work can and will have to will fit into life not the other way around.

Acknowledgments A good book to read on the future of work is *The New World of Work* by Peter Cheese, published by Kogan Page (2021).

References

ABC News. (2022, May 09) Retrieved 09 May 22 from https://www.abc.net.au/news/2022-05-09/parramatta-sydney-mobility-unlikely-to-recover-to-precovid-data/101040778

ABC News. (2022, July 21) Sophie Kesteven and Zoe Ferguson for this working life. Working from home can get lonely. Researchers have found a 'magic ratio' to balance it with office work. Retrieved 21 July 22 from https://www.abc.net.au/news/2022-07-21/hybrid-work-can-leave-us-feeling-lonely-and-disconnected/101227102

Australian Bureau of Statistics. Media release. (2021, December). Retrieved 21 December 21. https://www.abs.gov.au/media-centre/media-releases/more-40-cent-australians-worked-home

Australian Bureau of Statistics. Media release. (2022, February). Retrieved 01 March 22 from https://www.abs.gov.au/statistics/labour/jobs/job-mobility/latest-release

Australian Bureau of Statistics. (2022, October), *Labour Force*, Australia, ABS Website. Retrieved 10 November 22 from https://www.abs.gov.au/media-centre/media-releases/unemployment-rate-remains-35/30.1022

Australian Institute of Health and Welfare Annual Report. (2021, October). https://doi.org/10.25816/mmya-pc38

Australian Institute of Health and Welfare. Socialisation and Loneliness Report (2021). Retrieved 6 January 22 from https://www.aihw.gov.au/reports/australias-welfare/social-isolation-and-loneliness-covid-pandemic

BBC News. (2022, April 23). Hospitality: London's recruitment crisis causing mental health issues. Retrieved 23 April 22 from https://www.bbc.com/news/uk-england-london-61149218

BBC News. (2022, August 18). Why more people are working from home on Fridays. Retrieved 22 September 22 from https://www.bbc.com/news/business-62560520

Bendelta Survey. (2022). Retrieved 5 October 22 from https://www.bendelta.com

Bennett, A. A., et al. (2021). Videoconference fatigue? Exploring changes in fatigue after videoconference meetings during COVID-19. *Journal of Applied Psychology, 106*, 330–344. https://doi.org/10.1037/apl0000906

Bloom, N. (2021). *Hybrid is the future of work.* Retrieved 10 February 22 from https://siepr.stanford.edu/publications/policy-brief/hybrid-future-work

Bloomberg News Report. (2022, April 12). Retrieved 2 April 22 from https://www.bloomberg.com/news/articles/2022-04-12/one-or-two-days-in-the-office-is-the-sweet-spot-of-hybrid-work

Burns, R. (1993). *Managing people in changing times.* Allen and Unwin.

Deloitte. (2022). Women at work 22: A global outlook report. Retrieved 2 October 22 from https://www.deloitte.com/global/en/about/people/social-responsibility/women-at-work-global-outlook.html

Global Workplace Analytics. (2020). *Work from home experience survey.* Retrieved 24 November 21 from https://globalworkplaceanalytics.com/global-work-from-home-experience-survey.

Goodhire. (2022, October 27). Retrieved 01 November 22 from https://www.goodhire.com/resources/articles/state-of-remote-work-survey-2022/

HILDA (Household, Income and Labour Dynamics in Australia 2021) survey. Retrieved 06 January 22 from https://melbourneinstitute.unimelb.edu.au/__data/assets/pdf_file/0009/3963249/HILDA-Statistical-Report-2021.pdf

House of Commons Library. Research Briefing. (2022, August 09). Coronavirus: Impact on the labour market. Retrieved 12 September 22 from https://commonslibrary.parliament.uk/authors/brigid-francis-devine/

Ingoglia, C. (2022). At the intersection of vision and research. *Journal of Behavioral Health Services and Research, 49*(1):1–3. https://doi.org/10.1007/s11414-022-09786-4. Also see: https://www.washingtonpost.com/context/washington-post-kff-frontline-health-care-workers-survey-feb-11-march-7-2021/ba15a233-9495-47a9-9cdd-e7fa1578b1ca/

LinkedIn Workplace Culture Shifts Report (2022, January 26). Retrieved 04 May 22 from https://www.socialmediatoday.com/news/linkedin-publishes-new-report-into-workplace-culture-shifts-and-what-they/617801/

Mainstreets Insight Report. (2022). *Workplace and the future.* Retrieved 10 August 22 from https://mainstreetinsights.com.au/

Maslow, A. H. (1943). A theory of human motivation. *Psychological Review, 50*(4), 430–437.

Medallia Return to Work Report. (2021). Retrieved 17 November 21 from https://info.sense360.com/hubfs/210824_Sense360_Return%20to%20Work%20Insights_v2.pdf

Microsoft Work Trend Report. (2021). *The next great disruption is hybrid work.* Retrieved 17 November 21 from https://www.microsoft.com/en-us/worklab/work-trend-index/hybrid-work)

Min, H., Peng, Y., Shoss, M., & Yang, B. (2021). Using machine learning to investigate the public's emotional responses to work from home during the COVID-19 pandemic. *Journal of Applied Psychology, 106*, 214–229. https://doi.org/10.1037/apl0000886

Oakman, J., Kinsman, N., Stuckey, R., et al. (2020). A rapid review of mental and physical health effects of working at home: How do we optimise health? *BMC Public Health, 20*, 1825. https://doi.org/10.1186/s12889-020-09875-z

Office for National Statistics. Data and analysis from Census 2021. (2022, November 15). Retrieved 18 November 22 from https://www.ons.gov.uk/employmentandlabourmarket/peopleinwork

Oum, S., Kates, J., & Wexler, A. (2021). Global Health Policy economic impact of COVID-19 on PEPFAR Countries. Retrieved 03 March 22 from Retrieved 01 November 22 from https://www.kff.org/global-health-policy/issue-brief/economic-impact-of-covid-19-on-pepfar-countries/

OwlLabs and Global Analytic Sixth Annual Survey. (2022, November 24). Retrieved 01 November 22 from https://www.businesswire.com/news/home/20221024005224/en/Owl-Labs%E2%80%99-Global-Workplace-Analytics%E2%80%99-Sixth-Annual-State-Of-Remote-Work-Report-Uncovers-Latest-Remote-and-Hybrid-Work-Trends

PricewaterhouseCooper. (2021). *Remote Work Survey*. USA. Retrieved 27 November 21 from https://www.pwc.com/us/en/services/consulting/business-transformation/library/covid-19-us-remote-work-survey.html

Productivity Commission (2021). *Working from home*. Research paper, Canberra, Australia. Retrieved 27 November 21 from https://www.pc.gov.au/research/completed/working-from-home

Shockley, K. M., Gabriel, A. S., Robertson, D., et al. (2021). The fatiguing effects of camera use in virtual meetings: A within-person field experiment. *Journal of Applied Psychology, 106*, 1137–1155. https://doi.org/10.1037/apl0000948

The Burnt Chef Survey. (2022, February 24). Retrieved 29 June 22 from https://www.bighospitality.co.uk/News/Trends-Reports/The-Burnt-Chef-Project-launches-industry-survey-stress-mental-health-in-hospitality

The home office Life. Working from home UK statistics 2022. Retrieved 01 December 22 from https://thehomeofficelife.com/blog/work-from-home-statistics

The property council of Australia. (2022, February). Office occupancy results. Retrieved 29 March 22 from https://research.propertycouncil.com.au/blog/february-2022-office-occupancy-results-0

Trinka, H., & Fox, C. (2004). *Better than sex: How a whole generation got hooked on work*. Random House.

US Bureau of Labour Statistics. Monthly Report June 2021. Unemployment rises in 2020, as the country battles the COVID-19 pandemic. Retrieved 25 July 21 from https://www.bls.gov/opub/mlr/2021/article/pdf/unemployment-rises-in-2020-as-the-country-battles-the-covid-19-pandemic.pdf

US Census Bureau. (2022, September 15). Press Release Number CB22-155. The Number of People Primarily Working From Home Tripled Between 2019 and 2021. Retrieved 17 September 22 from www.census.gov/newsroom/press-releases/2022/people-working-from-home.html

Williamson, S., Colley, L., & Foley, M. (2020). Public servants working from home: Exploring managers' changing allowance decisions in a COVID-19 context. *Australian Journal of Public Administration, 79*(4), 601–607. https://doi.org/10.1177/1035304621105526

YahooLife UK report. Hannah Millington, (2022, May 16). Working from home ruining our health, report warns. Retrieved 18 May 22 from https://au.lifestyle.yahoo.com/working-from-home-health-eating-exercising-pandemic-105523368.html

CHAPTER 6

Isolation, Group Identity and Community

Non solum sed omnibus

Abstract This chapter discusses and reviews studies on the problems of social isolation and loneliness brought on by Covid restrictions involving quarantine, lockdown and movement restrictions which considerably reduced the bonds holding individuals, groups, communities and societies together. The nature of being a human being and possessing identity was under attack. The breakup of shared culture with some persons and groups being granted dispensation from the rules affecting everyone else headed society towards anomie. Fighting a global pandemic requires large-scale community cohesiveness. The role of group identity and community involvement is discussed to combat isolation and loneliness to regenerate society. Ways to reduce loneliness are offered such as Art therapy, and the issue of isolation in aged care homes is raised.

Keywords Loneliness · Isolation · Zero-sum game · Identity leadership · Community cooperation · Art therapy

The Disruption of Connections: Social Isolation and Loneliness

Breakdown of Society

Human resilience is closely linked to the depth and strength of interpersonal connections, including involvement in family, groups and communities. In contrast, simultaneous social isolation and loneliness appear to be a significant threat to our health and wellbeing. For humans, the absence of relationships

© The Author(s), under exclusive license to Springer Nature Singapore Pte Ltd. 2023

R. B. Burns, *The Human Impact of the COVID-19 Pandemic*,
https://doi.org/10.1007/978-981-99-1710-5_6

removes the essential conditions for the development of personal identity and the exercise of reason and recognition, the very nature of what the human being is. The natural channels of human expression and pleasure become depressed, with attendant impacts on mood and subjective wellbeing (Nardone & Speciani, 2019).

The quarantine and social isolation restrictions make us believe and behave '*as if*' other people are potentially dangerous to our health and health of our loved ones, and cultivate a new norm where proximity to fellow human beings is seen as a direct threat based on '*vulnerability-to-harm*'. Individuals are avoiding social relations not only by imposition but by choice, a decision caused by the fear of an invisible enemy and by the total uncertainty about what to do/not to do; we are witnessing the deterioration of interpersonal relationships (Pietrabissa & Simpson, 2020).

Although isolation and loneliness have been global experiences for many generations mainly impacting elderly widows/widowers, single persons, single mothers, refugees, etc., the pandemic changed things. Many more humans began to isolate themselves, either by government fiat or self-imposed, due to fear of contagion, firstly by country, then by city/region, ultimately by family. Some were left absolutely alone, and may, if up with technological developments, have had Alexa or Siri as their only companions. Human touch became a thing of the past, with people not knowing what was safe and what would put them at risk. They became driven by fear and emotion. Prolonged social isolation characterised by reduced social connections and contact generates a deep disconnect among those who live alone or cannot rely on an adequate social network, thus increasing the likelihood that depressive symptoms will emerge. Social isolation has been linked to cognitive impairment, reduced immunity, increased risk of cardiovascular disease, and ultimately, mortality (Heffner et al., 2011).

In many nations, restrictive measures are also creating rivalries and arousing discord between people. The Latin phrase '*Divide et impera*' (divide and rule) implies that a governing authority which exerts high levels of control not based on equity between people tends to fragment them. Grandiose leadership, for example, may create the seductive illusion of safety, with claims of invincibility and omnipotence as has been witnessed by leaders claiming '*I am saving you*', while offering relaxations of rules on the basis of '*star*' qualities to some groups or individuals like popstars and sports teams, leading to even greater grievances associated with inequalities that provide fuel for deeper divisions within society (O'Reilly & Hall, 2020).

People gain their sense of identity and self-worth from membership of groups such as church, sports, school, trades unions and work colleague groups. Shared behaviours, values and beliefs cement the individuals together providing mutual support, friendship and purpose. Destroy the possibility of these bonds within the group and individuals end up isolated, stressed, impulsive, addicted to drink or drugs, depressed and even suicidal, as they have no responsibility to others or even themselves. These are the chilling effects of lockdown, contact isolation, event banning, and highly restrictive rules about leaving one's residence that Covid has wrought for some as established routines of life were torn apart, particularly those living alone, or cooped up in small apartments with several children, coping with home schooling with limited skills or knowledge base, loss of access to peer, work place or other connectedness. No wonder alcohol sales have increased, domestic violence has risen, while mis-information alongside conspiracy theories has run rampant, all debilitating the smooth running of society. Imposing enforced isolation with the corollary of community group break down is a scenario for the breakdown of social cohesion. Even the over-riding group concept of Federalism has been damaged in Australia as States made their own rules. The current ethos is evolving towards '*anomie*' (or normlessness), a social condition in which there is a disintegration or disappearance of the norms and values previously common to society as people protest and refuse to accept mandates. Most societies globally have undergone a seismic shock. However, these social effects differed between major groupings of cultures.

Cultural Responses

A sense of the self as *independent versus interdependent* with others is a dimension of cultural variation. Western European and North American cultures that endorse individualism (Triandis, 1995) are considered independent, whereas many other cultures in Asia and Africa share a stronger commitment to collectivism such as country, tribe and family and are considered interdependent (Kitayama et al., 2009). While disease control policies are different across societies, some differences in the response to the pandemic may be better described as cultural, and many of those have a linkage to the dimension of individuality (Western societies) vs collectivism (Asian societies).

The priority given to obligations and duties in Asian societies may motivate individuals to remain committed to social norms while suppressing personal desires, thus accepting lockdown loneliness and isolation without rancour. In collectivist countries (like China, Singapore, and Japan), there was hardly any antagonism towards initial strong Covid response measures as people in collectivist cultures tend to more easily comply with rules protecting '*the greater good*', although the excessive imprisonment reported in China ventually evoked antagonism. They also tend to have strong social support structures for looking after elderly relatives and neighbours. Conversely, social norms and conventions in North America and much of Western Europe tend to positively value the expressivity of the self such as personal decision-making, and critical argument, making Government diktats rather unpopular and even unacceptable. (Kraus & Kitayama, 2019).

Another, closely related dimension of cultural variance is a society's '*tightness*' *vs* '*looseness*'. Research has found that tight cultures, such as those of Singapore, Japan and China, have very strict social norms and punishments for deviance, while loose cultures, in the West, have weaker social norms and are more permissive (Gefland et al., 2011). Cultures accustomed to prioritising freedom over security may have more difficulty coordinating a unified policy in the face of a pandemic leading to anti-vax rallies in the West. The cumulative evidence here suggests that very different strategies might be called for in varying cultural contexts in the fight against Covid.

The tendency to move into an *anomie ethos* is more apparent in individualistic democratic countries (such as Australia, UK and Canada) where there was far less acceptance of restrictive measures that impinged on freedom and personal responsibility, with imposed controls creating disruptive rallies and convoys against such measures and precipitating emotional and social distress among many in the general population, as social isolation led to people looking for new groups and purposes, for new bonds and values, to which to attach themselves, as old bonds became difficult to maintain in the restrictive environment of health public orders.

The internet has provided a new way of connectedness that does not require leaving the house, with a proliferation of extreme beliefs and norms across the spectrum from freedom libertarians to anti-vaxxers. Even this identity politics group development causes some individuals concern as they ponder whether they do actually belong with these extremists. But division plus repression can turn social cohesion into social disorder. If some extreme groups in society are less able to abide by the restrictions of Covid, and if, on top of that, they experience repressive sanctions when they violate these restrictions, then the potential for social disorder is greatly increased. Effective policing of a pandemic should only use enforcement as a last resort. Instead government organisations need to engage in dialogue with communities, understanding their situation, explaining and encouraging adherence (Reicher & Stott, 2020) as discussed in Chap. 4.

Shared Identity Is Fragile and Needs to Be Nurtured

The sense of developing anomie reflects that shared identity between members of the public is fragile and can easily be disrupted by leadership that sets people almost as tribes against each other in rhetoric or which favours some groups over others in practice. The context of lockdowns, controlled movement, loss of employment, coping with home schooling among other things have created cohorts who are less socially functional and almost group-less. This can impact on the influence of Government and hence to Government ability to steer a nation through a crisis. It is therefore critical to have good leaders who appeal to an inclusive sense of community and who provide the practical support needed to maintain a commonality of experience (Ntontis et al., 2020).

This was not achieved in situations where public health orders were not applied with equity or in a proportionate way with little clarity over providing exemptions for those seriously affected who offered little risk to the general public as happened over several years across some Australian States. An inclusive sense of community, '*we are all in this together*' approach is critically undermined by anything which smacks of '*one rule for us and another for them*' (Tyler & Blader, 2003), and this is what has happened in some countries where the general public was forced to bunker down for a time at home or in quarantine hotels, while other more *special* persons such as stars of films or sports fields were granted dispensation from the rules affecting everyone else (Chap. 10). A highly publicised example of government officials not following the rules they had set concerning movement and meeting restrictions surfaced in the 'Partygate' affair in the UK.

Shared identity is at the root of adherence to pandemic restrictions. The levels of adherence to lockdown in the UK and Australia were reasonable despite the fact that many were suffering emotional and economic distress. If they had been putting individual interest first many would have disobeyed since they had little to lose personally by going out. But they didn't and acted in terms of the collective interest and to ensure they didn't infect others and endanger the most vulnerable in the community (Duffy & Allington, 2020). Membership of social groups is a powerful prophylactic against a wide range of mental and physical disorders and did so during the pandemic. When we feel part of a group we can draw on the support of other group members, which increases the sense of coping and lowers stress. Thus despite problems working from home with Zoom-type meetings, schooling at home with online learning linking children and parents together, social media helped individuals keep in touch and chat with each other, and many people have retained social connectedness despite physically distancing self from others. The key challenge of the pandemic besides keeping healthy is to stay together while keeping physically apart.

Without good leadership, a pandemic can undermine shared identity and exacerbate social divisions. While disasters have the potential to bring people together and to unlock all the benefits of shared social identity, they also serve to spotlight and potentially exacerbate existing social divisions. The poor, the aged, the handicapped, the immigrant with inadequate language skills, those on the wrong side of the digital divide, and those who are discriminated against are all vulnerable and all suffer more, both during and after pandemics (see other material in Chaps. 4, 5, 7 and 8). These issues permeate the ethical and equity issues of the pandemic such as availability of vaccinations in aged care homes, high unemployment among certain groups, lack of computer and online facilities for home schooling, etc. Unless explicitly recognised and addressed, these divides will undermine shared identity and increase social tensions (Jetten & Peters, 2019). The aged care homes deaths in Australia and the UK are a glaring and poignant example of these inequalities.

Not a Zero-Sum Game. Self Gain Versus Cooperation

People often default to thinking that someone else's gain, especially someone from a competing group, implies a loss to themselves, and vice versa (Meegan, 2010). But this zero-sum thinking is not applicable with the nonzero-sum nature of pandemic infection, where someone else's infection is a threat to oneself and everyone else (Fosch et al., 2003). Zero-sum thinking means that while it might be psychologically compelling to hoard protective materials (sanitiser, masks, even vaccines) beyond what is necessary, doing so could be self-defeating as the infection will likely spread further as others have no protective materials and more rapidly becoming uncontrollable. Given the importance of slowing infections, it may be helpful to make people aware that others' access to preventative measures is a benefit to oneself.

Whereas reducing infections across the population is nonzero-sum, the provision of scarce healthcare resources to the infected does have zero-sum elements and considerable ethical implications. For example, when the number of patients needing ventilators exceeds capacity, healthcare providers are often forced to make life-for-life trade-offs. While some people are willing to sacrifice the elderly to save the young, there are cultural differences on this preference and considerable soul searching among Western society (Awad et al., 2018). Who is perceived to be making those decisions may also impact the public's and patients' trust. In experiments, people who make utilitarian judgments about matters of life and death are less trusted (Everett et al., 2016). Generally, trust in medical doctors who are less utilitarian in their ethical decision-making opting for the '*do no harm*' rule remains high compared to that for public health officials.

The behaviour of individuals living in communities tends to be regulated by moral norms and values (Tomasello, 2009), such as '*do no harm*', and recognising the nonzero sum condition of the pandemic. Those who do what is '*right*' are respected and publicly admired and modelled, while those who do what is '*wrong*' are devalued and socially excluded particularly if they have been involved in devising the excessive pandemic restrictions. Thus, politicians and health professionals must ensure that are visibly seen to be part of the responses and not making laws for others and ignoring the laws themselves (Partygate affair in the UK; film and sports persons in Australia). These mechanisms of social reinforcement and modelling encourage people to embrace and internalise shared guidelines, making them motivated to do what is considered right while avoiding behaviours that seem wrong, and which do not totally have to rely on legal agreements and formal sanctions (Ellemers & van den Bos, 2012).

Fighting a global pandemic requires large-scale cooperation. The problem is that, by definition, cooperation requires people to bear an individual cost to benefit other people. In particular, there is a conflict between short-term self-interest vs longer-term collective interest. Several techniques, such as sanctioning defectors or rewarding co-operators (Rand & Nowak, 2013), tend to increase cooperative behaviour in laboratory experiments using economic games. Providing cues that make the morality of an action salient such as having people read the Golden Rule before making a decision or asking them to report what they think is the morally right thing to do (the Golden Rule is the principle of treating others as one wants to be treated and is a maxim found in most religions and cultures). This has been shown to increase cooperation (Capraro et al., 2019). People are also more likely to cooperate when they believe that others are cooperating. Accordingly, interventions based on observability and descriptive norms are highly effective at increasing cooperative behaviour in economic games as well as in the field (Kraft-Todd & Rand, 2016). Again this suggests that leaders and the media can promote cooperation on health requirements by making these behaviours more observable and practical, emphasising the benefit to all.

Luckily in late 2022, as the shadows of anomie lift, more normality returns and old associations can be revived with the lifting of virtually all mandates. Perhaps the health officials in many Western nations were now well aware of the public's view of the draconian measures imposed over the last two years, as well as the over-riding of generally accepted ethical principles, and have binned ideas of irresponsible and ill-proportioned measures despite variants BA.2, 4 and 5 winging their way round the globe. Even 'Chairman' Dan Andrews, Premier of Victoria seems to have softened his former bunker approach. Of course, the autocratic Chinese response to this new variant has been to physically lockdown many millions of people in a number of major cities in 2022, but with their philosophy of collectivism, no norms have been offended and mute acceptance generally transpired until the citizens had had enough by November 2022.

The Known Effects of Loneliness and Social Isolation

> No man is an iland intire of itself; every man is a peece of the Continent, a part of the maine.
>
> John Donne (1673) Devotions 17. (Original spelling)

According to the Evolutionary Theory of Loneliness (Cacioppo & Cacioppo, 2018), social isolation and loneliness interact reinforcing and perpetuating each other over time. However, those who became socially isolated during the pandemic experienced greater loneliness feelings than those who had been previously persistently socially isolated (like elderly widows), as it was a novel experience to which the former had to adjust with immediate haste. This implied that social isolation during the pandemic seriously impacted the feeling of loneliness (Murayama et al., 2020).

There is a recognisable distinction between social isolation and loneliness:

- Social isolation is the state of having minimal contact with others.
- Loneliness is a subjective emotional reaction of negative feelings about having a lower level of social contact than desired.

Both are obviously linked but both may not co-exist on some occasions, in that a person obtaining meaning in their life from being deeply engaged in a hobby, interest or research may be socially isolated but not lonely, or a socially connected person may still feel lonely as their contacts at work within an individual work space or in the massive multilevel apartment block where they live, tend to be superficial with accidental meeting such as at the coffee dispenser or in the elevator. Since lockdown or social distancing policies may also lead to an increase in the prevalence of social isolation, it is difficult to distinguish the effects of lockdown or social distancing policies from the effects of social isolation on mental health when evaluating the results of studies in the area.

Loneliness an Emerging Issue Even Pre-Covid

To feel lonely is a reflection of being human. But it is a highly taboo subject, often inaccurately portrayed as a personal social deficiency by the uninformed. People who feel lonely often hide their feelings, find interacting with others stressful, and in coping with these feelings may unconsciously appear be more distant or uncooperative, sending an inaccurate signal to others. Many people who feel lonely socially withdraw; they might not turn up to social opportunities, or if they do, might try to avoid engagement, creating a self-fulfilling sequence.

Loneliness has been an emerging issue for many years in industrialised countries, prior to Covid with approximately one-third of the population affected, and one in 12 people affected at a severe level (Pietrabissa & Simpson, 2020). The detrimental effects on health and potential for premature mortality are increasingly recognised (e.g. Bzdok & Dunbar, 2020). Loneliness is associated with feelings of emptiness, sadness and shame, alongside the subjective perception that one is disconnected from others, and has been linked to depression, irritability and preoccupation with negative self-related thoughts, leading to a 26% increase in risk of premature death (Pietrabissa and Simpson op cit.). It can persist occur well beyond the predisposing context, even experienced when others are physically present. Loneliness has been linked medically to depression (Han & Richardson, 2010), increased cortisol levels (Miller et al., 2011), lowered immunity (Cole 2014), with increased length and frequency of hospital stays (Hawker & Romero-Ortuno, 2016). In spite of the clear risks associated with loneliness, treatments to date based on cognitive-behavioural principles have shown poor outcomes (Masi et al., 2011). Further, it appears that income and socio-economic status are no barrier to loneliness; given the right circumstances we are all equally at risk (e.g. Cacioppo et al., 2015; Holt-Lunstad & Smith, 2016). Other studies from around the globe reporting adverse effects on people's mental health due to loneliness and isolation include Holt-Lunstad et al. (2015), Ikeda et al. (2020), López-Castro et al. (2021) and Müller et al. (2021). Generally, overwhelming evidence on the association between social isolation and health status has been consistent across studies and countries.

There are a number of well-known existing risk factors for social isolation and loneliness with some living situations more likely to be associated with them than others, which amplifies the context for more severe impacts on social and mental stress when Covid restrictions are imposed. According to the 2016 Census of Population and Housing, 25% of Australian households are lone person households (Australian Bureau of Statistics (ABS), 2016). Living alone and not being in a relationship with a partner are substantial risk factors for both social isolation and loneliness (Relationships Australia, 2011). Relationship separation tends to result in an increase in loneliness across ages and genders; however, the effects are more pronounced for men than women. Recently separated men are over 13 times as likely to develop loneliness than married men, as opposed to twice as likely for separated women compared with married women. Single parents experienced the highest rate of social isolation. Unemployment, receiving income support (Relationships Australia, 2018) and lack of satisfaction with financial situation are also factors involved in the development of loneliness across age groups and gender. Loneliness can be self-reinforcing if it is associated with an experience of depression and anxiety, particularly around social interactions (Australian Psychological Society, 2018). All these risk factor situations make Covid impacts amplify loneliness and isolation difficulties into highly serious problems.

Reviews and Surveys on Isolation and Loneliness in the Covid Context

Evolutionarily, the formation of social bonds was fundamental to both human survival and to guarantee a healthy development. In normal circumstances, isolation and spatial distancing is unnatural for us. People crave social cues just like they crave food (Tomova et al., 2020). With the onset of Covid, social isolation and loneliness enforced or by choice is likely to be exacerbating what is already a significant issue for many individuals across the globe.

The Covid crisis via its influence on isolation and loneliness increases the risk of depression, anxiety and suicidal ideation which affect the individual's ability to solve problems, to set and achieve goals, to function effectively and to rebuild relationships, making recovery from the crisis even more difficult. People gradually lose any form of active response with an increasing tendency to complain, and rely completely on others in the management of themselves, all actions of delegation. Feeling safe and protected is a fundamental primary need of the human being to be able to move freely in the surrounding world, as well as the feeling of having control over the events of our own life. When all this fails, when the belief that whatever we do will not improve things begins to develop, a sense of '*learned helplessness*' takes hold, blocking any possibility of liberation or change.

Covid has been a natural social experiment and lockdowns made people more acutely aware of how critical meaningful social connection actually is. Many recent surveys suggest that Covid has made things far worse with Lim et al. (2020) in a multination study reporting that just over half (54%) of respondents felt more lonely since the start of the pandemic. Lim et al. (2022) found a recent significant rise in social anxiety derived from longitudinal survey data from the UK, USA and Australia into how social restrictions impacted loneliness, social anxiety and depression. The study tracked the impacts on isolated people from the onset of the pandemic right through to when the restrictions were lifted to determine how Covid social restrictions affected people's ability to feel meaningfully connected with others and the mental health symptoms this created.

The Lim et al. (2022) study showed Covid created a context where people became used to not interacting with others in person during lockdowns cocooned safely in their little world, but as social restrictions were easing fast, levels of social anxiety rather unexpectedly increased fastest, i.e. a negative correlation. The explanation suggested is that where a lengthy lack of social exposure has occurred, social anxiety severity increases as 'freedom' signalled danger to health (virus still present) combined with lost psychological skills in connecting with others. Easing social restrictions did not affect depression levels which remained fairly constant. Not being social face to face has been relaxing for some of us not having to self-present, and the idea of 'going back' into public again might be scary. Behaviours that were automatic to us pre-Covid now need to be reconditioned so we can regain our confidence in gathering in mingling and meeting socially.

The research also found that we generally misconceive loneliness as something that only happens to other people, particularly older people. When asked directly, Lim et al. (2022) found those aged 65 plus are the generation most likely to say they 'never' or 'hardly ever' feel lonely; it was being 18–25 years of age, unemployed, lower than average wealth, and living alone, that predicted higher loneliness, depression and social anxiety at the end of the restrictions, despite their presumed competences in operating internet social media. This shows that our sociocultural perceptions of loneliness are out of line with the reality. However, a greater proportion of young people live alone than other age groups, which leaves them more vulnerable to social isolation (Kabátek, 2020). The report found at least one in two Australians felt more lonely throughout the Covid pandemic, which may not be a big surprise to those who spent months isolating alone. Lim's research also revealed that one in five people in Australia say they don't have people they can regularly talk to or turn to, while three in ten say they never or rarely feel close to people. With restrictions of household visits, living within a family emerged as a protective factor for younger persons from experiencing loneliness during the pandemic (Lim et al., 2022).

Lockdown and isolation mandates made us aware of how critical social connections are to our happiness and wellbeing, something many of us may have taken for granted until we were severely restricted in social behaviours and routines. Many have simply got out of practice in being a friend. Those in Melbourne, for example, experienced two years of disembodied relationships and lost coffee catch-ups, shared gym activity or sales event shopping rituals that normally characterise friendships. There is now the anxiety of reconnecting. Yet friendships are important for overall mental health, often providing an essential protective layer to our lives. They also facilitate a reciprocal lived experience that helps people to realise the anxiety they are experiencing is natural.

COVID-19 Impact Monitoring Survey

In this Australian National University longitudinal COVID-19 Impact Monitoring Survey Programme (ANU 2022), participants were asked the question '*In the past week, how often have you felt lonely?*'. In the various survey waves conducted in 2020 and 2021 the overall loneliness rates have fluctuated in line with the extent and impact of Covid-related restrictions. Many people reported that they were experiencing more social isolation and loneliness as lockdown restrictions came into effect from March 2020. Although most regions of Australia reported improvements as lockdown measures began to ease in May, Victorians reported a relative worsening of loneliness between May and August 2020, associated with its 'second wave' of Covid cases. In April 2020, almost half (46%) of respondents reported that they felt lonely during the past week, and 40% reported an increase in the amount of time they felt socially isolated and lonely since March 2020. By May 2020, the proportion of respondents feeling lonely lowered to one-third (36%), a level that was reported in repeated surveys through to January 2021 (Biddle & Gray, 2021a) a consistency developed as many respondents accustomed themselves to the situation and used social media to engage in social contact.

In parallel with the changes in feeling lonely, social isolation also declined from the height of the initial Covid-related restrictions that were in place in 2020. The effect of lockdowns was made manifestly clear when in October 2020, before the second lockdown was lifted, Victorians were more than twice as likely to report experiencing loneliness (33%) as Australians residing in other states (13%) which had no second lockdown (ABS, 2020). In April 2020, almost half (49%) of Australian respondents said that they had not met with anyone socially since the onset of the pandemic, but by November 2020, this reduced to 6.8%, but was still higher than levels of social isolation reported prepandemic in February 2020 (2.0%) (Biddle et al., 2020a, 2020b).

Loneliness has had clear impact on both levels of psychological distress and life satisfaction during the pandemic. In a regression analysis (Biddle & Gray, 2021a, 2021b) that controlled for psychological distress levels in April 2020 found those reporting they felt lonely either some, occasionally or most of the time all had significantly higher levels of psychological distress in November 2020 compared to April 2020. This suggests that loneliness has been contributing strongly to levels of psychological distress.

Increased loneliness is also a strong predictor of psychological distress even when other factors like changes in employment status are controlled for. Prepandemic, men tended to report higher levels of loneliness than women (Relationships Australia, 2018). However, more women reported experiencing loneliness than men during the pandemic, a trend that remained consistent from May 2020 to October 2020.

Loneliness Is Bad for Physical and Mental Health

In pre-Covid studies, loneliness already had links to premature death, poor physical and mental health and general dissatisfaction with life (Relationships Australia, 2018). The spinoff restrictions from Covid have amplified these mental health problems as the loneliness persists over time and often experienced intensely particularly by those to whom it is a sudden and novel experience causing a stress response. These consequences observed in current research are unlikely to have reached their peak in the short term and will considerably outlive the current pandemic.

Overall, loneliness has amplified the full gamut of disorders no one wants: anxiety and panic, post-traumatic stress, depression and suicidal intentions, emotional distress, obsessive–compulsive symptoms, insomnia, digestive problems, development of dementia, premature death, poor health behaviours, increased smoking, alcohol and drug use, physical inactivity, and physiological effects, such as high blood pressure and weaker immune function. The Sepúlveda-Loyola et al. (2020) meta-analysis reviewed ten cross-sectional papers published on Pubmed, SciELO and Google Scholar databases 2019–2020 that addressed the impact of social isolation and distancing on mental and physical health in elderly persons, involving 20,069 non-institutionalised community living individuals, 58% women, from Asia, Europe and America. Consistently revealing no significant cultural differences, the main problems manifested were anxiety, depression, poor sleep quality and physical inactivity during the isolation period indicating that mental and physical health in these older persons were negatively affected during Covid isolating/ distancing restrictions. The authors argued for multicomponent programmes for this population during the confinement involving cognitive strategies and increasing physical activity levels using inter alia apps, online videos and telehealth.

Murayama et al. (2020) investigated the association of Covid pandemic social isolation with mental health among the general Japanese population using data obtained from a web-based nationwide survey conducted from August to September 2020 ($n = 28{,}000$; aged 15–79 years). Assessment of the participants' frequency of contact showed the prevalence of social isolation 21.2% in January 2020 (before the pandemic) increasing to 27.9% in August 2020 (during the pandemic). Mental health outcomes included psychological distress, suicidal ideation, loneliness and fear of Covid. Older people and men had the greatest increase in the prevalence of social isolation. People who became socially isolated during the pandemic had greater loneliness and fear of Covid infection than those who were consistently socially isolated before the pandemic. In other cross-sectional studies, stay-home orders contributed to higher depression and loneliness in the USA (Tull et al., 2020) and were associated with higher anxiety, depression, and loneliness in Germany (Benke et al., 2020).

In Australia, Rogers and Cruickshank (2021) also noted an overall association of lowered social contact with sustained decreases in feelings of wellbeing and life satisfaction, whereas more frequent social contact was associated with higher life satisfaction and overall health. These are not only a direct consequence of pandemic fear but also strongly driven by the effects of mandated prolonged social isolation, leading to increased numbers of people manifesting loneliness through the objective lack of interactions with others. The medical journal The Lancet recently published an article from which a clear and alarming picture emerges: periods of isolation, even less than 10 days, can have long-term effects, with a lasting presence of psychiatric symptoms, up to 3 years later (Brooks et al., 2020). Loneliness has been shown to increase the risk of early death by 26% (Gerst-Emerson & Jayawardhana, 2015). Loneliness is damaging to physical and mental health, but it's obverse, social interactions, isn't readily thought of as a preventative strategy for mental health.

Isolation and Loneliness Impact Social Desire and Social Competence

Since Covid brought widespread disruption to work and social lives, loneliness has soared. Unfortunately although half (54%) of Australians report experiencing greater loneliness since the start of the pandemic more than a third of 1000 surveyed felt less confident in participating in social activities even with friends (MainstreetsInsights Report, 2022). In the same research losing social relationship desire and competence skills during isolation manifested as a distressing step towards increasing loneliness particularly as half those surveyed chose to spend time on their own rather than go out.

One lady surveyed reported that she had only been out once the previous week and that was to buy milk, and that actually had gone onto her own unofficial lockdown. This is bordering on agoraphobia. Many others also claimed they tried to avoid touching others if possible for fear of infection. Covid has wrought major social change and although Australians believe they are largely social and outgoing (56%), almost half of Australians (48%) strongly/somewhat agree they choose to spend more time on their own as a result of Covid restrictions even when restrictions were removed. Australians are feeling less confident in their ability to organise and participate in social activities (35%) with 25% constantly focussing at a mobile screen when around others, avoiding or unwilling to join in conversation (Mainstreets Insights Report (op sit 2022). This highlights a worrying disconnect between how Australians would like to perceive themselves, as sociable and outgoing, and their the reality of their current social fitness in the post-Covid environment. It looks too as though the new Omicron strain has increased feelings of pessimism when we thought we may have been coming out of it all.

Mainstreets Insights Report (op sit 2022) also found that Australians are also less likely to use physical touch to greet each other than before the Covid pandemic. Only three in five Australians are shaking hands with others less (60%) and using physical greetings such as a hug less (58%) than they were before the Covid pandemic. A further one in two (48%) are using other physical contacts such as a high five less than they were before the Covid pandemic. While the Aussie spirit of helping out remains strong, the way it is expressed has changed with three in ten (30%) being less likely to hold the door open for others than before the pandemic. While many Australians are opting to use physical touch less than before the pandemic, showing kindness in other ways is still important to the fabric of Australian society. Despite a decline in hugging, shaking hands and high fiving, there are still other ways Australians believe people can show kindness to others, including asking 'are you ok?'(67%), helping people when we see a need (64%) and simply saying 'hi' to people when they see them (62%).

Health Impacts on Children from Not Going Outside

Quarantine and other social restrictions have meant that children were not allowed to play in outdoor areas and explore unstructured play, switching from a 'play-outside mode' to a highly restrictive 'play-indoor mode', which unfortunately increased the easy option of time spent gazing uneffortlessly at a TV screen or mobile. This inevitably produced a negative correlation between the increasing amount of screen use and delayed language development in younger children in a meta-analysis review (Madigan et al., 2020). Outside play exposure is known to reduce stress during early childhood in comparison to the those that did not have much access to similar outside stimuli (Wells & Evans, 2003). Children highly exposed to nature also present great health and physical development (development and refinement of locomotor skills, for example), improved self-control (reduces inappropriate in-class behaviours), better communication and social development (more complex language), besides benefits to cognitive development (multisensorial stimuli that raise curiosity and creativity) according to Kemple et al. (2016). Isolation mandates prevent all this, impeding essential elements of childhood development.

Sunlight exposures have also positive effects on human health through vitamin D synthesis, which is involved in several physiological functions. However, insufficient sunlight exposure along with a low status of vitamin D can be responsible for health issues and neuropsychiatric disturbances such as cardiovascular diseases, metabolic syndrome, hypertension, multiple sclerosis, asthma, type 1 diabetes, autism, Alzheimer's disease, schizophrenia and depression (Alfredsson et al., 2020). This list of potential health deficits again points to the crucial importance of appropriate external sunlight exposure even during lockdowns, particularly for childhood.

Effects of Social Media

The relationship between loneliness and social media as complex and depends on the individual and their life circumstances. Users of social media experiencing loneliness have reported increased use of social media to communicate with family and friends. Others argued that online socialising increased their levels of loneliness at switch off as these relationships are generally fragile and shallow (Boursier et al., 2020). The number of online friends appears less important than the quality and strength of the relationships. Numerous studies reveal that the pandemic has encouraged increased use of online communication tools, such as Zoom and Skype since face to face in person contact was significantly reduced by mandates or personal choice (e.g. Murayama et al. (2020). However, older people are generally less familiar with the internet, thus increasing their social isolation, with younger generations generally more adept in the uses of social media. This indicates that the pandemic may have widened the age disparity in social isolation. Social media use may also explain why social isolation during the pandemic was also associated with greater fear and threat from Covid (Scopelliti et al., 2021). The socially isolated were limited largely to deriving information and beliefs from social media offerings, the content of which tended to emphasise the worst aspects of the pandemic in an echo chamber engendering fear (more detail in Chap. 3 on fake news, conspiracy theory, etc.).

The Abandoned Neighbourhood: Experiencing the Bizarre

Covid with its lockdowns and isolation altered the familiar world to become unfamiliar and made outside different and strange to those who ventured out for allowable reasons like a bit of exercise or necessary shopping. This added for some an additional layer of anxiety and depression. Even without venturing beyond the front door, views of neighbourhood roads, streets, pavements, through house windows, abandoned by people, buses and cars, evoked unpleasant sensations that things were not right as places taken for granted suddenly morphed into new forms lacking the hustle and bustle of people going about their daily business. It was like viewing an apocalyptic film set (Bird & Green, 2021). Sensory deprivation of the visual and auditory derived from this uncanny condition of a formerly vibrant stimulating well-known neighbourhood allied with social isolation also led to some hearing voices and seeing visions to bring back the familiar. This occurs as the environment ceases to produce enough sensory input to the brain, which then commences to generate its own information from past experiences.

In creating these uncanny experiences, mental distress arose in many isolated and lonely persons due to the mismatch between current expectations of a place and past experiences of it. As well as coping with isolation and loneliness the new environment undermined confidence in the familiar and challenged prevailing assumptions that we are not in control of our environments as we had initially thought and it may never be the same.

Groups and Identity: Not Everyone Panics in a Pandemic

Disaster and 'Panic'

There is a common belief in popular culture that, when in peril, people panic, especially when in crowds, acting blindly and excessively out of self-preservation, potentially endangering the survival of all. This idea has been used to explain responses to the current outbreak, in relation to the notion of 'panic buying' and the zero-sum game. However while a few do act selfishly, cooperation and orderly, norm-governed behaviour is more common across a range of emergencies and disasters (Drury & Alfadi, 2019). There is already evidence that mutual aid groups among the public have become widespread in response to Covid. Indeed, in fires, earthquakes and floods, people are more likely to survive by reacting and working together than from not linking individual efforts together when responding to signs of danger.

The doomsday scenario of complete breakdown of social values and connectedness, involves the myth that **all people** are psychologically vulnerable, and in a crisis, crack. The myth suggests that in desperate and blind attempts at individual self-preservation, people turn a crisis into a tragedy with group values and support rendered asunder. But in reality, study of emergencies and disasters reveals that this is not what generally happens. The Elaborated Social Identity Model (ESIM) of crowd behaviour developed by Reicher et al. (1995) suggests that a common identity emerges among people as a result of a shared fate in the face of illegitimate attacks from an outgroup. This common identity can result in people helping and supporting each other, whether known or strangers (Quarantelli, 2001). Coronavirus functions in a similar way, positioning groups of people as being under attack from a common and indiscriminate enemy. If we look a little closer at the impacts of recent disasters throughout history people often respond in a calm orderly manner, they look after each other and try to find safety together whether it's crowd behaviour in emergency evacuations as in the recent floods in Australia March 2022, or the response of New Yorkers during and after the September 11th attacks, or embracing nationalism in the Ukraine in 2022.

There are repeated stories of altruism and cooperation, even when people themselves are at great risk. Psychological research suggests that being in an emergency can create a common identity among those affected. Emergencies appear to at least temporarily dissolve social division as the development of a common identity facilitates a degree of cooperative altruism even when among strangers in life-threatening situations. In a crisis the people are not the problem. To the extent that they come together under a shared identity, people develop a collective resilience which is the most precious of resources for confronting a challenge. Accordingly, the relationship between the Government and the public in a crisis (and beyond) needs to shift from paternalism to partnership. Rather than seeking to shepherd us, Government and its agencies should seek to scaffold the collective self-organisation of the public. In a crisis, such as the Covid pandemic, people faced with the same threat, share the same experience. This offers a sense of common fate which in turn is an important precursor of shared identity, the massive psychological move from thinking of ourselves in terms of '**I**' to thinking about '**we**'. When that occurs, each person facilitates reciprocal empathy and perspectives allowing the concerns of other individuals to become shared, with shared identity the immediate precursor of mutual support, coordination and positive direction of joint effort (Drury & Alfadhli, 2019). The whole becomes greater than the sum of the parts as a fertile conglomerate of motivation, helpfulness and performance.

This is where many people feel the anti-vaxxers have lost the plot. Perhaps it is your life to do whatever you want, but you are also now responsible for my life. It's not about '**you**' it's about '**we**'. Everyone needs to get their head around the '**we**' concept. It's about us all, and the shout of freedom cannot be an irresponsible demand to do what you want and impose your freedom actions on the freedom of others; freedom is essentially freedom of choice among options which all incur consequences, some minimal, others drastic, which we all must consider wisely as we choose.

In fact, the concept of 'panic' is becoming less used by researchers because it neither describes nor explains what people usually do in disasters (Quarantelli, 2001). Instead, the focus has shifted to factors that explain why people cooperate rather than compete in response to a crisis. One of these factors is an emerging sense of shared identity and concern for others, which arises from the shared experience of being in a disaster (Drury & Alfadhli 2019). This feeling can be harnessed by addressing the public in collective terms and by urging '**us**' to act for the common good.

Conversely, the sense of shared identity can be undermined by representing others as competitors. This can happen with images of empty shelves and stories of panic buying, which suggest that others are only looking out for themselves, thus prompting a desire for doing the same. Stocking up on supplies is adaptive in preparation for potential self-isolation. The use of the notion of panic can be actively harmful. News and media stories plus public announcements from senior medical professionals that employ the language of panic become self-validating as they create that phenomenon in their mistaken attempt to encourage each individual to keep safe. Fostering individualism and competitiveness undermines the sense of collective purpose which facilitates people supporting one another during an emergency. Appeals by politicians for people to 'come together' in emergencies need to be backed up with real practical attempts to engender and maintain such collective unity.

Proximity to Ingroup and Personal Space

The differences between the meaning and application of the concepts '*physical distancing*' and '*social distancing*' were explained in Chap. 1. Physical distancing behaviours we have all been required to adopt during the pandemic are often difficult to maintain because it is antithetical to a basic self-process, the comfort we feel with proximity to members of our ingroup, those who hold the same or similar beliefs, values and interests whom we can define as '*us*' or '*we*', and hence move to get closer. Experimental evidence for this is provided by the 'two chairs' study (Novelli et al., 2010), in which people chose to sit more closely to strangers but members of the same hypothetical ingroup than to those in an equivalent outgroup. These results have been replicated in numerous experiments, and complemented by field studies also showing that people try to get physically closer to fellow ingroup members, even if they are strangers.

While we often want to preserve '*personal space*', a little bubble around us, while studying in a library or sitting in a bus, on other occasions we deliberately seek to share common identity-space. As well as our personal identities, we have multiple social (or group) subidentities, the different '*we's*' shared with others and which become salient to us in different contexts such as religious worship, sporting/leisure activities, political allegiances, school/ playgroup entities. This explains why people often gravitate to the most crowded parts of crowd events like football matches, report a better 'atmosphere' in those locations, and can feel safer as others will come to their aid if needed, because '*they*' are '*us*'. In some groups, the norms for behaviour may encourage group members to touch those around them (when football fans hug strangers when their team scores a goal) or share personal items (when those at a music festival may share bottles of beer). The issue with Covid is how do we create and encourage new group norms like vaccination or mask wearing in order to make health-protective behaviours part and parcel of what it means to be one of the group and, conversely, to make risky behaviours like vaccination refusal or disobeying lockdown rules at odds with being a good group member?

The major way is to invoke higher-order group values (e.g. '*we look after each other'; or the Aboriginal version, 'get a jab for the mob*') in order to promote the new norms, that of shared identity. Messaging must allow expression of these norms within the group to demonstrate commitment to (and hence acceptance in) the group and its shared values (Chapter "Following Doctors' Orders: Persuasive Communication Delivery"). People should distance for their own good, for the greater good, for our public health, for keeping those we care about safe, to support our health and care workers, as a way of showing solidarity and being good citizens In Covid lockdown and other social distancing measures, our intimate home spaces have become retreats for personal protection. Daily routines have dissolved into short essential expeditions outside to garner supplies. Fleeting and socially distanced acts of kindness, such as a wave during a walk, may seem insignificant, but can reconnect people during a time of uncertainty, fear and dislocation. Even when largely confined to our houses, it is possible to reach out to others through community-focussed actions such as doorway applause for essential workers, musical recitals from balconies, placing soft toys in street-facing windows, issuing street newsletters, and writing inspiring chalk messages on the pavement. The numerous and creative ways we communicate messages of care, solidarity and a sense of community are a timely reminder that we are not alone and that the challenges of Covid require both personal and collective actions.

Cooperation: Aligning Individual and Community Interests

In imposing lockdowns, individuals began to realise just how much they had been part of their local and larger society, an aspect often undervalued in psychological wellbeing. It seems part of human nature for people to identify themselves with those who suffer such as neighbours, friends, relatives who are living through stressful events and emergencies. For instance, providing solidarity and humanitarian activities, food and medicine delivery for people who are unable to go to the supermarket. During isolation, many have used brief contacts with the simple question by phoning, emailing or even shouting through the letter box '*how are you*' provides an anchor for the others to express fears and emotions. In many ways Covid has affected the way people live interpersonal relationships. The lockdown was characterised as a different organisation of daily life, with an incrementation of time at home and a reduction of distance through digital devices.

The Covid pandemic as a turning point for understanding the importance of community making us look beyond self and family interest. Across the world, locked in their homes, people didn't wait for formal public services to look after their neighbours. Instead there has been the remarkable growth of informal community self-help, from neighbours checking on each other, to street level WhatsApp groups, to the formation of over 4000 mutual aid groups involving over three million people in the UK alone. In the UK, the pandemic brought people together with the mass mobilisation of community solidarity behaviours. The Brexit self-categorisations of division were quickly displaced as groups realised that shared, collective behaviour was the sole way to face a common enemy with groups and communities helping and supporting each other in ways that typically emerges from disasters such as warfare.

Such informal mutual aid groups have created local systems to ensure all neighbours, especially the aged, handicapped and single mother had access to food, medicine, social connection, emotional support. There are many tales of neighbours doing the shopping, taking prescriptions to the chemists, taking a non-car owner to a health checkup, etc. For example, Walker (April 2020) reports in the British Psychological Society Psychologist on a mutual aid group in East Worthing, Sussex with nearly 80 volunteers who have delivered essential food and medication to almost 100 local families in under two weeks mid 2020. This group set up a designated phone line, organised a daily rota and taken referrals to help people from pharmacies, GP surgeries and the local hospital, delivered school food packages to local pupil families. A temporary local foodbank made its target in less than a day, and a call by the local hospital for donations of folding beds for staff to sleep in at the local hospital received 250 emailed offers. This group have provided well organised and essential community support and care at breakneck speed from a standing start and is an example of what community spirit has done in many places. Such groups are an organisational expression of the shared identity that emerges in a crisis, and shared identity is at the root of mutual support among the public (Maki et al., 2019). The conundrum we call human nature readily rises to the occasion of a crisis and as readily slacks off when the living is easy.

Many of us have also discovered which workers really matter. It is the doctors, nurses and ancillary staff throughout the health service, child and aged care staff etc. It is the suppliers of energy, the food producers and distributors, waste and recycling, the funeral attendants, aged care workers, the postal workers and delivery drivers, who continue to go out on the streets daily to keep essential services going. Armies of people from organisations of all descriptions are pioneering new distributed ways of working. Centre and centre right governments have, in the face of Covid, made a left turn to policies and values that emphasise concern for the people. In the face of the threat to the economic and social wellbeing of their population from Covid, and the lockdowns, many governments including Australia, Japan and UK, seriously concerned by the anticipated suffering of their people, delivered the funds for to support the people. Wages for the majority of working and self-employed people were protected to some extent, welfare benefits were increased, all at the expense of increasing government debt. Suddenly, people mattered more than numbers. Community is at the heart of the motivation of most countries to enable '*we*' to trump '*I*'.

Social Connection Not Social Isolation

In the absence of a vaccine, one of the most vital strategies, now seen as not very effective, for slowing the pandemic is social distancing. However, distancing clashes with the deep-seated human instinct to connect with others. Even the term '*social distancing*' might imply that one needs to cut off meaningful interactions. As indicated in Chap. 1, the accurate term should be '*physical distancing*', to help highlight the fact that it is physical distance not social connection that is implied. Social connection is possible even when people are infected and physically separated. Social connection helps people regulate emotions, cope with stress and remain resilient during difficult times (Jetten & Peters, 2019). By contrast, loneliness and social isolation worsen the burden of stress and as noted above often produce deleterious effects on mental, cardiovascular and immune health (Hawkley et al., 2010). Older adults, who are at the greatest risk of severe symptoms from Covid, are also highly susceptible to the effects of isolation (Luo et al., 2012). Distancing threatens to aggravate feelings of loneliness and could produce negative long-term health consequences. As online interactions, both receiving and giving support, can also foster a sense of connection and bolster psychological well-being, special attention should be placed on helping people who are less familiar with these technologies to learn how to take advantage of digital connections to make human connections. However, passive use of social media may not contribute to one's sense of social connection. Instead, technologies that are informationally rich, and one on one at the same time, appear better suited to generating empathy and connection (Waytz & Gray, 2018).

Identity Leadership

Experimental studies clarify what leaders can do to promote trust leading to cooperation. A priority for leaders is to create a sense of shared social identity among their followers (Reicher et al., 2005). A large body of research suggests that people tend to prefer leaders who cultivate a sense that '*we are all in this together*' (Haslam et al., 2020). In part, such leadership gives people a sense of collective self-efficacy and hope. More importantly, though, it provides a psychological platform for group members to coordinate efforts to tackle stressors. Without leadership, there is a risk that people will avoid acts of citizenship and instead embrace a reverse philosophy of '*everyone for themselves*' (Haslam et al., 2020).

Leader behaviours that imply the leader is not prepared to share the burdens of followers can be corrosive to their ability to shape followers' behaviour. For instance, leaders who threaten people with sanctions as a way to deter undesired behaviour may make people feel distrust and paradoxically reduce their willingness to do as they are told. Leaders and authorities who treat people with respect, and who communicate that they trust people to do as they are told, tend to be more successful in eliciting cooperation (Mooijman et al., 2017). Building a strong sense of shared social identity can help coordinate efforts to manage threats and foster in-group commitment and adherence to norms. Modelling prosocial and selfless acts prompt observers to dispense kindness and generosity themselves. In this way, leaders can function as role models and motivate people to put their own values into action. Having respected politicians, celebrities and community leaders' model exemplary behaviours facilitates the promotion of prosocial behaviour and cooperation in crises like a pandemic.

Excessive efforts to foster a sense of national unity by promoting the image of the nation as handling the situation exceptionally well can backfire, especially if there is no objective basis for this such as an inflated belief in national greatness (i.e. '*collective narcissism*' de Zavala, et al., 2009). For instance, it emphasises a greater focus on defending the image of the country than on caring for its citizens (Cichocka & Cislak, 2020) as well as using the Freudian ego defence mechanism of projection perceiving out-groups(.g. other nations) as a threat and blaming them for in-group misfortunes (Cichocka et al., 2016). To increase people's willingness to take a pandemic seriously and engage with other nations to defeat it, citizens and leaders may need to accept that their country is at risk, and find ways to share resources and expertise across national boundaries. This is a theme echoed by the UN who are concerned that by not assisting less wealthy countries to ensure high vaccination rates and use high grade medical protections the virus will continue to circulate globally. It is not the individual country that is '*in it all together*' but ring fencing the whole world so that '*we*' the world's population are '*in it all together*'.

Social Inequality Between Groups

Inequalities in access to resources affect not only who is at greatest risk of infection, developing symptoms or succumbing to the disease, but also who is able to adopt recommendations to slow the spread of the disease. The homeless cannot shelter in a virus safe place, families in housing with limited water supply cannot wash their hands frequently, people who are detained by a state (e.g. in prisons, immigrant detention centres or refugee camps) may lack space to implement physical distancing, people without health insurance may delay or avoid seeking testing or treatment, people who rely on public transportation cannot avoid large crowds, and low-wage workers are often in occupations (e.g. service, retail, cleaning) where remote work is impossible and employers do not offer paid sick leave. Economic disadvantage is also associated with the pre-existing conditions associated with higher morbidity rates once infected, such as compromised immune systems, diabetes, heart disease and chronic lung diseases like asthma and chronic obstructive pulmonary disease. The economically disadvantaged will be most likely to be exposed to the hazard, most susceptible to harm from it and most likely to experience negative outcomes from it.

Issues of economic disadvantage intersect with issues of race and ethnicity. Members of minority communities (such as Aborigines in Australia, Latinos and American Indians/Alaska Natives in the US) are disproportionately found among the homeless, the detained, the workers in high public contact but low-benefit occupations, and those with prior health conditions that make them more vulnerable. Because their social networks tend to be ethnically grouped, members of minority communities who contract the disease may become vectors of transmission to others in their ethnic communities.

Another problem is that social position and cultural issues are also associated with levels of trust in social institutions, including the healthcare system. Racial and ethnic minority communities, in most parts of the world, have both historical and contemporary experiences of discrimination, leading to distrust

(Demaris et al., 1994). Members of these communities tend to be wary about the public health information they receive, less willing to adopt recommended safety measures and potentially more susceptible to '*fake news*'. This was a problem in Australia among some Aborigine communities, and suggests the need for more targeted public health information and for partnerships between public health authorities and trusted organisations that are internal to these communities.

We Need Friendship to Overcome the Stresses of Isolation

Given the restriction of quarantine and lockdowns that have been inflicted on many by governments worldwide and even self-imposed isolation by a substantial minority of particularly older people and single people who are too scared to venture out due to the unwise advice from leading politicians and medical professionals '*not to go out unless necessary*', it is probably not surprising that friendships have dissipated and loneliness is at an all-time high. But making new friends and, developing and maintaining them can be quite difficult. This is serious, because humans as social animals need friends. Loneliness can speedily and insidiously creep up around you. The research evidence reviewed earlier suggests chronic loneliness can be lethal, not only in mental distress but also in health status, the equivalent impact of 15 cigarettes a day on mortality rates. Loneliness itself has become an epidemic as Covid made it much harder to see friends and relatives with some feeling and experiencing cell like conditions, locked metaphorically, and some in reality, into their own homes. Instead of embracing new-found post-Covid freedom, the thought of re-immersing ourselves in crowded social settings, re-establishing and re-invigorating old friendships that have been left dormant during Covid, has become a source of anxiety.

Approaching some sort of new Covid-normal, it's worth taking stock of your friendships and assess whether you feel your social life is fine, or could use a little help. In the words of the Neighbours TV soapie, '*Everybody needs good neighbours*!' When researchers interviewed adults about making friends in a recent study, the most important challenge cited was a lack of trust. People found it harder to put their trust in someone new and fully invest in them as a friend compared to when they were younger. Perhaps that's why many people try to keep their circle of old friends as long as possible, given the trust they may have built up over many years. Women were more likely than men to say they didn't make new friends easily because they struggled to trust others.

Government Initiatives

Awareness of loneliness and social isolation as significant public health and wellbeing issues has increased in recent years, along with the development of targeted government and community support programmes for affected

Australians that have provided varying degrees of funding and support to local councils and community organisations for programmes to address the social isolation and loneliness of Australians. For example, the Australian Government funds a national Community Visitors Scheme, which supports local organisations to recruit volunteers who provide regular visits to Australians in receipt of Commonwealth-subsidised aged care services. The Seniors Connected Programme encompasses two activity streams: existing phone support service delivered by Friends for Good (FriendLine); and Village Hub projects across Australia, which bring older Australians together to support good mental and physical health. Although social isolation and loneliness are now well-recognised public health concerns, there is little research into what works to resolve them (Smith & Lim, 2020).

Some Things You Can Do if You Feel Lonely

- Understand that your feelings are normal and while they feel uncomfortable, they do not mean you are a 'lesser' person. All of us feel lonely at some point, and success is about managing loneliness effectively as we progress through our lives. Don't accept loneliness as inevitable. And while you might think everyone else is having a great social life, this is not so as loneliness is quite widespread.
- Learn to trust. As adults, we have greater self-awareness than children. While often a positive, it also means we're more aware of the risks of being evaluated by others, of being rejected, and of being hurt. If we've had previous rejections as friends or suffered a breach of trust, we may find it harder to be trusting of others in the future. To trust a new friend means opening ourselves up and being vulnerable, just as we do in closer relationships.
- Take small steps. You don't always have to make lots of close friends to feel less lonely. Build up over time.
- Connect with in your current network as this will probably be less threatening and consider how you can improve the quality of those relationships turning an acquaintance into a friend. When you do get to properly spend time with a friend or acquaintance, make the most of it. Avoid distractions, keep Instagram for the couch at home, and 'be present' with your new friend.
- Connect out as there are many others out there who feel lonely or who are looking to establish new connections—you're not alone. Take up an opportunity to connect in your community, where people may come together based on a shared interest.
- Willing to give time. It shouldn't surprise us that closer friendships take longer to build than casual acquaintances. US researchers have tried to quantify this, estimating it takes roughly 50 h of shared contact to move from acquaintances to casual friends. To be a close friend? More than 200 h. To make it start ten minutes a day may be all you need. Send a text, forward a meme, add to the group chat or give someone a quick

call. A coffee, cake and catch up session, enjoying an occasional event like a concert or sporting event, shopping spree, and even joking around can be just as important. Don't get caught up on how much effort, energy and time goes into building friendships.
- Volunteering. While having paid work and caring for others are important safeguards against loneliness, so is engaging in volunteer work and maintaining active memberships of sporting or community organisations also associated with reduced social isolation (Flood, 2005). During the pandemic, the proportion of adult Australians doing voluntary work in the previous 12 months decreased from 36% in late 2019 to 24% in April 2021. Those who stopped volunteering felt lonely more of the time in the previous four weeks than those who continued volunteering. In April 2020, 54% of Australians who stopped volunteering due to Covid and did not start volunteering again reported that they were lonely at least some of the time, which decreased to just over 40% in April 2021 (Biddle & Gray, 2021b).
- Get a pet for companionship and developing routine in your life. Pet ownership also facilitates social contact, for example, dog walking leads to contact with other dog walkers and act as a trigger for conversations to counter social isolation (Wood et al., 2015).

If You Know Someone Who Is Lonely

- Look around. It's not a rare occurrence with one in four Australians report feeling lonely at any given time. So, chances are high that there are people who are lonely in your network.
- Be present. Even when not physically together it is critical to building relationships and shown by checking in with the other by social media or a short phone call.
- Be open to opportunities to connect, like requests for conversation, or moments of interaction that don't seem important to you; they are likely to be important to the person reaching out to you. These interactions provide moments of comfort and relief to a lonely person.
- Be a non-judgmental listener. If someone reaches out to you, it is important to acknowledge how they feel and not to discount their experience. Don't try to impose your suggestions, but ask them what they think could work for them instead. Listening is essential towards helping someone who is experiencing loneliness.

Arts Therapy to Dissipate the Isolation Blues

Many psychologists and social workers have employed the 'Arts' to cultivate wellbeing and mental health, counter isolation and loneliness; it is particularly relevant under Covid restrictions. The 'Arts' can be interpreted here quite widely. It does include painting, but also a great range of activities from quilting, basket weaving, learning a musical instrument to play in a band, joining an informal choir, square dancing and pottery (and many more) but whatever the activity, it involves finding connection and meaning through creative endeavours. In full lockdown these can be done in isolation and shared through the internet like creating a group quilt with squares done by different people, or a small group of singers using Zoom, virtual museum tours, to online resources for home-based arts activities. The 'Arts' have been used to help prevent the development of depression, withdrawal and attention deficits in children dealing with isolation, DV and poverty, and to help grieving families come to terms with death.

Fancourt and Finn (2020) have assembled a wealth of evidence that underscores the positive impact that such activities can have on health, individual and collective wellbeing, and the development of a richer, meaningful life. They can improve our sense of self-worth, self-confidence, self-esteem and positive emotional expression/regulation, and reduce incidences/severity of depression, anxiety, stress, loneliness and suicidal ideation, enhancing wellbeing across a range of dimensions. 'Arts' in general thus be considered to be a social determinant of health, as research from youth music theatre, art therapy and beyond shows. Engagement in any of the 'Arts' has been found to promote social cohesion and conflict resolution through developing cognitive, emotional and social skills for constructive engagement with trauma, and by supporting empathy, trust, social engagement, collaboration and transformative learning.

This massive accumulation of benefits noted by Fancourt and Finn (2020) have come to the fore during the pandemic, with myriad arts and culture interventions that speak to wide-ranging aims, including helping children and adults respond adaptively to trauma, enhancing community cohesion and supporting children's home school education. It also points to the fact that 'Arts' will have an important role to play in supporting people to adjust to a 'new normal' once this crisis has passed, reducing isolation, strengthening social relationships and forging a sense of belonging. This is particularly apt given the increased isolation, separation, uncertainty and fragmentation, and decreased sense of self-efficacy, that characterised experiences during the pandemic.

While these benefits are well known, it raises serious ethical and equity questions. Are these interventions really accessible to all? Do they reach those who are marginalised and thus most at risk from the pandemic and its effects? The problem is that 'Art's' engagement in the past has been concentrated within a small sector of the population, regarded as an elite pursuit, leading to a participation gap which needs to be crossed to ensure that 'Arts' provision is available as a form of therapy to nourish all with trauma and disruption from the pandemic from a wide spectrum of different backgrounds. People of all abilities, incomes and educational levels are starting to engage with and appreciate the 'Arts', from rock painting, legalised graffiti sites, to comic drawing, to amateur dramatics, and local community talent music/voice shows; they might not be appreciated by arts experts, but they are greatly valued by those who produced them (https://tinyurl.com/IgniteHKP). There are two key issues behind the participation gap that currently impedes 'Arts' as a psychotherapeutic process. The first is a failure to acknowledge the widespread engagement among marginalised and deprived communities with undervalued, low status arts and crafts. The second is that social inequalities like funding prevent many people from accessing the Arts.

It is important, however, that the 'Arts' aren't seen as a mere 'sticking plaster' for trauma and inequality. Unfortunately the 'Arts' it can also be disruptive, troubling and unsettling in encouraging self-expression, and externalising noisy thoughts, e.g. children's 'death' concerns over Covid, while adults may have wondered what emotions Munch expunged in his painting The Scream, in which the agonised face in the painting has become one of the most iconic images of art, seen as symbolising the anxiety of the human condition. Art helps us connect with personal, subjective emotions, and through such a process, it enables us to discover our own interior landscape, helping to formulate the implications of self and daring to make 'real', but for some could be devastating.

Some social enterprises like the Element Project that produces creative arts projects with young people leaving the care system, and at-risk school students in the UK was based on group delivery in physical spaces. Under lockdown, they adapted and set up daily creative challenges, to be shared within a group of peers and co-creators with the creative drop-in turned into a weekly online session with games and collective artmaking. The process of making art has helped participants cope with what is going on both externally and internally.

Aged Care Isolation

As Omicron moved in, many Western countries including Australia have faced and are still facing a predictable tragedy in aged care. While the rest of the populations have been selfishly focussed on complaining about cancelled holidays, hours in testing queues, and days spent isolating at home or sick in bed, what's happening to the elderly in aged care has partially flown under the radar.

Over the last two years, there have been tens of thousands of elderly people sitting alone in their bedrooms in nursing homes around the developed world, some with Covid, some not tested or vaccinated sufficiently, while others are stuck there because of management's well-founded fears and strict imposition of visiting rules. Many have spent long months including for some the Christmas and New Year period isolated from family and friends for two consecutive years. This caused considerable stress through isolation and loneliness and added stress to their families navigating the external Covid world and many deaths of the elderly.

References

Australian Bureau of Statistics (ABS). (2016). 2071.0 *Census of Population and Housing: Reflecting Australia*. Retrieved 26 June 21 from https://www.abs.gov.au/ausstats/abs@.nsf/Lookup/2071.0main+features22016

Australian Bureau of Statistics (ABS). (2020). *Household Impacts of COVID-19 Survey*–October 2020 release. Retrieved 26 June 2021 from https://www.abs.gov.au/statistics/people/people-and-communities/household-impacts-covid-19-survey/latest-release.

Australian National University. Centre for Social Research & Methods. (2022). *COVID-19 Impact Monitoring Survey*. Retrieved 18 February 2022 from https://csrm.cass.anu.edu.au/research/publications/covid-19

Australian Psychological Society. (2018). *Australian loneliness report: A survey exploring the loneliness levels of Australians and the impact on their health and wellbeing*. Melbourne: APS. Retrieved 21 March 2021 from https://psychweek.org.au/wp/wp-content/uploads/2018/11/Psychology-Week-2018-Australian-Loneliness-Report.pdf

Alfredsson, L., Armstrong, B. K., Butterfield, D. A., et al. (2020). Insufficient sun exposure has become a real public health problem. *International Journal of Environmental Research and Public Health, 17*, 5014. https://doi.org/10.3390/ijerph17145014

Awad, E., et al. (2018). The moral machine experiment. *Nature, 563*, 59–64. https://doi.org/10.1038/s41586-018-0637-6

Benke, C., Autenrieth, L. K., Asselmann, E., & Pané-Farré, C. A. (2020). Lockdown, quarantine measures, and social distancing: Associations with depression, anxiety and distress at the beginning of the COVID-19 pandemic among adults from Germany. *Psychiatry Research, 293*, 113462. https://doi.org/10.1016/j.psychres.2020.113462

Biddle, N., Edwards, B., Gray, M., & Sollis, K. (2020a). PDF Tracking outcomes during the COVID-19 pandemic (August 2020a)—divergence within Australia. Australian National University: ANU Centre for Social Research and Methods. Retrieved 27 November 2021 from http://content.cass.anu.edu.au/https://doi.org/10.26193/ZFGFNE

Biddle, N., Edwards, B., Gray, M., & Sollis, K. (2020b). Tracking outcomes during the COVID-19 pandemic (Novmber 2020b)—counting the costs of the COVID-recession. Australian National University: ANU Centre for Social Research and Methods. Retrieved 27 November 2021 from https://csrm.cass.anu.edu.au/sites/default/files/docs/2020b/12/Tracking_wellbeing_outcomes_during_the_COVID-19_pandemic_November_2020b.pdf

Biddle, N., & Gray, M. (2021a). PDF Tracking outcomes during the COVID-19 pandemic (January 2021a)—cautious optimism. Australian National University: ANU Centre for Social Research and Methods. Retrieved 27 November 2021a from https://csrm.cass.anu.edu.au/sites/default/files/docs/2021a/5/Tracking_wellbeing_outcomes_during_the_COVID-19_pandemic_January_2021a.pdf

Biddle, N., & Gray, M. (2021b). Tracking wellbeing outcomes during the COVID-19 pandemic (August 2021): Lockdown blues. Australian National University: ANU Centre for Social Research and Methods. Retrieved 27 November 2021b from https://csrm.cass.anu.edu.au/research/publications/tracking-wellbeing-outcomes-during-covid-19-pandemic-august-2021-lockdown

Bird, J. and Green, D. (2021). Covid spaces and places: The uncanny, the weird, and the eerie. *Entanglements, 4*(2), 32–49. Retrieved 14 March 2022 from https://entanglementsjournal.org/covid-spaces-and-places/

Boursier, V., Gioia, F., Musetti, A., & Schimmenti, A. (2020). Facing loneliness and anxiety during the COVID-19 isolation: the role of excessive social media use in a sample of Italian adults. *Frontiers in Psychiatry, 11*, 586222 https://doi.org/10.3389/fpsyt.2020.586222

Brooks, S. K., Webster, R. K., Smith, L. E., et al. (2020). The psychological impact of quarantine and how to reduce it: Rapid review of the evidence. *Lancet, 395*, 912–920. https://doi.org/10.1016/S0140-6736(20)30460-8

Bzdok, D., & Dunbar, R. I. M. (2020). The neurobiology of social distance. *Trends in Cognitive Sciences*. https://doi.org/10.1016/j.tics.2020.05.016

Cacioppo, J. T., Cacioppo, S., Capitanio, J. P., & Cole, S. W. (2015). The neuroendocrinology of social isolation. *Annual Review of Psychology, 66*, 733–767. https://doi.org/10.1146/annurev-psych-010814-015240

Cacioppo, J. T., & Cacioppo, S. (2018). Loneliness in the modern age: An evolutionary theory of loneliness (ETL). In *Advance in experimental social psychology*, pp. 127–197. https://doi.org/10.1016/BS.AESP.2018.03.003

Capraro, V., Jagfeld, G., Klein, R., et al. (2019). Increasing altruistic and cooperative behaviour with simple moral nudges. *Science and Reports, 9*, 11880. https://doi.org/10.1038/s41598-019-48094-4

Cichocka, A., Marchlewska, M., & Golec de Zavala, A. (2016). Does self-love or self-hate predict conspiracy beliefs? Narcissism, self-esteem, and the endorsement of conspiracy theories. *Social Psychological and Personality Science, 7*(2), 157–166. https://doi.org/10.1177/1948550615616170

Cichocka, A., & Cislak, A. (2020). Nationalism as collective narcissism. *Current Opinion in Behavioral Sciences, 34*, 69–74. https://doi.org/10.1016/j.cobeha.2019.12.013

Cole, S. W. (2014). Human Social Genomics. *PLoS 10*, e1004601

Demaris, A., Yang, R., et al. (1994). Race, alienation and interpersonal mistrust. *Sociological Spectrum, 14*(4), 327–349. https://doi.org/10.1080/02732173.1994.9982075

de Zavala, A. G., Cichocka, A., Eidelson, R., & Jayawickreme, N. (2009). Collective narcissism and its social consequences. *Journal of Personality and Social Psychology, 97*(6), 1074–1096. https://doi.org/10.1037/a0016904

Drury, J., & Alfadhli, K. (2019). *Social identity, emergencies and disasters*. In R. Williams, S. Bailey & B. Kamaldeep et al. (Eds), *Social scaffolding*. London: Royal College of Psychiatrists.

Duffy, B., & Allington, D. (2020). The accepting, the suffering and the resisting: the different reactions to life under lockdown. The Policy Institute, Kings College London. Retrieved 04 June 2020 from https://www.kcl.ac.uk/policy-institute/assets/Coronavirus-in-the-UK-cluster-analysis.pdf

Element Project. Retrieved 20 September 2021 from www.elementproject.org

Ellemers, N., & van den Bos, K. (2012). Morality in groups: The social regulatory functions of right and wrong. *Social and Personality Psychology Compass, 6*(12), 878–889. https://doi.org/10.1111/spc3.12001

Everett, J. A., Pizarro, D. A., & Crockett, M. J. (2016). Inference of trustworthiness from intuitive moral judgement. *Journal of Experimental Psychology: General, 145*, 772–787. https://doi.org/10.1037/xge0000165

Fancourt, D., & Finn, S. (2020). What is the evidence on the role of the arts in improving health and well-being? A scoping review. *Nordic Journal of Arts Culture and Health, 2*, 77–83. https://doi.org/10.18261/issn.2535-7913-2020-01-08

Flood, M. (2005). *Mapping loneliness in Australia.* The Australia Institute.

Folch, E., Hernandez, I., Barragan, M., & Franco-Paredes, C. (2003). *American Journal of the Medical Sciences, 326*, 66–72. https://doi.org/10.1097/00000441-200308000-00003

Gelfand, M., Raver, J. L., Nishii, L., et al. (2011). Differences between tight and loose cultures; a 33 nation study. *Science, 332*, 1100–1104. https://doi.org/10.1126/science.1197754

Gerst-Emerson, K., & Jayawardhana, J. (2015). Loneliness as a public health issue: The impact of loneliness on health care utilization among older adults. *American Journal of Public Health, 105*, 1013–1019. https://doi.org/10.2105/AJPH.2014.302427

Han, J., & Richardson, V. (2010). The relationship between depression and loneliness among homebound older persons: Does spirituality moderate this relationship? *Journal of Religion & Spirituality in Social Work: Social Thought., 29*(3), 218–236. https://doi.org/10.1080/15426432.2010.495610

Haslam, S. A., Reicher, S. D., & Platow, M. J. (2020). *The new psychology of leadership: Identity, influence, and Power* (2nd ed.). Psychology Press.

Hawkley, L., & Cacioppo, J. T. (2010). Loneliness matters. *Annals of Behavioral Medicine, 40*, 218–227. https://doi.org/10.1007/s12160-010-9210-8

Heffner, K. L., Waring, M. E., Roberts, M. B., Eaton, C. B., & Gramling, R. (2011). Social isolation, C-reactive protein, and coronary heart disease mortality among community-dwelling adults. *Social Science and Medicine, 72*, 1482–1488. https://doi.org/10.1016/j.socscimed.2011.03.016

Holt-Lunstad, J., Smith, T., Baker, M., et al. (2015). Loneliness and social isolation as risk factors for mortality: A meta-analytic review. *Perspectives on Psychological Science, 10*, 227–237. https://doi.org/10.1177/1745691614568352

Holt-Lunstad, J., & Smith, T. (2016). Loneliness and social isolation as risk factors for CVD: Implications for evidence-based patient care and scientific inquiry. *Heart, 102*, 987–989. https://doi.org/10.1136/heartjnl-2015-309242M

Hawker, R., & Romero-Ortuno, R. (2016). Social determinants of discharge outcomes in older people admitted to a geriatric medicine ward. *Journal of Frailty and Aging, 5*(2), 118–120. https://doi.org/10.14283/jfa.2016.89

Ikeda, T., Cable, N., Saito, M., et al. (2020). Association between social isolation and smoking in Japan and England. *Journal of Epidemiology, 31*(10), 523–529. https://doi.org/10.2188/jea.JE20200138

Jetten, J., & Peters, K. (2019). *The social psychology of inequality.* Springer.

Kabátek, J. (2020). Jobless and distressed: the disproportionate effects of COVID-19 on young Australians. University of Melbourne: Melbourne Institute—Applied Economic & Social Research. Retrieved 05 October 2021 from www.apo.org.au.

Kemple, K. M., Oh, J., Kenney, E., & Smith-Bonahue, T. (2016). The power of outdoor play and play in natural environments. *Childhood Education, 92*, 446–454. https://doi.org/10.1080/00094056.2016.1251793

Kitayama, S., Park, H., Sevincer, A. T., et al. (2009). A cultural task analysis of implicit independence comparing. N. America, W. Europe and E. Asia. *Journal of Personality and Social Psychology, 97*(2), 236–255. https://doi.org/10.1037/a0015999

Kraft-Todd, G., & Rand, D. (2016). Adaptive foundations of heroism: Social heuristics push advantageous everyday ethical behavior to heroic extremes. In S. T. Allison, G. Goethals & R. Kramer (Eds), *Handbook of heroism and heroic leadership*. London, UK: Routledge.

Kraus, B., & Kitayama, S. (2019). Interdependent self-construal predicts emotional suppression in Asian Americans. *Biological Psychology, 146*, 107733. https://doi.org/10.1016/j.biopsycho.2019.107733

Lim, M. H., Eres, R., & Vasan, S. (2020). Understanding loneliness in the twenty-first century: An update on correlates, risk factors, and potential solutions. *Social Psychiatry and Psychiatric Epidemiology, 55*, 793–810. https://doi.org/10.1007/s00127-020-01889-7

Lim, M., Qualter, P., Thurston, L., et al. (2022). A global longitudinal study examining social restrictions severity on loneliness, social anxiety, and depression. *Front. Psychiatry, 13*, 818030. https://doi.org/10.3389/fpsyt.2022.818030

López-Castro, T., Brandt, L., Anthonipillai, N. J., et al. (2021). Experiences, impacts and mental health functioning during a COVID-19 outbreak and lockdown: Data from a diverse New York City sample of college students. *PLoSone, 16*, e0249768.

Luo, Y., Hawkley, L. C., Waite, L. J., & Cacioppo, J. T. (2012). Loneliness, health, and mortality in old age: a national longitudinal study. *Social Science and Medicine, 74*(6), 907–914.https://doi.org/10.1016/j.socscimed.2011.11.028

Madigan, S., McArthur, B. A., Anhorn, C., et al. (2020). Associations between screen use and child language skills: A systematic review and meta-analysis. *JAMA Pediatrics, 174*(7), 665–675. https://doi.org/10.1001/jamapediatrics.2020.0327

Mainstreets Insights Report Retrieved 26 February 2022 from https://mainstreetinsights.com.au/wp-content/uploads/2022/01/MI_Relational-Wellbeing_Report_22Jan2022.pdf

Maki, A., Dwyer, P. C., Blazek, S., et al. (2019). Responding to natural disasters: Examining identity and prosociality in the context of a major earthquake. *British Journal of Social Psychology., 58*(1), 66–87. https://doi.org/10.1111/bjso.12281

Masi, C. M., Chen, H. Y., Hawkley, L. C., & Cacioppo, J. T. (2011). A meta-analysis of interventions to reduce loneliness. *Personality and Social Psychology Review, 15*, 219–266. https://doi.org/10.1177/1088868310377394

Meegan, D. (2010). Zero sum bias. *Frontiers in Psychology, 1*, 191. https://doi.org/10.3389/fpsyg.2010.00191

Miller, G. E., Chen, E., & Parker, K. J. (2011). Psychological stress in childhood and susceptibility to the chronic diseases of aging: Moving toward a model of behavioral and biological mechanisms. *Psychological Bulletin, 137*(6), 959–997. https://doi.org/10.1037/a0024768

Mooijman, M., Hoover, J., Lin, Y., Ji, H., & Dehghani, M. (2017). When protests turn violent: The roles of moralization and moral convergence. *Nature Human Behaviour, 2*(6), 389–396. https://doi.org/10.31234/osf.io/4bvyx

Müller, F., Röhr, S., Reininghaus, U., & Riedel-Heller, S. (2021). Social Isolation and Loneliness during COVID-19 Lockdown: Associations with depressive symptoms in the German old-age population. *International Journal of Environmental Research and Public Health, 18*(7), 3615. https://doi.org/10.3390/ijerph18073615

Murayama, H., Okubo, R., & Tabuchi, T. (2020). Increase in social isolation during the COVID-19 pandemic and its association with mental health: Findings from the JACSIS study. *International Journal of Environmental Research and Public Health, 18*, 8238. https://doi.org/10.3390/ijerph18168238

Nardone, G., & Speciani, L. (2019). Mangia, muoviti, ama. Firenze: Ponte alle grazie. National Institute of Allergy and Infectious Diseases. Researching Ebola in Africa. Retrieved 18 August 2020 from https://www.niaid.nih.gov/diseases-conditions/researching-ebola-africa

Novelli, D., Drury, J., & Reicher, S. (2010). Come together: Two studies concerning the impact of group relations on personal space. *British Journal of Social Psychology, 49*, 223–236. https://doi.org/10.1348/014466609X449377

Ntontis, E., Drury, J., & Amlôt, R., et al. (2020). Endurance or decline of emergent groups following a flood disaster. *International Journal of Disaster Risk Reduction, 45*. https://doi.org/10.1016/j.ijdrr.2020.101493

O'Reilly, C. A., & Hall, N. (2020). Grandiose narcissists and decision making: impulsive, overconfident, and skeptical of experts-but seldom in doubt. *Personality and Individual Difference* https://doi.org/10.1016/j.paid.2020.110280

Pietrabissa, G., & Simpson, S. (2020). Psychological consequences of social isolation during COVID-19 outbreak. *Frontiers in Psychology, 11*. https://doi.org/10.3389/fpsyg.2020.02201

Quarantelli, E. L. (2001). Sociology of Panic. In N. J. Smelser & P. B. Baltes (Eds.), *International encyclopedia of the social and behavioural sciences* (pp. 11020–11023). Pergamon Press.

Rand, D. G., & Nowak, M. A. (2013). Human cooperation. *Trends in Cognitive Sciences, 17*(8), 413–425. https://doi.org/10.1016/j.tics.2013.06.003

Reicher, S., Spears, R., & Postmes, T. (1995). A social identity model of deindividuation phenomena. *European Review of Social Psychology, 6*(1), 161–198. https://doi.org/10.1080/14792779443000049

Reicher, S., Haslam, S., & Hopkins, N. (2005). Social identity and the dynamics of leadership: Leaders and followers as collaborative agents in the transformation of social reality. *The Leadership Quarterly, 16*(4), 547–568. https://doi.org/10.1016/j.leaqua.2005.06.007

Reicher, S., & Stott, C. (2020). Policing the coronavirus outbreak: Processes and prospects or collective disorder. *Policing. A Journal of Policy and Practice, 14*(3), 569–573. https://doi.org/10.1111/bjso.12398

Relationships Australia. (2011). Issues and concerns for Australian relationships today: Relationships Indicators Survey 2011. Canberra: Relationships Australia. Retrieved 16 June 2021 from www.relationships.com.au

Relationships Australia. (2018). Is Australia experiencing an epidemic of loneliness? Findings from 16 waves of the Household Income and Labour Dynamics of Australia Survey. Canberra: Relationships Australia. Retrieved 16 June 2021 from www.relationships.com.au

Rogers, S. L., & Cruickshank, T. (2021). Change in mental health, physical health, and social relationships during highly restrictive lockdown in the COVID-19 pandemic: Evidence from Australia. *Peer J, 9*, e11767. https://doi.org/10.7717/peerj.11767

Scopelliti, M., Pacilli, M. G., & Aquino, A. (2021). TV News and COVID-19: Media influence on healthy behavior in public spaces. *International Journal of Environmental Research and Public Health, 18*(4), 1879. https://doi.org/10.3390/ijerph18041879

Sepúlveda-Loyola, W., Rodríguez-Sánchez, W., Pérez-Rodríguez, P., et al. (2020). Impact of social isolation due to COVID-19 on health in older people: Mental and physical effects and recommendations. *The Journal of Nutrition, Health & Aging, 24*, 938–947. https://doi.org/10.1007/s12603-020-1469-2

Smith, B., & Lim, M. (2020). How the COVID-19 pandemic is focusing attention on loneliness and social isolation. *Public Health Research & Practice, 30*, e3022008.

Tomasello, M. (2009). *Why we cooperate.* MIT Press.

Tomova, L., Wang, K., Thompson, T., et al. (2020). The need to connect: Acute social isolation causes neural craving responses similar to hunger. *Nature Neuroscience, 23*(12), 1597–1605. https://doi.org/10.1038/s41593-020-00742-z

Triandis, H. (1995). *Individualism and collectivism.* Westview Press.

Tull, M. T., Edmonds, K. A., Scamaldo, K. M., et al. (2020). Psychological outcomes associated with stay-at-home orders and the perceived impact of COVID-19 on daily life. *Psychiatry Research, 289*, 113098. https://doi.org/10.1016/j.psychres.2020.113098

Tyler, T. R., & Blader, S. L. (2003). The group engagement model. *Personality and Social Psychology Review, 7*(4), 349–361. https://doi.org/10.1207/S15327957PSPR0704_07

Walker, C. (2020, April 16). What is remarkable about what we've achieved is that it's unremarkable. *British Psychological Society. The Psychologist*, *33*, Summer 2020. Retrieved 19 October 2021 from https://thepsychologist.bps.org.uk/volume-33/summer-2020/what-remarkable-about-what-weve-achieved-is-unremarkable

Waytz, A., & Gray, K. (2018). Does online technology make us more or less sociable respect. *Psychological Science, 13*, 73–491. https://doi.org/10.1177/1745691617746509

Wells, N. M., & Evans, G. W. (2003). Nearby nature: A buffer of life stress among rural children. *Environment and Behavior, 35*, 311–330. https://doi.org/10.1177/0013916503035003001

Wood, L., Martin, K., Christian, H., et al. (2015). The pet factor—Companion animals as a conduit for getting to know people, friendship formation and social support. *PLoS ONE, 10*(4), e0122085. https://doi.org/10.1371/journal.pone.0122085

CHAPTER 7

Impacts on Students, Teachers and Education Delivery

Abstract This chapter investigates the impact of the pandemic on the delivery of education services which were disrupted at all levels of education globally with most institutions closed during quarantine, lockdown periods and contact isolation periods. Education systems were ill prepared for the experience. Teachers lacked competence in designing and utilising distance teaching methods and technology. Students at all levels also reported difficulties in using the technology, carrying out tasks to time and missed personal contact with teachers and peer group, all of which contributed to increased stress over and above the concerns about Covid. Student success and management of distance learning were also affected by personal psychological characteristics needed for success in the minimally supervised context such as self-regulated learning and intrinsic motivation. The digital divide in many countries led to educational disengagement. Distance education critically altered student, parent and teacher education experiences in adverse circumstances of the Covid restrictions particularly in terms of their wellbeing and imposed stress of coping with what to them was a novel learning mode. Domestic violence increased in the confined home context while special needs children and their parents were deprived of contact with professional support. Some parents actually enjoyed the experience of teaching their young children at home so that a significant trend to home schooling has occurred in developed countries.

Keyword Distance education · Teacher wellbeing · Digital divide · Student distress · Domestic violence · Home schooling

© The Author(s), under exclusive license to Springer Nature Singapore Pte Ltd. 2023
R. B. Burns, *The Human Impact of the COVID-19 Pandemic*,
https://doi.org/10.1007/978-981-99-1710-5_7

Implications of the Covid Pandemic for Education

There is no doubt that the pandemic has caused unprecedented disruption to all spheres of human life and consequently to all levels of education worldwide. From late March 2020, 191 countries instigated nationwide school closures affecting approximately 91.3% of students, around 1.5 billion students worldwide had their education disrupted by nationwide school closures, and were effectively confined to home (UNESCO, 2020a). Making the situation worse was that the closures and openings were repeated at irregular intervals as the contagion alternately increased and decreased only to increase again in response to new variants. Education plays a particularly significant role in children's and adolescents' health and wellbeing, and any interference with it, particularly a fluctuating one, interrupting developing routines, has a lasting impact on their lives as adults.

The effects of Covid on children, students and parents are not from the disease itself but from the consequent lockdowns and school closures of educational establishments disrupting education provision at all levels. The positive news is that Covid spares children from the more deleterious health issues that impact adults. The negative element is the mental health and educational effects on students of all ages. The Australian Institute of Health and Welfare Annual Report (2021) reported more children using crisis helplines than in the previous year with significant increases in hospital visits for self-harm and suicidal thoughts in NSW and Victoria. The anxiety and panic generated by earlier often misinformed hype about climate change provided a fertile bedding environment ready for mulching in the Covid threats nourishing amplified feelings of helplessness, hopelessness and disconnection. Due to the mild presentation of very contagious Omicron in children, there are likely to be 3 to 4 times as many cases than reported and a swathe of children will return with immunity especially as vaccination is ramped up for primary school children. High school adolescent vaccination in Western nations was generally over 80% by late 2022, and therefore, there is little reason to close schools down again.

The UK, EU, Australia and many other countries started returning students into school early 2022, adding masks, highly monitored sanitation like hand cleansing and frequent use of RATs as support strategies. The biggest problem initially was the absenteeism of some teachers and classroom aides due to their own infection or isolation requirements. Strategies involving considerable flexibility has seen education continue by combining classes, supervised class attendance using online teaching, as achieving academic work in school has positive psychological benefits by maintaining routines of schooling and facilitating social interaction with peers and teachers. Many countries adopted online methods to ensure continuity in learning; however, this raised concerns over how students would be educationally, emotionally and socially impacted by online learning and how to support vulnerable students from socially and financially disadvantaged backgrounds to continue their education. Adapting to Covid turned into a massive international educational and social experiment with little time to plan and execute that not only has caused loss of learning throughout lockdown but also possessed power to diminish educational opportunities in the long term as well as generating mental distress among the students and their families.

An Australian national survey by Orygen and Mission Australia, between April and August in 2021, when the Delta wave of Covid was in full swing, collected data from 20,000 young respondents during 2021's pandemic and lockdowns whose studies were disrupted, found lockdowns caused high psychological distress to 70% of students affected. Of more than 3000 young people who rated their mental health and wellbeing as poor, over three quarters (76.5%) indicated the pandemic had a negative impact on their mental health. Over the past two years, the report claims, young people have borne the brunt of the effects of Covid and have faced a multitude of unique challenges—socially, financially, their education and potential employment. Researchers noted this led to increased rates of stress, loneliness and a perceived loss of control over their lives for these groups of young people. Gender diverse young people were twice as likely to report adverse mental health effects than their peers.

Between 12 and 27 March 2020, a survey of educators from 89 countries identified the following priorities (Reimers & Schleicher, 2020):

- Ensuring continuity of academic learning for students,
- Supporting students who lack skills for independent study,
- Providing support for teachers (medical, mental health, professional development),
- Ensuring integrity of the assessment process,
- Defining new curricular priorities and
- Providing social services to students and their families.

Among the concerns that arose from the priorities above identified by this same international group of educators include (Reimers & Schleicher, 2020):

- Threats to the health and safety of students, families and educators,
- Disruptions to the continuity of learning,
- Limited access to social services and other forms of support for student and families,
- Negative effects on students' perception of the value of study,
- Drastic reductions in face-to-face teaching and instruction time,
- Teachers' preparedness and skill sets to support digital learning,
- When and how to reopen schools.

These priorities and concerns present a gargantuan task for national education providers, educational institutions and their staff. There could be no *'one-size-fits-all'* approach to provide nations with the best way of proceeding as schools' systems and cultural nuances demand a sensitive formulation of plans, structures, methodologies and delivery consonant with what is likely to work in each place. The process was termed in some quarters as *'trying to fly the plane while still building it'*.

So while the global responses to the pandemic are generally similar, they have been evolving and fluid as local experience informed modifications. Although countries generally mandated a mass school shutdown, some schools remained open for students from essential worker families and disadvantaged backgrounds. This partial continuance enabled learning in small targeted groups as well as providing safe sanctuary for those who needed a regulated and secure environment. As the full school closures started, it was accepted that if it were to be a long-term strategy, a range of barriers, such as long-term educational disengagement, digital exclusion, poor technology management and increased psycho-social challenges, would create disadvantage that would continue long after school reopening, which would be experienced by many students from more vulnerable backgrounds. The pandemic has made visible and exacerbated the multiple and profound educational divisions that already exist globally (Beaunoyer et al., 2020; Chandra et al., 2020).

Some children in Victoria missed out on a full two years face-to-face education in their last two years in primary and older ones in their first two years in high school. These students are reporting increasing anxiety, more medicated, trying to adjust to face-to-face teaching, being asked questions and missing individual support, with social media with its addition of bullying, eating disorders and instructions on self-harm. Isolation has shown positive correlations with unhealthy eating, lack of exercise and for the youngest children poor development of language skills. Even many of those at school have disengaged from extra-curricular activities and sports as social reconnections are found difficult to undertake (See this issue extended for adults in Chap. 6).

All the Covid-related challenges are exacerbated among the vulnerable (Ambrose, 2020), who are routinely disadvantaged by social injustice based on the mal-distribution of power, money and resources (Xafis, 2020). They include, those living in poverty, residents of rural/remote communities, indigenous peoples, those experiencing job and housing insecurity, people experiencing chronic mental illness, disabilities, or dependence on substances and migrant workers (Xafis et al., 2020). The suspension of childcare services due to isolation measures exacted the highest toll on families who were already struggling, and these families are most likely to experience severe, long-term deleterious effects.

Another serious issue just coming to light is that during Covid lockdowns (Melbourne spent 262 days in lockdown), there was a significant increase in children being exposed to online extremist material. The lockdowns increased conducive conditions for radicalisation while reducing protective factors. Unsupervised home-based online usage and absence of after school activities provided far right and Islamic messages to infiltrate causing increased emotional response and mental health issues as well as distorted thinking and behaviour.

Even the steps taken to protect the family, such as frequent hand washing, maintaining physical distance and wearing personal protective equipment, were out of reach for some. Such issues were not limited to countries that lack an infrastructure for water, energy, finances and health and education services. Wealthy countries, such as the USA, are home to young children living in extreme vulnerability, including those who are hungry, neglected and abused. Many of the services that these children depended upon, such as healthy meals, social services and educational interventions, came to a halt with quarantine, lockdown and physical distancing measures.

Also, for children living in extreme adversity, early childhood programmes frequently had been their only respite from home, but children lost their safe havens. Even among children whose basic needs are routinely met, educational vulnerability persists. Preschool and children in early primary grades are most vulnerable as they often do not respond to online learning and are at a critical time of social, cognitive and intellectual development. Not all parents accepted the switch to online learning; a study in China found that parents resisted or even rejected it because they felt it was ineffective, that their young children were not sufficiently independent as learners to benefit from it, and that the parents themselves had neither the time nor expertise to accept a teaching role (Dong et al., 2020). Social-emotional vulnerability is another concern for young children. Early childhood is a critical period for learning how to deal with powerful emotions and to build skills that support positive interactions with others.

A study conducted in Italy found that mothers with children in the 0–5 age group found it especially difficult to balance the demands of home and work (Del Boca et al., 2020). Parents and families have been thrust into the role of teacher under difficult conditions. If the family is home to more than one child, home schooling responsibilities multiply quickly because every day, Monday through Friday, new assignments related to each subject area from various teachers representing different programmes keep coming in. Family members often have little or no training in supporting young children's learning and possess few resources, but even these limitations are not the hardest part. Yu et al. (2022) found parents had more effect on children's home school learning during closure if the parents had strong psychological control involving showing concern providing reinforcement, caring behaviours, improving expectations of success, and inducing increased levels of competency feelings. These are fairly standard techniques for improving performance and intrinsic motivation, but many parents do need training to know how to apply them adroitly and coping with several children amid all the Covid upheaval is a big ask for many parents to achieve.

The most daunting task, according to a study conducted in Italy with parents whose children were on the autism spectrum, is motivating children to learn and to complete assigned tasks (Espinosa et al., 2020).

Even the things that could be used as rewards for children were suddenly off limits, such as playing with friends or going on an outing. Thus, parents during lockdown described having difficulties with balancing responsibilities, motivating their children, accessing online materials and producing satisfactory learning outcomes (Garbe et al., 2020). To further compound learning losses, many young children have been deprived of a year or more of regular interactions with groups of peers that normally promote social and emotional development.

Impacts on Pre- and Early Primary School Children and Their Parents

Young children require stability and security for healthy physical, emotional and mental growth and development but significant changes to expected daily routines caused by Covid have impacted heavily on many young children and their parents during this critical phase of development. Research on the indirect psycho-social impact of the pandemic on young preschool children is limited, but some evidence is emerging from international studies, much of which has been summarised in a report by the Centre for Community Child Health (2022)/for the Commonwealth of Australia Department of Education, Skills and Employment. These international studies each paint a similar picture across the board of the effects of restrictive public health measures and their impact on children and their family dynamics. They demonstrate that maintaining routines like continuing attendance at early learning centres in the UK where centre closures were more substantial than in Australia, was a bonus. Pascal et al. (2020) reported greater negative impacts on their child's social and emotional development who were deprived of attending, than parents of children who continued attending and also expressed concerns about the impact of lockdowns on children without access to green spaces, about children's ability to assimilate back into early childhood education, and the social-emotional support they would require. Another UK study of children 8–36 months examined growth in language and executive functions (i.e. working memory, flexible thinking and self-control) and found that receptive vocabulary growth (the number of words a child can understand) was greater in children who continued to attend early childhood centres (Davies et al., 2021).

A further UK study surveyed early years providers from 35 settings in Yorkshire, UK. Providers particularly noted that children with developmental needs were missing out on assessments and other professional support, and that referrals for speech and language and the need for individual support plans had increased (Bowyer-Crane et al., 2021). Scottish parents reported worsening child behaviour and/in some cases worsening of child's mood, with some 4–7 year olds scoring very highly for emotional difficulties, conduct problems and hyperactivity/inattention (Watson et al., 2020). In China, Jiao et al. (2020) found children aged 3–6 years were more likely than older children to show problem behaviour including clinginess and fear about family members contracting the virus. Other smaller studies of young children from a range of countries also concur noting high levels of stress, anxiety, behavioural difficulties and hyperactivity/inattention (Di Giorgio et al., 2021).

A US study reveals a dramatic drop in IQ for children born during pandemic compared to children born prepandemic. In the decade preceding the pandemic, the mean IQ score hovered around the expected mean of 100 on standardised tests for children aged between three months and three years of age, but for 672 healthy children born during the pandemic that score declined to 78 (Deoni et al., 2021). It appears that the isolation, limited stimulation and less socialisation enforced by Covid-19 public health guidelines, deprived many infants of normal developmental experiences, while home environments became more stressful and unstable. Whether these lower cognitive scores will have a long-term impact is presently unclear.

One cross-national study compared responses from parents in an existing Western Australian cohort with responses from parents in an existing Bradford cohort (UK) about the initial impact of Covid on children 0–4 years. Parents from both cohorts provided similar responses regarding their worries and challenges during the lockdown period. Most concerns were related to financial insecurity and employment, anxieties about contracting Covid, educating and caring for children, the impact of Covid on society, child development and wellbeing, child and parent mental health, not seeing friends and family (Gibson et al., 2021). As Western Australia did not experience the same lockdown restrictions as the UK (and the eastern states of Australia), future waves of data collection from these cohorts will provide important insights into the impact of different isolation and confinement measures (compared to children who did not experience these measures).

There were increased reports of child abuse, neglect and exploitation throughout the pandemic (Australian Institute of Health and Welfare Report 2021; Chanchlani et al., 2020; Merrill et al., 2021). The lockdown has also contributed to increased rates of intimate partner violence, which can produce anxiety and trauma responses in children (Singh et al., 2020). In the first month of the pandemic in the UK, there was a significant increase in admissions for suspected abusive head trauma (Kuehn, 2020). As restrictive public health measures imposed less attendance at ECEC and health services and therefore fewer child interactions with adults outside the home, these statistics may not reflect the actual scale of levels of abuse resulting from the pandemic (Kang & Jain, 2020).

A BBC investigation found child speech delays increase due to lockdowns in the UK (BBC News, 2022). The number of five and six year olds who need speech and language support at school had risen by 10% in England over 2021 and may be partly due to lockdown limiting social interactions. The BBC's Shared Data Unit's analysis found that the number of children in year 1 who needed help with their language use increased more than most other areas of special educational needs. A total of 42,341 children required extra support in 2021/22, up from 38,560 in 2020/21. This is the year group which started reception after the first lockdown and had considerable disruption to their early years learning. Covid restrictions affected some children's development by limiting socialising and new experiences, which helps them learn new words. Pupils who had experienced disrupted early years learning—preschool to reception—struggled once they reached year 1 as they had missed opportunities for play-based learning. Children struggling with speech and language may end up being incorrectly 'labelled' with having mental health or behavioural problems. There have been similar rises in Scotland, with children needing communication support increasing by 20% in the last two years.

The speech and language problem in the UK was also highlighted in the Ofsted Chief Inspector's Report (2021) where young children's development, following the pandemic, was 'particularly worrying', with many lingering challenges, noting babies in nurseries with 'limited vocabularies' and struggling to understand facial expressions based on inspections of 70 early years providers. The report suggested face masks were having a negative impact on young children's language and communication skills. They have been unable to see lip movements or mouth shapes as regularly. All they've seen is parents and a house, not interacting in local parks, or seeing their friends, or going to birthday parties.

Pandemic restrictions have also created a lockdown generation of Covid kids at least in Australia who can't catch or throw a ball. The two-year loss of community sport and school PE represented a large part of a child's lifetime, and it was where they develop motor skills. Beyond learning to hop, skip, jump, run, catch and throw, these places teach children important social skills and help them develop broader physical literacy. In Victoria, Australia's most locked down state, more than half of all five to nine-year-olds, or 82,000 children, had to cease playing community sport, a lockdown-forced hiatus that has created a generation of kids with poor motor skills a Victoria University report (2022) revealed.

Pandemics are related to increased rates of improper nutrition and dramatic changes in children's play. In a longitudinal study of 14 countries (including Australia), children spent 55 min more per day in sedentary screen time and 81 min less per weekday outdoors during Covid-19 restrictions. The risks for children with additional healthcare needs (e.g. developmental and behavioural issues) are even greater, with limited access to health care, school and support services, including early intervention (Scibberas et al., 2020).

The estimated achievement gap between disadvantaged and advantaged students grows at triple the rate during remote learning compared with onsite learning with the value of gross domestic product lost from one-third of a year of remote learning estimated to be US$871 billion in Australia. Recent data suggest that children born during the pandemic may already be demonstrating reduced cognitive performance (Deoni et al., 2021).

Goldfeld et al. (2022) using data from the Australian Early Development Census conducted the previous year (2020) that measured five areas of child development: physical health and wellbeing; social competence; emotional maturity; language and cognitive skills; and communications skills and general knowledge, for the first time since 2009, found the percentage of children who were 'on track' in the five areas had decreased. Increased screen time and less outdoor activity, due to Covid restrictions, could have also affected development. They bore the brunt of the indirect impacts. These developmental losses were worse for lower income, lower resourced families and predict the inequality between communities before the pandemic will increase.

Considering all these aspects of children's lives, the potential impacts on young children and parents are substantial, with impact areas able to be grouped under three broad categories (Goldfeld et al., 2022):

- Child-level factors such as poorer mental health, poorer child health development and bonding, poorer academic achievement; changes to routine,
- Family-level factors such as poorer parent mental health, poverty and job losses, increased household stress, increased abuse and neglect, food insecurity, poorer maternal and newborn health, lack of physical activity and increased screen time contributing to obesity, weaker language development, exposure to domestic violence, parental mental illness and child abuse and
- Service-level factors that affect children involving school closures, reduced access to health care and support services, closure of sport activities reducing activity and social skill levels, inadequate technology skills for learning, connection and health care.

In summary, this small sample of research reviewed suggests there is increasing international concern about the likely disproportionate impact of the current pandemic on younger children and their family dynamics experiencing adversity, widening existing disparities in child health and developmental outcomes, with many children facing a generation-defining disruption from indirect impacts. As the early home environment is a key indicator of future outcomes for young children, this places them at considerable risk of negative health and developmental outcomes. At greatest risk will be young children who already have developmental needs. This is compounded by disrupted early childhood centre attendance and by the removal of personal, social and therapeutic supports with the increased likelihood of parental stress spelling current and future harms. Children bore the brunt of indirect impacts, and those impacts have been shown to be greatest on lower income, lower resourced families and the inequality existing before the pandemic will likely increase.

Consequences for Older School Students

In Australia, the challenges wrought by Covid have compounded the already identified risks for vulnerable young people. Data from the Australian Bureau of Statistics (ABS) show that as of 2019 there were 3,948,811 students enrolled in 9503 schools. Mass school closures thus impacted nearly four million Australian students from time to time over the last two years. There is little research available yet given the time factor from the end of closures, but the potential effects are likely to be dramatic with the gap for students from more socially disadvantaged backgrounds likely to be exacerbated by the very speedy global mass movement to online and off-site education which resulted in considerable learning opportunity variations and increased risk for students in households experiencing economic disadvantage (Chandra et al., 2020).

School closures and lockdown in the face of Covid-19 will have affected children of all ages in myriad ways. In particular, the lack of face-to-face contact with peers, less chance for play, interrupted education and potential for domestic abuse will be felt for some time. Empson (2020) asked '*what do children think is normal?*'. Initially, some children saw the lockdown as new and exciting, but gradually, some younger children have become more emotional and some of the older children are playing new games which involve killing the coronavirus. Empson (op cit.) wrote that the mental health implications of coronavirus would be profound, especially for the most vulnerable members of society; she suggested psycho-social recovery would take at least 18–24 months for many households.

There is a mistaken assumption that children's emotions do not run as deep as those of adults and that children can be expected to recover more readily from adversity than mature individuals. This perspective tends to minimise the effects of change and crisis on young children, assumes that they are oblivious to and therefore unconcerned about bad situations, and expects them to be exceptionally resilient. For some families, quarantine resulted in parents spending significantly more time in the company of their children and witnessing, first-hand, worrisome changes in behaviour (Evans et al., 2020). Families could see for themselves that young children are actually quite vulnerable as support networks like childcare, peer group and schooling became victims of lockdowns and social distancing. The Covid crisis may have informed the general population that children's social and emotional developments are perhaps as important as their schoolwork and acknowledge the inherent vulnerability in the young.

Many parents wanted their children back to school as they become more fearful of the mental health hazards of keeping children at home than the risk of them catching the Covid-19 virus. Many parents despaired whether classroom would reopen for the academic year 2022. On the other hand, some families were reluctant to send children to school at the peak of the early 2022 Omicron pandemic as they have been conditioned to fear. Before Christmas, hundreds of Covid cases in a single day were of really serious concern and ballooned to over 50,000 cases a day as schools were due to reopen in the new reset context, with politicians and epidemiologists saying it is OK as they try to peak out Omicron and reduce it to endemic levels.

In a letter to the Australian Prime Minister, premiers and chief ministers mid-January 2022, signed by 26 of the nation's most eminent paediatricians, infectious disease researchers and child and adolescent psychiatrists, insisted that it was safe to allow schools to be open for face-to-face learning in February, the normal start of the new school year after the long summer Xmas holidays. Their argument was based on Australian data that confirmed Covid is a mild disease in children, that the few hospitalisations are short-lived, and that the overwhelming majority of children recover from the virus without adverse effect. The letter continued by stating there is no medical case for face-to-face learning to be suspended awaiting the vaccination of 5–11-year-old children, although all children should be offered access as soon as practical as a delay in returning to in-person learning puts children's mental health at risk, with additional increases in the risk of child abuse, obesity and delayed social and emotional development. The danger of long-term chronic high-fat diet (so-called comfort food), induced by social isolation stress and lack or exercise, produces anxiety and depression-like behaviours in children as well as increased food intake and weight gain (Mengin et al., 2020). Therefore, schooling was seen as an antidote offering activities, exercise, peer companionship with less need and opportunity for comfort food. The association of high-fat diets and social isolation during development has been noted to lead to structural synaptic changes, impacting learning and memory later in adult life such (Cavaliere et al., 2019).

Some senior disease specialists are adamant; young children are less likely to catch and spread the virus because prepubescent children lack the ACE2 receptor, a protein the coronavirus latches on to infect human cells, and therefore that schools can reopen safely. For teachers, having lunch together in the staff room is more of a danger than the classroom in all probability, and if necessary a short-term 'hybrid' teaching model combining classroom and home schooling could be effected. This would be a stopgap measure to allow teachers who are isolating at home to teach and for children who are at school to learn. Realistically, Covid is here for years and the issues are not going to go away so unless you're going to become a hermit, there is little else you can do than now start to live 'normally'. If bars are open, how can we justify closing schools?

In economic terms, school closures are a negative factor increasing the workforce absenteeism rate by 50%, as parents are compelled to stay home to look after children. Schools open means shops open, means hospitals are open. It means essential services and supply chains operate. Childcare and schools are essential to improving workforce participation and where possible should be the first to open and last to close with face-to-face learning prioritised. State leaders in Australia have agreed that no vulnerable child or child of an essential worker is 'turned away' from classrooms, implying that whenever schools and childcare have to be shut down, a skeleton staff will have to be on duty to supervise onsite children of essential workers and those in need of support.

As always, the Australian states are each going their own way: Victoria and NSW were adamant and opened schools on schedule early February 22 but Queensland postponed term one by two weeks, with year 11 and 12 students remaining on remote learning a week before other kids head back to class. South Australia staggered return dates for different year levels. All states claimed that schools were 'made' Covid safe through a combination of vaccination, mask wearing, physical distancing, strict hygiene practices, frequent cleaning of schools and ventilation, all important ways to stop the spread of Omicron in schools, combined with RAT testing of teachers exposed to the virus.

The opposite side of the coin is a concern for teacher wellbeing by the Australian Education Union (2020), which is furious that teachers are being treated like 'babysitters' so their parents can go to work. The vast majority of children would not be fully vaccinated for some months after return to school and that deeply concerned teacher union members because Omicron was highly transmissible. The union urged teachers to stay home if they don't feel safe working in classrooms and remote learning would have to continue. To be told the reason schools need to be open is for workforce considerations, rather than prioritising the safety of both teachers and education of young people at home was offensive to many teachers.

Teachers globally, burnt out by two years of on–off remote teaching, threatened classroom boycotts unless governments did more to protect them in their workplace. If teachers are essential and must go to work, they must be provided with the essential tools like RATs that are needed to ensure their safety and the safety of students in their care. Vaccine mandates are exacerbating the problem in Australia, with roughly one in ten teachers refusing or unable to get the jab and therefore not allowed to teach face to face. It is unlikely any schools will mandate Covid vaccines for pupils as it is unreasonable to punish a child and deprive them of an education because their parents made a decision about vaccination.

Research on Consequences of School Closure

Drane et al. (2021) provide a thorough scoping review of the Covid implications for students of a mass school closure across Australia, particularly focussing on consequences for approaches to managing unanticipated school closures and what existing literature related to young people learning outside-of-school could offer as prognosis for the long-term educational impacts of navigating the Covid disruption including psycho-social and emotional repercussions, and on technology availability and learning, several major issues emerged from this review.

1. Disengagement from Education

The teacher–student relationship is often the major driver for student engagement. During mass school closures, all three components of student engagement, viz. behavioural, emotional and cognitive, are disrupted. To maintain some semblance of student engagement with their education requires immediate and constructive teacher online feedback. This necessary feedback may not be feasible when students have limited or no access to computers, or Internet, and are in home isolation, restricting their ability to connect online and 'see' their teachers (Drane et al., 2021).

This absence of positive interactions and feedback from their school community for some disadvantaged students may influence their engagement and emotional wellbeing for some time to come even after return to normal schooling. School connection is a protective factor for many students and associated with a reduction in risk-taking behaviours, as well as maintaining school attendance and academic achievement (Simpkins et al., 2015). For some really disadvantaged students, school is the only constant (and for a few, safe place) in their lives.

While parents did their best during 'house schooling', it was a difficult engagement for both child and parent with many of the latter ill equipped to offer academic help and often trying to manage several children's needs at once. Many children are reported to want a return to their friends and teachers. With many children missing up to half their face-to-face teaching hours in the last two years due to various lockdowns, there is an academic impact to add to mental distress and social isolation effects. Unfortunately, these impacts fall disproportionately on disadvantaged children and will increase the socio-economic divide. Remember too that this is not just affecting the 'normal' child but has a more massive effect on children already disadvantaged with physical impairment, learning and behavioural problems. The response to this risk of educational disengagement is to sustain meaningful communication between schools and families.

2. The Digital Divide

The 'everything is online now' slogan does not acknowledge those without such resources. Reliable Internet access and hardware, the fundamental requirement of online teaching is not within reach for many families, even in a wealthy country such as the USA (Li, 2022). A US Pew Research Centre survey conducted late January–early February 2021 estimated that five million children and nearly one-third (31.4%) of families with children ages 6–17 with family incomes below $50,000 do not have a high-speed Internet; this group represents about 40% of all families with school-age children in the USA.

Similarly in Australia, according to the Australian Bureau of Statistics (ABS 2018a, 2018b), on average, 13.2% of Australian households do not have access to the Internet. More than 90% of households in advantaged areas have an Internet connection, but less than 40% of households in disadvantaged or remote geographical areas are connected (Drane et al., 2021). Approximately, 471,600 households from the lowest quintile of household income (i.e. the lowest 20% of the population) have no access to the Internet, and approximately 621,800 households in the lowest quintile do not have access to a laptop or desktop computer. This data points to numerous disadvantaged students with insufficient access and connectivity making it difficult for them to continue their learning online (Drane et al., 2021).

The above evidence from wealthy countries illustrates the digital divide that exists between students from low and high socio-educational backgrounds as the most disadvantaged do not have access to and possess all the skills to use communication technologies. The *Digital Inclusion Index* measures digital inclusion in three discrete ways (access, affordability, and digital ability). Inadequate technology access is related to financial resources. This indicates that the digital divide in other less wealthy countries is far greater. For example, in Nigeria as a whole, employment and income were closely associated with Internet usage as access to the Internet is very costly and can only be afforded by those employed with a substantial level of income (Adeleke, 2020). The study showed that there were obvious disparities in Internet usage between the north and south as well as urban and rural areas of Nigeria. There were noticeable high values for Internet usage in major cities like Lagos, Kaduna, Kano and Abuja but minimal use in rural areas. Nigerians spend an average of N 2141 to access the Internet which is equivalent to 12% of the current national minimum wage. It has been reported that prices need to drop by 97% to become affordable for Nigerians (Quartsz, 2016). This is replicated to varying degrees all over Africa.

Another problem is that the proportion of income required for Internet expenditure in Australia has increased faster than actual increases in income (Thomas et al., 2021). This seriously affects those on lower or fixed incomes and becomes more concerning at a time when an estimated 10% of the population has lost income since the pandemic started due to lockdown and small business closures. The Digital Inclusion Index report (2021) highlights the increase in amount of household income spent on Internet services from a base of 1.00% in 2014 to 1.18% in 2019 (Thomas et al., 2021) further impacting the ability of households to maintain Internet costs when there has been a loss of income due to the pandemic. Additionally, households experiencing financial hardship may only be able to access the Internet via mobile-only plans which have lower download limits, and once these limits are exceeded, additional costs are imposed, resulting in students having limited Internet download for educational purposes compared to being on fixed line. The use of such mobile-only plans is reported in 30.7% of households in the lowest income quartile (Thomas et al., 2021). The digital divide is a multifaceted concept characterised not only by differences in hardware ownership (i.e. laptops, computers) but also by differences in access and connectivity to the Internet as well as the cost, which places an additional burden on households already experiencing financial strain (Drane et al., 2021).

To redress the digital divide during the Covid pandemic, Drane et al. (2021) report that many countries recognised the necessity to employ a variety of methods to provide student learning during school closure. For example, delivery of hard copy teaching resources to disadvantaged homes has been operating in a number of countries, e.g. Portugal. Educational content via two television channels, combined with learning resources available in both hard and soft copy, has been provided by the New Zealand (NZ) government. In response to poor Internet connectivity, especially in rural and remote regions the Queensland government has used television for teaching purposes, with material included to engage with parents to assist them in home schooling their children. Several countries have implemented loans of electronic equipment, such as laptops or tablets (Chandra et al., 2020). In addition to differing teaching mediums, the United Arab Emirates, in an attempt to assist the practical application of online teaching, opened a technical support hotline for teachers and students devised to offer free support for individuals facing difficulties with technology (UNESCO, 2020b).

Recently, a low-tech non-smart phone has been deployed to help students learning remotely during Covid and enabling students in developing nations to continue learning effectively involving a combination of text messages and weekly, one-on-one, 20 min phone calls with tutors. With limited Internet access and expensive data costs of online learning programmes in Botswana, online learning wasn't an option when the schools closed there. After a successful pilot in Botswana during pandemic-driven school closures, where 4500 families accessed the initial trial, resulting in a 31% lift in numeracy which equates to about one year of learning increase for about [$100] spent, it has moved to further trials in another five countries involving more than 20,000 school students across five countries: Uganda, Kenya, Philippines, Nepal and India (ABC News, 2022).

It is claimed that phone-based learning could facilitate disadvantaged developed nations' children in remote areas as in Australia with capacity to plug gaps, especially when students are offline for relatively brief periods, if for example they're unwell, their Internet drops out or if they're cut off due to extreme weather. The mobile phone is one way to set up a substitute system quickly. While the gold standard is of course quality in-person, real-time learning, there are occasions such as natural disasters where we need to rollout useful technological responses adapted to the conditions, as online learning is not necessarily the saviour when it comes to maintaining learning during disruptions.

Clearly, nations recognise there is a digital divide issue and are addressing the problem in their own particular and creative ways. The reason for these losses is that many families lack the physical spaces, technology and other resources to support learning at home. Additionally, many parents and caregivers lack the time needed to support their children's learning. This is occurring irrespective of socio-economic status, with full-time waged and sole parent-waged families reporting difficulties. Further, parents who have lower levels of educational attainment, or have limited capability with technology, face particular challenges in facilitating children's learning at home. The gap in digital inclusion across many nations means that online learning is not possible, or suitable, for all students. In addition to the learning losses, many families, especially those in vulnerable groups, are confused and stigmatised by the current policy positions.

A number of misconceptions exist around the technology competencies of students who are often assumed to be digitally *savvy*, but their technology use at home is typically for personal use and not for learning purposes. As technological skills vary among young people, many may not meet the required level of proficiency for learning online (Drane et al., 2021). In using online technology far more when at home, there will be greater exposure to inappropriate material as well as an increased risk of cyberbullying unless parents take more notice of what their children are doing.

Distance learning has implications for student educational experiences including home distractions, often ineffective supervision and limited interaction with peers. Even for pupils of essential workers and those with special needs who attended school had many lessons still delivered online, in mixed aged classes not in class groups, with supervision from any staff available. In summary, challenges to online learning include poor Internet access, home environments unconducive to online learning, student difficulties with self-discipline and self-directed learning, lack of professional development for teaching staff and means of supporting not only students' academic learning outcomes, but also their social and emotional development (Zhu & Liu, 2020a, 2020b, 2020c). Thrust into emergency remote teaching, a survey of K-12 educators indicated that even they struggled to find high-quality tools, locate curated content aligned with standards and curriculum, use digital tools effectively, communicate with students at a distance, support student engagement/persistence and adapt teaching material to the conditions and needs of particular students (Rasmitadila et al., 2020; Trust & Whalen, 2020).

In a UK study of secondary school students perception of on line teaching experience during Covid, Walters et al. (2022) found that concentration, engagement, ability to learn and self-worth from learning were all significantly lower for online learning than classroom learning These differences were more marked in pupils with specific learning difficulties. In particular, dyslexics' slowness to read text makes synchronous learning environments difficult to manage. A case study of young children in the South Pacific region during the pandemic, one young child poignantly captured the difference between online and in-person teaching by asking, 'When are we going to have the real school?' (Dayal and Tiko, 2020). Covid has changed education at every level, from infant care to postdoctoral study. Unprecedented long-term closure of schools and suspension of face-to-face teaching during the Covid crisis surely has reduced opportunities to learn for students, particularly those of young children. In terms of social-emotional development, most children have lost the equivalent of a year or more of interaction with peers in group settings.

3. Emotional Wellbeing and Anxiety

As schools made the shift to online learning, supporting students' social and emotional wellbeing became imperative. Although some students were faced with online learning issues attributed to technology use, there were also emotional challenges associated with change, the shift to off-site learning. The emotional consequences related to school closures cannot be underestimated (Drane et al., 2021). Anxiety disorders are the most common mental, emotional and behavioural problems among young Australians. Specifically, 13.9% of children and adolescents normally experience a mental health disorder, including 6.9% experiencing anxiety (Australian Institute of Health and Welfare, 2016). As students lost school connectedness due to being physically distanced from school, or having to maintain a social distance from teachers and peers, there was a sense that adults and/or peers in their school were no longer concerned about them as an individual or concerned about their learning. As such, psychological distress such as anxiety and depression has increased during the pandemic disruption (Holmes et al., 2020).

Lowered perceived ability to learn and engage with online learning was also associated with lowered mental wellbeing. Mental health problems rose in the UK for 5–16 year olds from 11 to 16% over the two years of the epidemic. Anxiety seemed engendered by the sudden change in working environment. This has been particularly noted by Bagnall et al. (2022) who investigated the effects of the multiple challenges derived from simultaneous changes facing pupils transiting from primary to secondary school in a Covid context, the biggest disruption to education in history. From the beginning of the new school year late August 2020–January 2021, school attendance due to closure dropped over 80% in the UK. Pupils faced the negotiation of these two key events (transition and school closure) in conditions of rapid change and reduced support. This study highlights a range of valuable strategies that were used to meet children's needs pre and post-transition as on and off periods of school closure imposed home learning and the use of various online techniques.

Generally, online learning appears to have had a negative effect on learning. The opportunity to ask questions, share opinions or disagree with points are all fundamental to learning. Communication benefits of face-to-face teaching and peer group learning are often not available with online teaching minimalising learning opportunities and social skill development such as self-confidence and collaborative skills.

As schools often provide a safe haven for many students, remote learning with its social and physical isolation may deny them this emotional refuge and in some cases may place a child in a degree of limited safety. The burden of acting as home educator is thrust on parents at the same time as many experience psychological distress from personal disruptions due to Covid such as unemployment and financial strain, further exacerbating psychological distress (Drane et al., 2021). The expectation that parents assume the role of educator within the household is one that many parents may not be equipped for physically, intellectually or emotionally (Burke & Dempsey, 2020). The challenge of navigating this has required communities to step up to supply support for families, e.g. Western Australian police, prisoners and local businesses supplied furniture and computers to Mt Barker Community College students so they could study at home.

Strategies to ameliorate these socio-emotional and psychological distress issues for both students and parents have included utilising existing student mentoring programmes already established in many districts. For example, the Australian Indigenous Mentoring Experience (AIME) programme has successfully mentored young people in both primary and high school settings for over a decade (O'Shea et al. 2020) and was used in this context; and e-mentoring programmes, established in many universities, have supported prospective or commencing students.

Schools and school systems are generally becoming aware that flexibility in both structure of content and delivery must vary according to different circumstances avoiding a *one-stop-shop* approach to remote education and recognise that bespoke strategies may be necessary to cross the digital divide and facilitate connectedness with teachers enabling engagement and teacher awareness of when things may be going sadly wrong in the emotional, social and physical distress areas to ensure equity for all students. Drane et al. (2021) emphasise that this pandemic risks are exacerbating existing educational inequities and subjecting students and their families particularly those in vulnerable settings, to an increased risk of adverse social, emotional and behavioural outcomes.

It is generally expected that the worry and depression from lockdown and home schooling would create further problems on return to school as learning gaps, deteriorated social relationship skills add to the compendium of problems. A recent report from the Centre for Independent Studies questions this assumption. Using a longitudinal study plus overseas data, the effects educationally and psychologically have been less than envisaged. In lockdown capital Victoria, the NAPLAN results revealed students had made close to the amount of progress that they would have made in a typical year. The psychological damage of home learning was less severe, although some children did express feelings of loneliness with follow-up data suggesting the best remedy to address loneliness and the milder problems is simply return to the classroom environment.

Despite the emotive appeals about children's safety, experts on child health have repeatedly reassured parents that the risk of serious health outcomes is very low for young people who contract Covid. In fact, they've consistently warned school closures cause more harm than the virus, particularly for disadvantaged students. In Australia, Murdoch University Children's Research Institute research review (2022) found lockdowns and remote learning denying much face-to-face relationships are adding to existing issues of bullying, helicopter parents, over scheduled lives and bombardment of online information. Children need training in resilience, basic life and social skills and coping strategies. Children have suffered from school closures during the pandemic, and it is essential to keep schools open by taking proportionate, evidence-based responses to outbreaks. The benefits to children and families of having children in school far outweigh the alternative. School is a foundation for wellbeing for many years into the future.

Competence Problems in the Switch to Distance Learning for Students

Simonson and Berg (2016) define distance learning (also called remote learning) as a form of education in which the main elements include physical separation of teachers and students during instruction and the use of various technologies to facilitate student–teacher and student–student communication. Previous studies on distance learning conclude that it can be just as effective as face-to-face teaching (Means et al., 2013). However, Covid is a new and challenging situation with respect to distance learning, as mandatory school shutdowns due to a pandemic or natural catastrophe have never before been necessary at such a large scale. It became therefore particularly important to investigate how students could best cope with this new situation and how students who perceived themselves as competent differed from those who did not.

Student Attributes for Success

While the school closures provided many challenges for teachers in preparing material and delivering online and for parents monitoring that work was done being and assisting their offspring to master the material, students also found themselves in a novel situation. While face-to-face teaching, and fixed routines like timetables had regulated most aspects of school life and learning time, students were now far more on their own, controlling and organising their own learning activities and time management with autonomous self-regulation the theme of their lives within and outside the education context. Two major attributes both considered important factors for learning success in 'normal' face-to-face settings are (Dent & Koenka, 2016; Fortier et al., 1995):

- *Self-regulated learning* (SRL) involving planning, monitoring and adapting one's thoughts, feelings and actions in a cyclical process to attain a personal goal (Zimmerman, 2000) and
- *Intrinsic motivation* that is doing of an activity for its personal satisfaction and feelings of mastery rather than for some external consequence. When intrinsically motivated, a person is moved to act for the fun or challenge entailed rather than because of external rewards, or pressures. It's the difference between reading a book for amusement or reading a book in order to study for a test in which you feel obliged to do well or learning a new language because you want to travel, not because your job requires it.

These two attributes gain considerable additional relevance when students face a situation such as distance learning with decreased external structure and guidance. Furthermore, intrinsic motivation, goal setting and SRL are all influenced by the student's own perceived competence in applying these processes, that is, by the learner's feeling of being able to handle given tasks (e.g. Cho et al., 2011). A lack of both intrinsic motivation and of self-regulation has been associated with higher passive procrastination which is the act of delaying or postponing a task or set of tasks, which obviously is detrimental impediment to academic outcomes (Howell & Watson, 2007).

Passive procrastination in the academic context means delaying school-related tasks even when faced with negative consequences (Steel & Klingsieck, 2016). Procrastination is also related to higher levels of anxiety in students , and it has been proposed that both anxiety and depression would make students more vulnerable to repetitive negative thoughts about past events, which in turn increases levels of procrastination (Constantin et al., 2018). Distance learning in comparison with regular face-to-face lessons is characterised by greater flexibility in scheduling, the opportunity to individualise learning processes, the potential to enhance SRL skills and the easy distribution of information (Means et al., 2013). However, this can present both advantages and disadvantages, especially for younger students as the greater flexibility available in distance learning places high demands on the learner's ability to regulate their learning and motivation (Adam et al., 2017) and on parental supervision, interest and ability to 'teach' when students had difficulty understanding. All this poses an increased risk of passive procrastination.

Possession of SLR, IM and a lack of procrastination are essential in order to succeed when there is much less supervision and daily routine learning and studying under Covid imposed conditions of distance learning. Pelikan et al. (2021) investigated how differences in these three personal characteristics affected performance in a large sample of around 19,000 Austrian students after the switch to distance learning in March 2020. Pelikan et al. (2021) separated students based on their self-reported perceived competence, which allowed them to create two extreme groups of still considerable sample size. This final sample of 2652 secondary school students answered closed questions regarding SRL, IM and procrastination as well as open-ended questions about challenges, successes and need for support in distance learning. Students were also requested to rate themselves in terms of their perception of their own competence as being high vs. low in SRL, IM and procrastination. The objective was to determine whether the novel distance education scenario plus the accumulation of negative life events during this pandemic period has increased the risk of academic underperformance as well as deteriorated mental health.

Results showed highly statistically significant differences between high and low self-belief competence groups (Pelikan et al., 2021). Students who not only believed but also experienced themselves as highly competent used SRL strategies (goal setting and planning, time management, metacognitive strategies) more often and were more intrinsically motivated than students with lower perceived competence. They also procrastinated less. Gonzalez et al. (2020) also found that the confinement affected academic performance of Spanish students strongly positively if they adopted intrinsic motivation when facing the new and unknown scenario that the confinement procedures are formed which enabled students to work more continuously and uninterrupted. In both these studies, it could very well be that the coping mechanism employed by students plays a key role in determining the direction of academic performance. Coping strategies have been classified depending on their functionality to solve or evade the challenges: adaptive coping behaviours lean towards acknowledging the stressors, analysing the situations, seeking support, and making efforts to solve the problems. In contrast, maladaptive coping behaviours lean towards avoiding the problems, withdrawal, and substance use to evade the sources of stress, all forms of procrastination (delaying tactics).

In a recent study, Zhoc et al. (2022) provide additional support for the notion that how well a student managed their emotions and wellbeing influences their engagement with online learning. Cognitive reappraisal by which emotions were lessened by evaluating the situation and lessen its emotional impact was strongly related to effective online earning.

Freyhofer et al. (2021) showed that maladaptive coping strategies and loneliness play a significant role on academic outcomes through the mediation of procrastination in undergraduate management students during the pandemic. Maladaptive coping strategies in the form of denial, substance use, behavioural disengagement and frustration increased the levels of anxiety and depression after the lockdown restrictions started. Higher levels of depression leads to increased levels of procrastination, impacting academic performance negatively. This suggests that depression and not anxiety prevents people from taking effective actions towards a better performance.

Furthermore, Pelikan et al. (2021) in qualitative analysis of their data revealed that although all students face similar challenges (e.g. independent learning, time and task management, learning on the computer, lessening of contact with teachers and peers), students who perceived themselves as highly competent at employing those skills coped better and registered less need for support. Most students reported in the qualitative part of the study that they did miss face-to-face communication with teachers in real life as well as online, stating difficulties with understanding instructions and assignments and that they needed more detailed explanations, particularly when learning new content. Moreover, most students stated that they had difficulty contacting teachers, a lack of feedback from teachers, and were getting no or delayed responses. Consequently, they didn't know whether their performance was sufficient. Some students also indicated that they would like to have more contact with their peers, either in order to support each other in school-related efforts or simply because they missed their friends.

Difficulties concentrating and avoiding distractions as well as a lack of motivation and self-discipline were mentioned more often in the low perceived competence group. While learning independently and without support was difficult for both groups, it was even more challenging for students who perceived themselves as lacking competence in SRL and IM. Some students indicated that their home learning environment was suboptimal, as they had to share a room with siblings or were otherwise distracted while studying. Difficulties arose for many students with respect to the learning platforms, either because there were too many different platforms that had to be checked, running the risk of overlooking important information or assignments, or because the platforms didn't work. Some students reported technical issues due to malfunctioning soft or hardware or because they lacked the necessary technical equipment for digital learning (e.g. they had to share a computer with another family member or had no access to a printer). Students also mentioned that they didn't have sufficient knowledge to accomplish all necessary tasks (e.g. receiving and handing in digital assignments) and that they weren't accustomed to working in front of a screen for prolonged periods of time and were easily distracted and exhausted (Pelikan et al., 2021).

Students who perceived themselves as less competent tended to struggle in dealing with general anxiety and uncertainty resulting from the situation and maintaining a healthy learning life balance. Students also indicated that being in close quarters with their family led to increased stress and arguments.

Overall, from the Pelikan et al. (2021) study, students who perceived themselves as highly competent differ in their use of self-regulated learning strategies, their intrinsic motivation and passive procrastination from students who perceive themselves as less competent. The latter who perceived themselves as lacking competence described fewer successes in learning independently, experiencing more anxiety and uncertainty than students from the high perceived competence group. Students across the board asked for more contact with teachers and peers found technical issues intruding into their studies and often found home conditions suboptimal for study. Conditions under which learning should take place did raise common problems. In general, the qualitative analysis revealed that even though all students faced similar challenges in distance learning, students who perceived themselves as highly competent were better able to cope with the situation.

Implications for Distance Learning

The Pelikan et al. (2021) provides some useful guidelines for distance teaching under adverse circumstances.

- Fostering SRL needs to be a priority in online teaching, by helping students set goals and schedule their time within the teaching programme or else supporting their monitoring by asking prompting questions. Helping students to set and reach achievable goals allows them to experience increased perceived competence, which in turn also boosts intrinsic motivation and learning success.
- Introducing learning buddies may serve to foster social relations between students encouraging each other to follow through on their plans and provide some of the social support most students missed.
- Students from both the high and low perceived competence groups expressed a desire for clear and comprehensive instructions for tasks and assignments. Teachers should provide detailed instructions, offer explanations when necessary and be available for questions.
- Better co-ordination among teachers regarding deadlines and delivery intervals may relieve some of the stress students reported. Additionally, providing timely and respectful feedback can support students' self-efficacy and motivation as well as the teacher–student relationship.
- Students expressed a need for social contact, which was particularly impaired during the lockdown. Increasing social interaction by providing opportunities for video conferences/tutorials, virtual learning groups, study buddies) as well as asynchronous (e.g. forum discussions) communication may promote distance learning success.
- Teachers need to be prepared and supported in their switch to distance learning as online teaching is not merely about transferring normal lessons into a digital environment.

Teachers' Wellbeing in the Shift to Distance Learning

Teachers, like medical staff, have been globally confronted with increased demands and limited resources since March 2020 as school closure and lockdowns were mandated and therefore not exempt from impacts on their own mental health and wellbeing (*MHWB*). However, the dominant focus around *MHWB* in schools has largely been on students coping with education at home with teachers' experiences and needs being less widely heard or considered. Understanding teachers' *MHWB* is important because poor *MHWB* can lead to teachers exiting the profession with teacher shortage exacerbating the demands on those remaining and also impacting student outcomes. Teachers across the world needed to adapt quickly to the demands of continued delivery of education often without all the resources necessary, as they attempted to look after the ongoing education programmes and welfare of students in spite of the pandemic, all of which has had consequences for their *MHWB*.

A sudden shift in the working environment while needing to maintain personal responsibility at home has taken a toll on the MHWB of many teachers all around the world (Kraft et al., 2020). Anxiety surrounding the pandemic and lack of administrative support seem to be important predictors of teacher burnout (Pressley, 2021), with many teachers reporting symptoms of stress, anxiety, and depression, e.g. in Portugal (Alves et al., 2021); Spain (Ozamiz-Etxebarria et al., 2020); Poland (Jakubowski &Sitko-Dominik, 2021); Finland (Poysa et al., 2021); and Australia (Dabrowski, 2020). These findings from a range of nations highlight the need to study teachers' MHWB in this challenging period, to provide improved understanding of how some of the impacts could be mitigated in any future situation.

England has been affected by falling teacher retention levels for over a decade (Kim et al. (2022), while lesson planning, teaching, and assessment as well as caring for pupils with empathic feedback and support during the pandemic have increased the normal challenges for many teachers at the same time as teacher retention rates continued to fall. The impact of this combination on teachers' mental health and wellbeing (*MHWB)* has become of great concern in the UK as well as internationally, but there is little data on teacher wellbeing during the pandemic under the demands of imposed distance teaching approaches when there was significant pressure and limited time to think about, design and operate new online systems.

Various pandemic-related events and changes have affected teachers' lives In England. Teachers were regularly requested to implement and work within the bounds of last-minute governmental decisions when school closures for most pupils started on 20 March 2020. A month later, April was the time of lowest *MHWB* in the education population. Moreover, with a see saw of reopening and closing, over 2020 and 2021, as in many other countries, teachers at all levels of responsibility in the UK experienced not only constant changes in their work, from which they recounted a mixture of stories of joy and sense of achievement, but also many of sadness and frustration (Kim & Asbury, 2020).

A major problem, as in many other nations including Australia, was that teachers had to plan and facilitate the execution of home instruction taking into account the digital divide between pupils resulting from a lack of adequate digital technology and/or reliable Internet connection, both at school and in the home context where students struggled to work. The prevalence of this divide in the UK was reported just before the pandemic onset where by only 12% of 11–18 year olds in the UK had a laptop, desktop, or tablet to access the

Internet at home. The UK government, in response, has provided 1.3 million laptops and tablets to disadvantaged pupils during the pandemic. But teachers still had to respond in a variety of ways to continue teaching their pupils, ranging from sending paper workpacks home, to delivering almost fully online teaching (Bayrakdar & Guveli, 2020).

Kim et al. (2022) followed 24 UK primary and secondary school teachers' *MHWB* experiences across three time points (April, July and November 2020) using a longitudinal approach focussing on the effects of job demands (aspects of the job that can be physically or psychologically costly) and job resources (aspects of the job that can buffer the effects of job demands and promote achievement and growth) with teachers reporting across the three time points. Generally, the teachers' *MHWB* declined throughout the pandemic, especially for primary school leaders with six job demands contributing negatively to teachers' *MHWB* (i.e. uncertainty, workload, negative perception of the profession, concern for others' wellbeing, health struggles and balancing multiple roles). Another UK study (TeacherTapp, 2021) covering a slightly longer timescale than Kim et al (2022) examined the proportions of teachers self-reporting scores of 8 and above on a 10-point measure of work-related anxiety between October 2019 and January 2021. They found high peaks, marking high prevalence of anxiety, in March (as school lockdown began), in May (when June school reopening announcements were made), and in January 2021 (as a third national lockdown and second partial school closure was announced). Moreover, the peaks were higher for head teachers (e.g. 40% on 12 May 2020 and 54% on 5 January 2021) than classroom teachers (e.g. 11% on 19 May and 28% on 5 January 2021). These two studies are suggestive of increasing levels of pressure and a need to understand the experiences of teaching professionals, including senior leaders, in more depth.

Given the importance of teachers' *MHWB*, particularly during the pandemic when they are under new forms of pressure, policymakers and senior education managers need to support school staffs' *MHWB* by engaging in more collaborative communication and ensuring greater accessibility to sources of required quality equipment and social support. These discussions and provisions will be crucial in supporting teachers, and thereby the educational system, both during and after the pandemic, and enhance our understanding of the impact of sudden changes on the teaching profession and how we should move forward.

Covid Effects on Post-School Education and Scholarship

Universities and colleges have all been hard hit. Universities went online, gap years were cancelled, and remote working added previously unheard of challenges to practical and work experience requirements for entering some professional workforces. Industries most decimated by lockdowns, such as hospitality and the retail in Australia, are also largely staffed by young, casual workers, often post-school students but because they receive Centrelink's student allowance, they aren't eligible for government disaster relief. So they're thrust to a situation where they can't support themselves, they can't pay rent, so not only is it financially impacting them, it's a huge mental toll.

There is little doubt that has resulted in drastic changes to university teaching and scholarship. Higher education globally has also suffered lockdowns forced to implement distance education almost overnight. The switch to digital communication also required faculty to be available over a wide daily time period to cover student enquiries, etc., from normally large classes, even across three or four time zones in some places in Australia and the USA, disturbing the balance of staff life between work and family. It was assumed that the home study would become the replacement university study, so all faculty could simply be online from their residence, permitting a continued professional presence, including some who were parents with responsibility for home schooling too.

In a study of 1148 academics in the UK, Watermeyer et al. (2020) reported that college/university staff felt they had been dropped with little warning into an almost continual presence on a digital interface not only for scheduled Zoom type tutorials but also round the clock question fielding and support for the weaker students. This for most was an unwelcome intrusion and experience affecting not only the faculty member but also the rest of the family. They were also suddenly faced with the immediate necessity of recording lectures and placing them online for student access and working out how to operate practical and written examinations/assessment procedures. Many college-level instructors without training in online course design resorted to whatever was available and familiar, such as TED Talks, YouTube videos, and massive online open courses (*MOOCs*) as well as 'leaning on' instructional technology colleagues for time-consuming help during a short lead in period when everyone was scrambling to salvage the semester and figure out ways to engage their students from a distance (Bloom et al., 2020).

Yet digital solutions were not without their drawbacks, and some of them were related to security issues (Szente, 2020). Some hackers crashed online class meetings, awkward images were illegally introduced into the material by hackers, and sometimes confidential materials became public. Faculty members had difficulty ensuring the integrity of assessment processes on tests, projects and papers. Institutions with better infrastructures for already existing online distance learning had an obvious advantage, as did the tech-savvy faculty members, who navigated the transition more easily. The most formidable problem was providing practical work experience and internships (Kidd & Murray, 2020; Marinoni et al., 2020). Simulations had various limitations, field placements were unavailable, and opportunities to observe trainee nurses working with patients or early childhood educators teaching were virtually impossible given lockdowns, isolation and social distancing.

As with school students, higher education systems around the world have enforced campus closures to combat the pandemic and these measures have also threatened undergraduate students' basic psychological needs for relatedness, competence and autonomy and the development of intrinsic learning motivation successful learning outcomes. Janke et al. (2022) compared data between the 2018 cohort 1 of prepandemic students and the 2019 cohort 2 affected by closure. Cohort 2 manifested negative developmental trends for competence, relatedness (particularly peer relationships) and intrinsic learning motivation which were not evident in cohort 1. This highlights the importance of preplanning for the amelioration of these personal damaging side effects should closure ever be required again in order to minimise risks of drop out, failure, loss of self-esteem and motivation, as closure and compulsory online learning come with psychological costs among all age groups of students.

Internationally, mental health problems account for about one-third of the world's disability among adults, and these issues escalate during deadly disease outbreaks (Otu et al., 2020). Even before the pandemic, there was a mental health crisis in college students (Shackle, 2019). Forced isolation compounded students' problems because the university experience fundamentally altered for many students, especially undergraduates who were unable to experience a unique life stage of social learning and development and removed the possibility of higher education as a socially immersive and participatory learning experience (Watermeyer et al., 2020). For many students, worries about health and safety made it difficult to concentrate on studies, academic enthusiasm waned and declining hopes of future employment undermined persistence at programme completion.

During Covid lockdowns and quarantines throughout the world, the mental health issues of university and college students were exacerbated (Aristovnik et al., 2020). Among international students, the circumstances frequently were even worse (Stewart et al., 2021). Travel bans were instituted, campus housing faced shutdowns, finances depleted, and visa restrictions became problematic. International students had travelled great distances expecting to be immersed in a new culture and hoping to develop greater proficiency in another language, only to find themselves isolated and working from a computer. In a qualitative study of faculty and students involved in international university programmes, students used the words 'painful', 'heartbroken' and 'crestfallen' to describe their experiences during the lockdown (Peters et al., 2020).

As student support services were curtailed or even discontinued, faculty members were available 24/7 through digital means and were contacted frequently on non-academic issues by needy, stressed, anxious, fearful and panic-stricken students. In one university known to the author, a large number of returning students in February 2022 who unfortunately developed a positive test after arrival were isolated and locked down in several halls of residence and academic staff 'invited to volunteer' to deliver food and other essentials daily to their rooms! This level of assuming responsibility for students' welfare often exceeding their expertise and training, as well as what might be reasonably asked of them, plus associated contractual and legal obligations worried many staff. Nevertheless, respondents in a study of 30,383 students from 62 countries during the first wave of the Covid crisis in early 2020 rated faculty members as the most satisfactory source of support (Aristovnik et al., 2020).

The need to provide more support to their own family members, restructure course delivery, revise policies/programmes/planning, attend to students' needs and support distressed colleagues brought about 'Zoom fatigue' (as it did in employees working from home in Chap. 5), such a pervasive phenomenon that *National Geographic* published an article explaining why the online meetings were so dissatisfying (Sklar, 2020). Online iteration somehow fails to offer the main benefits of face-to-face events which according to Bloom et al. (2020) is the electricity of real-time idea exchange, the expansion of possibilities that come with open debate, plus the connectivity of human warmth and emotion.

Scholarly work has suffered too, so much so that some institutions had to extend research period plans; data collection and analysis were postponed or even abandoned, and some lost support personnel, such as research assistants. Repurposing home offices into online college classrooms, normally places to home school children, impacted on having a time and place to complete scholarly work (Cutri et al., 2020). Annual conferences were forced to cancel these important events in the lives of scholars. The networking and collaborative projects that often are initiated at these gatherings were greatly diminished and some scholarly publishers operating on slim profit margins, faltered and failed.

Wellbeing of Students

Nearly half (46%) of Australian children and students of all ages are at risk adverse effects on their educational outcomes, nutrition, physical movement, social and emotional wellbeing by being physically disconnected from educational establishments. It is already clear that nationally that children and young people are experiencing learning losses. This means that there will not be the expected cognitive gains for these students over the period of learning at home. These losses will cause a delay in cognitive gain and achievement in some students and result in others being lost to the education system. The impacts are particularly evident in:

- The early years, which are critical years for learning, with an established body of research demonstrating the return on investments made in these years,
- Vulnerable students for whom learning loss is difficult to recover,
- Students who are at risk of disengaging or who have disengaged, noting that the longer they are away from school the higher the likelihood that they will never adjust or re-engage,as in now occuring.
- Students from Culturally and Linguistically Diverse (CALD) backgrounds and

- Students undertaking vocational and technology subjects who have been unable to undertake all their required practical or workplace-based components.

More broadly, despite the best efforts, a great many teaching staff have not previously had to develop the specialist skills required to develop and deliver online learning and are required to upskill very quickly, exacerbating the challenge of sustaining the rate of learning and level of engagement.

Children with Special Educational Needs and Disabilities (SENDs)

UK studies reveal that young people with special educational needs and disabilities (SENDs) and their families have been particularly hard hit by the pandemic isolation as sibling conflict perpetrated against siblings with special educational needs and disabilities by other siblings rose considerably during lockdown and school closure (Toseeb et al., 2020a). During the first lockdown, many support networks like speech and language therapy, occupational therapy, mental health support, or specialist school provision were abruptly broken. Parents suddenly had to care for and educate their children all day every day without usual support systems, creating many unmet needs. As a result, young SENDs people and their parent carers experienced high levels of psychological distress during the first UK lockdown (Asbury et al., 2021). An accumulation of such psychological distress is a risk factor for intra-familial conflict, with harsh parenting increasing during the pandemic, likely a result of increased stressors experienced by parents (Lee & Ward, 2020).

In a longitudinal study, Toseeb (2022) investigated sibling conflict in SENDs families during and after the first lockdown in the UK when routines and support networks were almost abandoned. Online questionnaires were completed by 504 parents at four time points between 23 March 2020 and 10 October 2020. As lockdown progressed, SENDs children were more likely to be picked on or physically hurt by their siblings compared with earlier stages of the lockdown. At T1 (beginning of UK lockdown), over half of young people with SENDs were picked on or hurt by their siblings at least once (i.e. any response other than 'never'). At T2, the victimisation rate increased to two-thirds and reached nearly three quarters of the sample by T3. However, at T4 (i.e. when schools fully reopened for face-to-face teaching), there appeared to be a slight decrease in the rate of victimisation of young people with SENDs.

These rates of sibling conflict during the first Covid lockdown in the UK were troublingly high. At their highest level (the third month of lockdown), three out of four of young people with SENDs were being picked on or hurt by their siblings and four out of five were picking on or hurting their siblings on purpose (according to parent and carer reports). At T4, one in five young people were being picked on or hurt by their siblings on most days and one in three picked on or hurt their siblings on most days. These findings have implications for the protection of SENDs children in future pandemic-related lockdowns (Toseeb et al., 2020b). Spending extended periods of time at home together in close proximity with rising stress in all family members providing fuel for expressed aggression, frustration, quarrelling, annoyance, etc., has a not unexpected negative effect on sibling relationships in families but becomes devastating when SENDs are involved. This is supported by the finding that once schools had fully reopened, sibling conflict rates decreased. The scale of the problem, however, should be cause for alarm given that persistent sibling conflict is associated in any case with poor outcomes in the short and long term (Liu et al., 2020; Lopes et al., 2019), specifically in young people with SENDs.

While direct comparisons were not made to typical families, it is likely that the effects observed occurred there but were much more pronounced for families of young people with SENDs due to loss of support from specialist agencies on a daily basis and with rates of social and mental health difficulties tending to be higher than in typical families. In other studies with this sample, parents did report being overwhelmed by having to deal with their child with SENDs all day every day without support and that they suffered psychological distress as a result (Asbury et al., 2021). Taken together, the findings appear to be in line with previous work suggesting that increases in parental distress during the Covid pandemic are associated with increases in conflict within the family (Lee & Ward, 2020). There are vital implications and a signal for many nations in this study for support and planning to assist SENDs families in any future school closures when normal support systems are also in abeyance.

Should Parents Be More Worried About Mental Health Than Covid?

Transitions from primary to secondary school and on to university have always been stressful. So too are the transitions between face-to-face schooling and home distance learning which for many have been traversed several times as peaks and hollows of the contagion reversed policies several times. During this time of sudden changes and uncertainties, the skills it takes to cope with transitions should be embedded into the school curriculum. This would facilitate the transitions caused by Covid. These transitions included having the knowledge that change is part of a typical lifespan, that coping mechanisms used in previous transitions can help cope with future change and understanding the various, strong, emotions which can emerge at times of change. Resources on supporting children and young people, for the public and professionals, have been created by the British Psychological Society (BPS) Covid-19 response group.

The strategies for return to education should include many of the following:

- Safety protocols in place for physical reconnection of a significant number of students and professional staff, as required such as social distancing, hand washing,

- Where full-time reconnection of a significant number is not going to be possible for safety or logistical reasons plan for a blend of online and physical presence through a week,
- Encourage universal full-time onsite attendance for preschool to year 2 nationally,
- Utilise direct and personalised invitations to specific vulnerable school students and their families/carers to see those students attend school and complement this group with invitations to a balanced cohort of students to reduce stigmatisation of specific groups and 'normalise' attendance,
- Invest in targeted and personalised learner engagement for students who are not physically attending and who cannot access online learning, are not engaging in learning or are at risk of disengaging over the short and long term,
- Invest in, and support, teachers to manage the increased workload of teaching both offline and online by providing additional staffing on a short-term basis and with provision for teachers to have time for professional learning to enhance skills in, and implement, online pedagogy for skills and expertise in the creation of non-school-based learning strategies, such as high-quality online content, lower technology radio, as well as television content,
- As soon as health restrictions permit, there is an urgent need to reconnect all students to the context of the school with rapid investment to develop significant capability in schools to deliver education both online and onsite,
- Resources to facilitate learning in the home, e.g. a national hotline for parents supporting their children's learning.

Home Schooling

Some Australian families are now considering home schooling as a permanent option due to the pandemic. In Australia, current data suggest that many students who missed many months schooling particularly during long lockdowns in Victoria and New South Wales are not returning to school during 2020 and 2021. Similar to the *'great resignation'* in the employment field, there is a sort of *'great withdrawal'* in the education field. In NSW, the number of students switched to permanent home schooling by parents rose 28% in 2021, while in Victoria 20% more students were enrolled to learn at home. Even in Queensland which was spared long lockdowns, registrations for home schooling oared by 88% for high school age and by 36% for primary children in 2021. Thus, a small minority of children may never return to the formal school system. There are numerous reasons offered by parents and children for this move to home schooling.

- Firstly, some families were scared to return children to school in case they contracted and brought home the virus to younger siblings and vulnerable grandparents.
- Secondly, there are two groups of parents concerned about 'vaccinations'; one group doesn't want their children vaccinated, objecting to vaccine mandates imposed for school attendance, while the other group doesn't want their children associating with others until all are vaccinated.
- Thirdly some students just refused to go back to school.
- Finally, some parents of younger children felt they did a better job during lockdown than the teachers who sent home boring worksheets day after day. While driven initially by Covid, some of the parents actually found they enjoyed home schooling, found their offspring happier and more relaxed under home tuition and both really enjoyed the extra time together. Others found their children did better at home with individual attention, are able to see where their children are at and understand their current needs particularly those suffering ADHD or anxiety.

So a variety of issues about disruptive lockdowns on their children's education, worries about children's' heath, and some parents enjoyed the teaching time with their children witnessing and experiencing their child's skill and knowledge development are all driving the shift.

Home schooling is not always a totally rosy picture and does possess some negative implications. Parents who now want to move over to home schooling as a deliberate decision after experiencing the process during Covid have to abide by rules and regulations of home schooling. Parents also need to recognise that schools are able to offer a far wider range of other benefits such as physical and social development in dance, music, art and sports. Professor Sciberras (2022) at Deakin University in a Herald Sun news story (Jan 20) (May02) suggests parents ask themselves eight questions before home schooling their children and indicates that research finds 30% of parents educating children at home lost $30,000 income a year, creating a big lifestyle change as more one-on-one learning and family time is required. Thus, there is a considerable loss of income to set against being your child's teacher.

References

ABC News. (2022, August 13). COVID-19 caused millions of school closures. Here's the low-tech solution that is keeping kids in developing nations learning. Retrieved August 13, 2022 from https://www.abc.net.au/news/2022-08-13/phone-learning-developing-nations-covid-19/101326670

Adam, N. L., et al. (2017). Self-regulated learning and online learning: A systematic review. In H. Badioze Zaman, P. Robinson, A. F. Smeaton, ... & N. Mohamad

Ali (Eds.), *Advances in visual informatics*. 10, 645, 143–154. Springer International Publishing. https://doi.org/10.1007/978-3-319-70010-6_14

Adeleke, R. (2020). Digital divide in Nigeria: The role of regional differentials. *African Journal of Science, Technology, Innovation and Development*. https://doi.org/10.1080/20421338.2020.1748335

Alves, R., Lopes, T., & Precioso, J. (2021). Teachers' well-being in times of Covid-19 pandemic: Factors that explain professional well-being. *International Journal of Educational Research and Innovation, 15*, 203–217. https://doi.org/10.46661/ijeri.5120

Ambrose, A. H. (2020). Inequities during COVID-19. *Pediatric, 146*(2), e20201501. https://doi.org/10.1542/peds.2020-1501

Aristovnik, A., Keržič, D., Ravšelj, D., et al. (2020). Impacts of the COVID-19 pandemic on life of higher education students: A global perspective. *Sustainability, 12*(20), 8438. https://doi.org/10.3390/su12208438

Asbury, K., Fox, L., Deniz, E., Code, A., & Toseeb, U. (2021). How is COVID-19 affecting the mental health of children with special educational needs and disabilities and their families? *Journal of Autism and Developmental Disorders., 51*, 1772–1780. https://doi.org/10.1007/s10803-020-04577-2

Australian Institute of Health and Welfare (AIHW). (2016). *National drug strategy household survey. Detailed findings*. Report no.: PHE 214. Retrieved June 20, 2021 from https://www.aihw.gov.au/reports/

Australian Bureau of Statistics (ABS). (2018a). Schools Report. Retrieved June 20, 2021 from https://www.abs.gov.au/statistics/people/education/schools/2018a

Australian Bureau of Statistics (ABS). (2018b). Internet usage report. Retrieved June 20, 2021 from https://www.abs.gov.au/statistics/industry/technology-and-innovation/internet-activity-australia/latest-release

Australian Education Union. (2020). Retrieved October, 17 2020 from https://www.facebook.com/couriermail/posts/queensland-teachers-say-they-are-being-treated-like-glorified-babysitters-and-sa/10157649827702702/

Australian Institute of Health and Welfare. (2021). *Australia's welfare report*. Retrieved January 04, 2022 from https://www.aihw.gov.au/reports/australias-welfare/child-protection

Bagnall, C., Skipper, Y., & Fox, C. (2022). Primary-secondary school transition under Covid 19. *British Journal of Educational Psychology, 92*, 1011–1033. https://doi.org/10.1111/bjep.12485

Bayrakdar, S., & Guveli, A. (2020). Inequalities in home learning and schools' remote teaching provision during the COVID-19 school closure in the UK. *British Sociological Society*. https://doi.org/10.1177/0038038522112244

BBC News Report. (2022, November 07). Child speech delays increase following lockdown. Retrieved November 8, 2022 from https://www.bbc.com/news/education-63373804

Beaunoyer, E., Dupéré, S., & Guitton, M. J. (2020). COVID-19 and digital inequalities: Reciprocal impacts and mitigation strategies. *Computers in Human Behavior, 111*, 106424. https://doi.org/10.1016/j.chb.2020.106424

Bloom, D. A., Reid, J. R., & Cassady, C. I. (2020). Education in the time of COVID-19. *Pediatric Radiology., 12*(20), 8438. https://doi.org/10.1007/s00247-020-04728-8

Bowyer-Crane, C., Bonetti, S., Davies, C., et al. (2021). Early years settings and the COVID-19 pandemic. Research briefing. Retrieved December 04, 2021

from https://www.niesr.ac.uk/wp-content/uploads/2021/10/Early%20Years%20Survey.pdf
British Psychological Society. COVID19 Response Group. Retrieved June 16, 2020 from https://bps.org.uk/coronavirus-resources
Burke, J., & Dempsey, M. (2020). Covid-19 practice in primary schools in Ireland report. *Maynooth: National University of Ireland Maynooth.* Retrieved October 15, 2021 from https://www.maynoothuniversity.ie/education/news/covid-19-practice-primary-schools-report
Cavaliere, G., Trinchese, G., Penna, E., et al. (2019). High-fat diet induces neuroinflammation and mitochondrial impairment in mice cerebral cortex and synaptic fraction. *Frontiers in Cellular Neuroscience, 13*, 509. https://doi.org/10.3389/fncel.2019.00509
Centre for Community Child Health (2022, January) Royal Children's Hospital Melbourne. The impact of the COVID-19 pandemic on children in Australian early childhood education and care. Retrieved April 04, 2022 from https://www.rch.org.au/ccch/
Chanchlani, N., Buchanan, F., & Gill, P. (2020). Addressing the indirect effects of COVID-19 on the health of children and young people. *Canadian Medical Association Journal., 192*, E921–E927. https://doi.org/10.1503/cmaj.201008
Chandra, S., Chang, A., Day, L., et al. (2020). Closing the K–12 digital divide in the age of distance learning. *Common Sense Media, Boston Consulting Group.*
Cho, Y., Weinstein, C. E., & Wicker, F. (2011). Perceived competence and autonomy as moderators of the effects of achievement goal orientations. *Educational Psychology, 31*, 393–411. https://doi.org/10.1080/01443410.2011.560597
Constantin, K. et al. (2018). Anxiety, depression and procrastination among students. *Journal of Rational Emotive & Cognitive Behaviour Therapy, 36*, 15–27. https://doi.org/10.1007/510942-077-0271-5
Cutri, R. M., Mena, J., & Whiting, E. F. (2020). Faculty readiness for online crisis teaching: Transitioning to online teaching during the COVID-19 pandemic. *European Journal of Teacher Education., 43*, 523–541. https://doi.org/10.1080/02619768.2020.1815702
Dabrowski, A. (2020). Teacher wellbeing during a pandemic: Surviving or thriving? *Social Education Research., 2*(1), 35–40. https://doi.org/10.37256/ser.212021588
Davies, C., Hendry, A., Gibson, et al. (2021). Early childhood education and care (ECEC) during COVID-19 boosts growth in language and executive function. *Infant and Child Development, 30*(4), e2241. https://doi.org/10.1002/icd.2241
Dayal, H. & Tiko, L. (2020). When are we going to have the real school? *Australasian Journal of Early Education, 45*, 336–347. https://doi.org/10.1177/1836939120966085
Del Boca, D., Oggero, N., Profeta, P., & Rossi, M. (2020). Women's and men's work, housework and childcare, before and during COVID-19. *Review of Economics of the Household, 18*, 1001–1017. https://doi.org/10.1007/s11150-020-09502-1
Dent, A. L., & Koenka, A. C. (2016). The relation between self-regulated learning and academic achievement across childhood and adolescence: A meta-analysis. *Educational Psychology Review., 28*, 425–474. https://doi.org/10.1007/s10648-015-9320-8

Deoni, S. C., Beauchemin, J., Volpe, A., et al. (2021). Impact of the COVID-19 pandemic on early child cognitive development: initial findings in a longitudinal observational study of child health. medRxiv 2021.08.10.21261846

Di Giorgio, E., Di Riso, D., Mioni, G., & Cellini, N. (2021). The interplay between mothers' and children behavioral and psychological factors during COVID-19: An Italian study. *European Child and Adolescent Psychiatry, 30*(9), 1401–1412. https://doi.org/10.1007/s00787-020-01631-3

Digital Inclusion Index. Retrieved June, 10 2022 from https://www.digitalinclusionindex.org.au/category/2021/

Dong, C., Cao, S., & Li, H. (2020). Young children's online learning during COVID-19 pandemic: Chinese parents' beliefs and attitudes. *Children and Youth Services Review*. https://doi.org/10.1016/j.childyouth.2020.105440

Drane, C., Vernon, L., O'Shea, S., et al. (2021). Vulnerable learners in the age of COVID-19: A scoping review. *The Australian Educational Researcher, 48*, 585–604. https://doi.org/10.1007/s13384-020-00409-5

Empson, J. (2020, May 18). British psychological society psychologist. What do children think is 'normal'? Retrieved July 09, 2020 from https://thepsychologist.bps.org.uk/what-do-children-think-normal

Espinosa, F., Metko, A., Raimondi, M., et al. (2020). A model of support for families of children with autism living in the COVID-19 lockdown: Lessons from Italy. *Behavior Analysis in Practice, 13*(3), 550–558. https://doi.org/10.1007/s40617-020-00438-7

Evans, S., Mikocka-Walus, A., Klas, A., et al. (2020). From "it has stopped our lives" to "spending more time together has strengthened bonds": The varied experiences of Australian families during COVID-19. *Frontiers in Psychology, 11*, 588667. https://doi.org/10.3389/fpsyg.2020.58866

Fortier, M. S., Vallerand, R. J., & Guay, F. (1995). Academic motivation and school performance: Toward a structural model. *Contemporary Educational Psychology., 20*, 257–274. https://doi.org/10.1006/ceps.1995.1017

Freyhofer, S., Ziegler, N., de Jong, E. M., & Schippers, M. C. (2021). Depression and anxiety in times of COVID-19: How coping strategies and loneliness relate to mental health outcomes and academic performance. *Frontiers in Psychology, 12*, 682–684. https://doi.org/10.3389/fpsyg.2021.682684

Garbe, A., Ogurlu, U., Logan, N., et al. (2020). COVID-19 and remote learning. Experiences of parents with children during the pandemic. *American Journal of Qualitative Research, 4*, 45–65. https://doi.org/10.29333/ajqr/8471

Gibson, L. Y., Lockyer, B., Dickerson, J., et al. (2021). Comparison of experiences in two birth cohorts comprising young families with children under four years during the initial COVID-19 lockdown in Australia and the UK: A qualitative study. *International Journal of Environmental Research and Public Health, 18*(17), 9119. https://doi.org/10.3390/ijerph18179119

Goldfeld, S., O'Connor, E., Sung, V., et al. (2022). Potential indirect impacts of the COVID-19 pandemic on children: A narrative review using a community child health lens. *Medical Journal of Australia, 216*, 364–372. https://doi.org/10.5694/mja2.51368

Gonzalez, T., De la Rubia, M., Hincz, K. P., et al. (2020). Influence of COVID-19 confinement on students' performance in higher education. *PLoS ONE, 15*(10), e0239490. https://doi.org/10.1371/journal.pone.0239490

Herald Sun newspaper Melbourne. (2022, May 01). Retrieved May 02, 2022 from www.heraldsun.com.au/news/victoria/pandemic-restrictions-created-generation-of-kids-who-cant-throw-or-catch-research/news-story/d1a84aa9998f190bac47932b1671d712?amp=&nk=7821a2680004942988b479c7329f51b7-1667729285)

Holmes, E. A., O'Connor, R. C., Perry, V. H., et al. (2020). Multidisciplinary research priorities for the COVID-19 pandemic: A call for action for mental health science. *Lancet Psychiatry, 7*, 547–560. https://doi.org/10.1016/S2215-0366(20)30168-1

Howell, A. J., & Watson, D. C. (2007). Procrastination: Associations with achievement goal orientation and learning strategies. *Personality and Individual Differences., 43*, 167–178. https://doi.org/10.1111/bjep.12450Kim

Jakubowski, T. D, & Sitko-Dominik, M. (2021). Teachers' mental health during the first two waves of the COVID-19 pandemic in Poland. *PLoS ONE, 16*, e0257252. https://doi.org/10.1371/journal.pone.0257252

Janke, S., Messerer, L., & Daumiller, M. (2022). Motivational development in times of campus closure: Longitudinal trends in undergraduate students' need satisfaction and intrinsic learning motivation. *British Journal of Educational Psychology, 92*(4), 1582–1596.

Jiao, W. Y., Wang, L. N., Liu, J., et al. (2020). Behavioral and emotional disorders in children during the COVID-19 epidemic. *Journal of Pediatrics, 221*, 264–266. https://doi.org/10.1016/j.jpeds.2020.03.013264-266

Kang, K. T., & Jain, N. (2020). Child abuse and neglect in the covid-19 era: A primer for front-line physicians in British Columbia. *British Columbia Medical Journal, 62*(7), 238–240.

Kidd, W., & Murray, J. (2020). The Covid-19 pandemic and its effects on teacher education in England: How teacher educators moved practicum learning online. *European Journal of Teacher Education., 43*, 542–558. https://doi.org/10.1080/02619768.2020.1820480

Kim, L. E., & Asbury, K. (2020). "Like a rug had been pulled from under you": The impact of COVID-19 on teachers in England during the first six weeks of the UK lockdown. *British Journal of Educational Psychology., 90*, 1062–1083. https://doi.org/10.1111/bjep.12381

Kim, L. E., Oxley, L., & Asbury, K. (2022). "My brain feels like a browser with 100 tabs open": A longitudinal study of teachers' mental health and well-being during the COVID-19 pandemic. *British Journal of Educational Psychology., 92*, 299–318. https://doi.org/10.1111/bjep.12450

Kraft, M., Simon, N., & Lyon, M. (2020). Sustaining a sense of success. Anneberg Institute at Brown University. https://doi.org/10.263000/35nj-v890

Kuehn, B. M. (2020). Surge in child abuse harm during COVID-19 pandemic reported. *JAMA, 324*(7), 621. https://doi.org/10.1001/jama.2020.14433

Lee, S., & Ward, K. (2020). Stress and parenting during the coronavirus pandemic. Retrieved January, 08 2021 from https://www.parentingincontext.org/uploads/8/1/3/1/81318622/research_brief_stressandparenting_during_the_coronavirus_pandemic_final.pdf

Li, F. (2022). Disconnected in a pandemic: COVID-19 outcomes and the digital divide in the United States. *Health Place, 77*, 102867. https://doi.org/10.1016/j.healthplace.2022.102867

Liu, X., Peng, C., Yu, Y., et al. (2020). Association between sub-types of sibling bullying and mental health distress among Chinese children and adolescents. *Frontiers in Psychiatr., 11*, 368. https://doi.org/10.3389/fpsyt.2020.00368

Lopes, P. P., Relva, I. C., & Fernandes, O. M. (2019). Psychopathology and sibling violence in a sample of Portuguese adolescents. *Journal of Child and Adolescent Trauma, 12*, 11–21. https://doi.org/10.1007/s40653-017-0194-4

Marinoni, G., Van't Land, H., & Jensen, T. (2020). The impact of Covid-19 on higher education around the world: IAU global survey report. Paris: International Association of Universities. Retrieved 19 January 2021 from https://www.iau-aiu.net/IMG/pdf/iau_covid19_and_he_survey_report_final_may_2020.pdf

Means, B., Toyama, Y., Murphy, R., & Baki, M. (2013). The effectiveness of online and blended learning: a meta-analysis of the empirical literature. *Teachers College Record, 115*(3), 1–47. Online at: http://www.sri.com/sites/default/files/publications/effectiveness_of_online_and_blended_learning.pdf

Mengin, A., Alle, M. C., Rolling, J., et al. (2020). Psychopathological consequences of confinement. *Encephale, 46*, 43–52. https://doi.org/10.1016/j.encep.2020.04.007

Merrill, K., William, T., Joyce, K. M., et al. (2021). Potential psychosocial impact of COVID-19 on children: A scoping review of pandemics & epidemics. *Journal of Global Health Report., 4*, e2020106. https://doi.org/10.29392/001c.18229

Murdoch Children's Research Institute. Report (2022, January 01). Indirect impacts of COVID-19 pandemic take significant toll on children Retrieved March 16, 2022 from https://www.mcri.edu.au/news-stories/indirect-impacts-covid-19-pandemic-take-significant-toll-children

Ofsted Chief Inspector's Report (2021, December 07). Retrieved March 27, 2022 from https://www.gov.uk/government/news/ofsted-annual-report-we-must-do-all-we-can-to-make-sure-this-generation-is-not-denied-its-opportunities

Orygen and Mission Australia. https://www.orygen.org.au/About/News-And-Events/2022

O'Shea, S., Delahunty, J., & Gigliotti, A. (2020). Consumer or collaborator: Exploring a 'students as partners' approach to delivering effective support and outreach programs. In K. Megan, & H. Huijser (Eds.), *Student support services: Exploring impact on student engagement, experience and learning*. Springer.

Otu, A., Charles, C. H., & Yaya, S. (2020). Mental health and psychosocial well-being during the COVID-19 pandemic: The invisible elephant in the room. *International Journal of Mental Health Systems., 14*, 1–5. https://doi.org/10.1186/s13033-020-00371-w

Ozamiz-Etxebarria, N., Berasategi, N., Idoiaga, N. et al. (2020). The Psychological state of teachers during the COVID-19 crisis: The challenge of returning to face-to-face teaching. *Frontiers in Psychology, 11*. https://doi.org/10.3389/fpsyg.2020.620718

Pascal, C., Bertram, T., Cullinane, C., & Holt-White, E. (2020). COVID-19 and social mobility. Impact Brief #4: Early Years. The Sutton Trust. Retrieved July 16, 2021 from https://dera.ioe.ac.uk/35885/1/Early-YearsImpact-Brief.pdf

Pelikan, E. R., Lüftenegger, M., Holzer, J. et al. (2021). Learning during COVID-19: the role of self-regulated learning, motivation, and procrastination for perceived competence. *Zeitschrift für Erziehungswissenscha, 24*(2), 393–418. https://doi.org/10.1007/s11618-021-01002-x

Pessley, T. (2021). Factors contributing to teacher burnout during COVID-19. *Educational Researcher, 50*(5). https://doi.org/10.3102/0013189X211004138

Peters, M. A., Wang, H., Ogunniran, M. O., et al. (2020). China's internationalized higher education during COVID-19: Collective student autoethnography. *Postdigital Science and Education, 2,* 968–988. https://link.springer.com/content/pdf/10.1007/s42438-020-00128-1.pdf

Pew Center Report. (2021). Retrieved September 26, 2021 from https://www.pewresearch.org/fact-tank/2021/04/02/7-of-americans-dont-use-the-internet-who-are-they/

Pöysä, S., Pakarinen, E., & Lerkkanen, M. K. (2021). Patterns of teachers' occupational well-being during the COVID-19 pandemic: Relations to experiences of exhaustion, recovery, and interactional styles of teaching. *Frontiers Edu*cation, *6*, 699785. https://doi.org/10.3389/feduc.2021.699785

Quartz, J. (2016). Nigeria's mobile data are prices are finally starting to come down. Retrieved October 20, 2021 from https://qz.com/africa/691930/nigeria-could-be-on-the-verge-of-a-mobile-data-price-revolution/

Rasmitadila, A. R., Rachmadtullah, R., Samsudin, A., et al. (2020). The Perceptions of primary school teachers of online learning during the COVID-19 Pandemic period: A case study in Indonesia. *Journal of Ethnic and Cultural Studies, 7*(2), 90–109. https://doi.org/10.29333/ejecs/388

Reimers, F. M., & Schleicher, A. (2020). A framework to guide an education response to the COVID-19 Pandemic of 2020. OECD. Retrieved May 07, 2021 from https://read.oecd-ilibrary.org/view/?ref=126_126988-t63lxosohs&title=A-framework-to-guide-an-education-response-to-the-Covid-19-Pandemic-of-2020

Sciberras, E. (2022, January 20). Eight questions to ask yourself before home schooling your kids. Retrieved March 30, 2022 from https://www.heraldsun.com.au/smart/news-story

Sciberras, E., Patel, P., Stokes, M. A. et al. (2020). Physical health, media use, and mental health in children and adolescents with ADHD during the COVID-19 pandemic in Australia. *Journal of Attention Disorders, 26*(4), 549–562. https://doi.org/10.1177/1087054720978549

Shackle, S. (2019, September 27). The way universities are run is making us ill: Inside the student mental health crisis. *The Guardian*. Retrieved February 02, 2020 from https://www.theguardian.com/society/2019/sep/27/anxiety-mental-breakdowns-depression-uk-students?utm_source=pocket-newtab

Simonson, M., & Berg, G. (2016). Distance learning. Retrieved August 27, 2021 from https://www.britannica.com/topic/distance-learning

Simpkins, S. D., Fredricks, J. A., & Eccles, J. S. (2015). Families, schools, and developing achievement-related motivations and engagement. In J. E. Grusec, & P. D. Hastings (Eds.), *Handbook of socialisation: Theory and research* (pp. 614–636). Guilford Press.

Singh, P., Singh, S., Sohal, M., et al. (2020). Psychological fear and anxiety caused by COVID-19: Insights from twitter analytics. *Asian Journal of Psychiatry, 54*, 102280. https://doi.org/10.1016/j.ajp.2020.102280

Sklar, J. (2020). 'Zoom fatigue' is taxing the brain. Here's why that happens. *National Geographic*. Retrieved July 07, 2020 from https://www.nationalgeographic.com/science/2020/04/coronavirus-zoom-fatigue-is-taxing-the-brain-here-is-why-that-happens/

Steel, P., & Klingsieck, K. (2016). Academic procrastination: psychological antecedents revisited. *Australian Psychologist, 51,* 36–46. https://doi.org/10.1111/ap.12173

Stewart, D. W., Davoren, A. K., Neumeister, J. R., et al. (2021). Graduate schools respond to COVID-19: Promising pathways to innovation and sustainability in stem education (White Paper). *NORC/University of Chicago. NORC COVID Executive Summary 2021st*

Szente, J. (2020). Live virtual sessions with toddlers and preschoolers amid COVID-19: Implications for early childhood teacher education. *Journal of Technology and Teacher Education, 28*(2), 373–380. Retrieved January 08, 2021 from https://eric.ed.gov/?=EJ257409

TeacherTapp. (2021). Lockdown 2.0: What do we know so far? *TeacherTapp*. Retrieved April 13, 2022 from https://teachertapp.co.uk/lockdown-2-0-what-do-we-know-so-far/

Thomas, J., Barraket, J., Wilson, C. K. et al. (2021). Measuring Australia's digital divide: The Australian digital inclusion index 2019. Melbourne: *RMIT University and Swinburne University of Technology, for Telstra*. https://doi.org/10.25916/phgw-b725

Toseeb, U. (2022). Sibling conflict during COVID-19 in families with special educational needs and disabilities. *British Journal of Educational Psychology, 92*, 319–339. https://doi.org/10.1111/bjep.12451Toseeb

Toseeb, U., Asbury, K., Code, A., et al. (2020a). Supporting families with children with special educational needs and disabilities during COVID-19. *PsyArXiv*. https://doi.org/10.31234/osf.io/tm69k

Toseeb, U., McChesney, G., Oldfield, J., & Wolke, D. (2020b). Sibling bullying in middle childhood is associated with psychosocial difficulties in early adolescence: The case of individuals with autism spectrum disorder. *Journal of Autism and Developmental Disorder, 50*, 1457–1469. https://doi.org/10.1007/s10803-019-04116-8

Trust, T., & Whalen, J. (2020). Should teachers be trained in emergency remote teaching? Lessons learned from the COVID-19 Pandemic. *Journal of Technology and Teacher Education, 28*(2), 189–199. Retrieved May 15, 2021 from https://www.learntechlib.org/primary/p/215995/

UNESCO. (2020b). World education blog. UNESCO. Retrieved April 09, 2022 from https://gemreportunesco.wordpress.com/2020b/03/24/how-are-countries-addressing-the-covid-19-challenges-in-education-a-snapshot-of-policy-measures/

UNESCO. (2020a). COVID-19 educational disruption and response. UNESCO. Retrieved April 09, 2022 from https://en.unesco.org/news/COVID-19-educational-disruption-and-response

United Nations. (2020). Policy brief: The impact of COVID-19 on children. Retrieved April 09, 2022 from https://unsdg.un.org/resources/policy-brief-impact-covid-19-children

Victoria University Report. (2022). Lockdown-forced hiatus that has created a generation of kids with poor motor skills. Retrieved November 02, 2022 from www.heraldsun.com.au/news/victoria/pandemic

Walters, T., Simkiss, N., Snowden, R., & Gray, N. (2022). Secondary school students' perception of on-line teaching experience during Covid 19. *British Journal of Educational Psychology, 92*, 843–860. https://doi.org/10.1111/bjep.12475

Watermeyer, R., Crick, T., Knight, C., & Goodall, J. (2020). COVID-19 and digital disruption in UK universities: Afflictions and affordances of emergency online migration. *Higher Education, 81*(3), 623–641. https://doi.org/10.1007/s10734-020-00561-y

Watson, M., Sarica, S., Parkinson, J., et al. (2020). COVID-19 Early Years Resilience and Impact Survey (CEYRIS). In E. M. Westrupp, C. Bennett, Berkowitz, et al. (Eds.) (2021), Child, parent, and family mental health and functioning in Australia during COVID-19: comparison to pre-pandemic data. *European Child Adolescent Psychiatry*, 1–14. https://doi.org/10.1007/s00787-021-01861-z

Xafis, V., Schaefer, G. O., Labude, M. K., et al. (2020). The perfect moral storm: Diverse ethical considerations in the COVID-19 pandemic. *Asian Bioethics Review, 12*, 65–83. https://doi.org/10.1007/s41649-020-00125-3

Xafis, V. (2020). 'What is inconvenient for you is life-saving for me': How health inequities are playing out during the COVID-19 pandemic. *Asian Bioethics Review, 12*, 223–234. https://doi.org/10.1007/s41649-020-00119-1

Yu, X., Chen, Y., Yang, C., et al. (2022). How does parental involvement matter for children's academic achievement during school closure in primary school? *British Journal of Educational Psychology, 92*(4), 1621–1637.

Zhoc, K., Cai, Y., Yeung, S. S., & Shan, J. (2022). Subjective wellbeing and emotion regulation strategies: How are they associated with student engagement in online learning during Covid-19? *British Journal of Educational Psychology, 92*(4), 1537–1549.

Zhu, X., & Liu, J. (2020). Education in and after Covid-19. Immediate responses and long-term visions. *Postdigital Science and Educational, 2*(3), 95–9. https://doi.org/10.1007/s42438-020-00126-3

Zimmerman, B. J. (2000). Attaining self-regulation: A social cognitive perspective. In M. Boekaerts, P. R. Pintrich, & M. Zeidner (Eds.), *Handbook of self-regulation* (pp. 13–39). Academic Press. https://doi.org/10.1016/B978-012109890-2/50031-7

CHAPTER 8

Personal Pandemonium: Stress and Mental Health

Abstract A review of the effects of Covid on individual stress and mental health is offered, indicating the major immediate and long-term concerns for all age groups of society across many nations. An outline of what stress is and how it affects the body physiologically and emotionally is provided. The stress appears to derive from fear of the infection but more so from the drastic change in life due to public health orders and the overwhelming of health services. Rises of anxiety and depression levels are noted worldwide as are the increased burnout of healthcare staff. Domestic violence and suicidal intentions show considerable increase over previous years. The thrust towards online medical and psychological support has proved beneficial. Activities to reduce stress conclude the chapter.

Keyword Stress · Mental health · Domestic violence · Online support · Coping strategies

Stress

Stress and mental health are sometimes the hidden harmful impacts from Covid triggering a lot of trauma and anxiety around the world. When something is encountered that is new, unexpected or potentially threatening, like the virus, imposing rapid change on how we live, it is like a fire alarm, alerting us to potential problems and mobilising resources to deal with it. The result is a change in the general level of arousal or activation, which can range from high levels, under stress and fear, to low levels when the environment makes

© The Author(s), under exclusive license to Springer Nature Singapore Pte Ltd. 2023

R. B. Burns, *The Human Impact of the COVID-19 Pandemic*,
https://doi.org/10.1007/978-981-99-1710-5_8

no demands at all. But with increasing demand, human performance breaks down.

We often think of stress as being a largely mental state; but stress is not just a thought in our heads but a physical response in our body to a perceived threat. Thousands of years ago, this stress kept us alive by flooding our bodies with cortisol and adrenaline in large enough amounts to escape attacking animals or tribes, enabling flight or fight. In modern times, our most stressful life events are much different, but our bodies respond the same way and sometimes that can lead to mental distress and illness.

A working definition of stress is '*any demand perceived by the individual that requires some kind of physical or emotional readjustment*'. Cox (1981) advanced views in which stress is seen as the lack of compatibility between the demands of the environment and what one feels capable of in responding to that demand. This model would seem to be eminently acceptable as stress is an individual experience, i.e. '*I make my own stress by the way I view and interpret the events in my life*'. Selye (1976) acknowledged that stress impacts each individual differently. What one person considers to be a severely stressful situation, another person may experience as only mildly distressing.

For example, in one experiment, psychologists attempted to study the stress reaction in soldiers undergoing combat training using live ammunition. They were surprised at the apparently low levels of stress associated with the combat training. The trainees simply refused to believe that the army would place them in a position where they could get hurt. They believed (falsely) that being perched precariously in a tree with bullets whizzing all around ('sniper training') must be safer than it seems or the army would not permit it.

The study of stress has had a long history in psychology, including Selye's (1976) General Adaptation Syndrome (*GAS*) exposition and studies of the effects of the accumulation of stress events by Holmes and Rahe (1967).

Biochemical Responses to Stress: The General Adaptation Syndrome (GAS)

Often, we are first alerted that a situation is threatening by one of the many side effects of stress; our heart rate increases, we may feel shaky or faint, we become aware of goosebumps on the skin and need the toilet, among other physical symptoms. While conducting experiments relating to hormone production, Selye noticed that his subjects showed a similar set of side effects regardless of the type of life-threatening stimulus that researchers presented to them. He became the first scientist to identify collectively these side effects as all being the result of '*stress*', a term that did not even exist until 100 years ago.

Selye (op cit.) termed this collection of responses the G*eneral Adaptation Syndrome* (*GAS*), a specific three-stage sequence of biological reactions, *alarm, resistance and exhaustion* that constitutes the body's standardised response to stress, which prepare, or adapt, the body for danger so that we are ready to stand a better chance of surviving it. This system evolved to cope well in paleolithic times with sudden and brief stressors, such as escaping attack by a predatory sabre toothed tiger. But the biological reactions don't seem designed to handle continuous or chronic stress such as accumulating and lasting complex of impacts like fear of contagion, social isolation, unemployment, travel restrictions, children's home education added to those of normal everyday stressors like work pressures, relationship pressures, crowding, noise and crime.

All this creates lasting detrimental effect of ongoing and increasing stress that keeps many people unable to escape from the third stage of exhaustion with concomitant stress-induced health problems. Struggling with prolonged stress in the exhaustion stage drains physical, emotional, and mental resources to the point where your body no longer has strength to fight stress. Feeling your situation hopeless, fatigue, burnout, depression and anxiety set in. This prolonged mental stress also raises the risk for chronic high blood pressure, stroke, and heart disease, as well as a higher risk for infections and cancer due to a weaker immune system. The longer you have to deal with stress, the more harmful it is to your health.

Life Events

The first systematic attempt to qualify the degree of stress associated with various events in life was developed by Holmes and Rahe (1967). Studies of personal histories suggest that physical and emotional disorders tend to cluster around periods of major change in a person's life. The Covid outbreak is typical event that caused major changes in most peoples' lives.

Psychiatrists Holmes and Rahe decided to study the links between stress and illness by examining medical records of over 5000 patients and focussed specifically on which of 43 common life events they'd experience in the previous two years. That allowed Holmes and Rahe to work out the relative 'weights' or stressfulness (called *Life Change Units*, or *LCUs*) of different events. These 43 life events were placed in order of scale of impact by the units assigned to each event to form *The Life Change Stress Index* (Holmes & Rahe, 1967). This survey works via a point accumulation score which then gives an assessment of risk, i.e. the point at which someone's combined stress load was likely to put them at risk. Among the top eight events on the scale of impact are '*death of spouse—100 units*', '*death of family member—63 units*', '*personal illness—53 units*' and '*job loss—47 units*'. All these stressful life events are relevant for many families in the current Covid context.

Studies using the *Life Change Stress Index* have found a consistent relationship between the number of stressful events in a person's life and the person's emotional and physical health. When the life change units for each event impacting are added and reach 200 plus, more than half the people had health and mental stress issues within a year; a score of 300 or more predicts an 80% chance of health breakdown the following year. The most stressful event on the scale is the death of spouse, a loss that requires an obvious major adjustment to life. In a UK study, 4500 widowers were observed for 6 months after bereavement, and in addition to high rates of ill health and depression, these men had a mortality rate 40% higher than expected for their age (Bowling, 1987). The more critical the changes in an individual's life, the greater the effort it takes to adapt; this exhaustion effort is presumed to lower the body's natural resistance to disease.

What is the explanatory link between life events and stress? Firstly, many life events are undesirable (e.g. death of a relative), but they also have a second element, which is the impact of change; just the fact that something has altered. What matters most as a stressor is change per se and not undesirability, particularly if the change requires major psychological readjustment or reformulation of identity as involved in becoming a widow, or becoming unemployed, or the sudden life impacting changes of imposed quarantine and isolation. Obviously, these occurrences affect self-image and perceived ability to cope with what had been the accepted routines of life. If we lose our job, or a relative who was very close to us, or we end up isolated learning to live in a different world on the wrong end of a border shutdown, our identity structure becomes fractured, and we now have to rethink ourselves. Such changes require major psychological readjustment and that is what we find most difficult to cope with.

Two Important Personality Factors

Two personality factors that seem to have an influence on how stressful a person will judge an event are *low self-concept* and *external locus of control.*

Low self-concept persons generally have a poor opinion of themselves, lack confidence, feel incompetent, have low resilience and hold many negative beliefs about themselves. Thus, many events that occur in their lives are perceived and interpreted as more stressful than a person with a *high self-concept* who believe in their ability to cope and see life as a source of potential opportunity (Burns, 1982).

Locus of control refers to the degree of control a person thinks they have over what happens to them. Those with an *external locus* believe what happens to them is out of their control and determined by external agencies such as powerful others or outside events. Stressors therefore have much more influence on their thinking and behaviour increasing the stress of the event in that they may feel absolutely helpless believing nothing they can do will alter the outcome.

Both low self-esteem and external locus of control can develop into *learned helplessness*. This obviously can occur with harmful and distressing situations like those met with in many aspects of the pandemic. Depression and anxiety can also emerge frequently as significant symptoms characteristic of the person with learned helplessness when they believe they have no control. This combination of anxiety, depression and believing in an inability to have some control over the environment can even lead to suicidal thoughts. '*I might as well give up'* or *'all I can see ahead is continuing upset in my life that I don't want'*. Lockdowns, restriction of movement, isolation, loneliness, job loss and mask wearing in various combinations can wear people down as they can't see how it will change and control of these issues is all in the hands of '*the authorities*' not themselves.

Stress Itself Is a Cause of Stress

Once emotional responses start to build up by repetition to some event, the response will generalise to other events. It is like child developing a fear of a neighbour's dog, which leads to a fear response to any dog seen nearby, or even any four-legged animal, in other words, a *generalised conditioned response.* The person starts responding automatically in terms of the emotion rather than a sensible rational appraisal of the event. So a person with low self-esteem will constantly feel under pressure since every event can become a cue for the activation of the sense of inferiority and inability to cope.

Psychological stress soon converts to physiological stress (see Selye above). For example, anxiety over fear of catching Covid can produce muscular tension which brings tiredness and fatigue. This defeats a vicious circle creating less resistance to bugs leaving the person with less vitality to cope. As well as anxiety and depression, another major stress reaction is anger when authorities issue rulings which we perceive as unfair but cannot alter. This anger and resentment may not be able to be expressed and builds up creating peptic ulcers, headaches, asthma and other psychosomatic illness. Obviously, there are considerable differences between individuals in what they each perceive as stressors depending on their previous life experiences and their learned expectations of ability to cope.

Burnout

This is another important stress response work-related illness first noticed by Freudenberger (1974). It was only in the 1980s that evaluation criteria for the syndrome became available, through the design of a standard measurement instrument, the *Maslach Burnout Inventory or MBI.* Burnout is a progressively developed psycho-social syndrome, the result of a relationship with the environment that the person appraises as significant for their self-concept, identity and wellbeing but where the demands tax or exceed available coping resources. A person will be psychologically vulnerable to a specific situation if they do not possess sufficient coping resources to handle it adequately, and if at the same time, they place considerable importance on the threat implicit in the consequences of this inadequate handling. This can be very relevant in a medical situation like Covid with its heavy demands on medical and nursing staff where, in many countries, resources are not commensurate with the demands, leaving staff emotionally and psychically exhausted, with diminished personal accomplishment at work, doubting their own capacity to carry out tasks and to interact with clients for whom they have a duty of care, feeling unhappy or dissatisfied with the results obtained, ultimately tacitly acknowledging they are not doing a good job and eventually unable to continue working.

Types of Illness Caused by the Most Stressful Life Events

The types of illness that top stressors can cause are not particularly surprising. They include

- High blood pressure, heart disease, severe asthma and increasing mental illness, including schizophrenia.
- *Depression and anxiety* : Stress increases the chances of developing depression and anxiety by as much as 80%.
- *Obesity*: Excess levels of cortisol, the stress hormone that floods our body during stress causes fatty deposits around the mid-section when stress becomes chronic.
- *Diabetes*: Stress raises the glucose levels of those with Type 2 diabetes directly. It also seems to increase desire for unhealthy foods and lowered levels of physical activity.
- *Gastrointestinal disorders*: Stress doesn't cause ulcers. It can, however, make gastrointestinal issues worse such as chronic heartburn (or gastroesophageal reflux disease, *GERD*) and irritable bowel syndrome *(IBS)*.
- *Accelerated ageing*: Chronic stress can accelerate the pace of ageing and may be due to stress effects on telomeres, a structure at the end of each chromosome protects against deterioration of that chromosome. Stress shortens telomeres, in effect offering less protection.

It is important to recognise that there are healthy levels of stress that motivate performance and that stress can be caused by happy events, such as readjusting your life upon marriage or the birth of a child. *The issue is not with stress itself but how you perceive and deal with it.*

Threats to Quality of Life and Human Wellbeing

Without a doubt, quality of life and wellbeing worldwide have been impacted by the sweeping changes that government and individuals were forced to make within the context of the Covid crisis. Clearly, coping with a world pandemic on a daily basis over an extended period of time can compromise physical and mental health. As the World Health Organization (2020) notes, '*Fear, worry, and stress are normal responses to perceived or real threats, and at times when we are faced with uncertainty or the unknown. So, it is normal and understandable that people are experiencing fear in the context of the COVID pandemic*'. Schimmenti et al. (2020) classified fear into four types that characterise experiences with Covid, viz. (1) ravages to the body, (2) worries about significant others, (3) intolerance of uncertainty and (4) agonising over action/inaction. It is important to understand that anxiety and fear are also associated with grief (see Chap. 9), which is normal and expected following any significant loss or change (Fegert et al., 2020). Worldwide, human beings are not only mourning the loss of life as they knew it but also are experiencing anticipatory loss, defined as the expectation that additional, future losses will occur.

While people often view trauma in the context of one-off disasters such as the Grenfell Tower fire, a tsunami in S. E. Asia, a cyclone hitting the Queensland coast, or '9/11', Covid unfortunately is not a one-off traumatic event. Its effects, medically, economically and psycho-socially, will last for many years, impacting on every aspect of our lives and providing exposure to ongoing trauma with intergenerational impact. The current global pandemic is unprecedented in recent history. The effect this crisis will have on both population mental health, and on frontline healthcare workers in short and long term is striking, with large numbers of research studies across the world revealing similar devastating effects. There is considerable anxiety about potential exposure to infection among the general population and healthcare workers, plus psychological distress about potential and actual loss of loved ones, employment, lockdowns/isolation, home schooling and financial strain in the broader population.

This distress may be further exacerbated in individuals who have experienced prior life traumatic events which have left them vulnerable. In the longer term, grief and trauma are likely to emerge as financial and social impacts become entrenched amplifying the risk of highly increased levels of depression and suicidality. A recent meta-analysis by Bueno-Notivol et al. (2021) estimated that compared to the prevalence of depression in 2017, the current crisis has produced an increase up to seven times the levels of depression in the general population. Furthermore, the changes to normal life have become a major source of anxiety due to mobility restrictions, reduced social connections, fear for access to supplies, loss of family incomes, loss of loved ones, financial strain, social isolation, communication of conspiracy theories and fear for individuals' health conditions and that of their families and are all well-documented correlates of mental health problems (Jakovljevic et al., 2020).

Reports of the mental health impacts of previous severe health epidemics have focussed primarily on disease survivors (e.g. of SARS and Ebola). Almost invariably, these studies show survivors actually experience greater psychological distress post-epidemic (*PTSD*) than others from affected communities. Risk for psychological distress may also be great for people employed in occupations that potentially expose them to infection and in those who have friends or family members who have been infected and some bereaved.

The Impact of Covid on Prevalence of Psychological Disorders Among Adults

Studies from a range of countries that have examined psychological disorders during the pandemic have reported common results in that affected individuals show mental trauma symptoms such as emotional distress, anxiety, depression, stress, mood swings, irritability, insomnia, attention deficit hyperactivity disorder, post-traumatic stress and anger (Brookes et al., 2020; Rubin & Wessely, 2020). Those who follow Covid news the most experience more anxiety (Neria & Sullivan, 2011) because most Covid news is distressing and sometimes associated with rumours, often untrue, which amplify anxiety levels with constant exposure. Misinformation and fabricated reports about Covid can exacerbate depressive symptoms in the general population (Zhou et al., 2020). The publication of the latest positive most accurate information by medical professionals, such as the number of people who have improved and the progress of medications and vaccines, avoiding negative data, can reduce anxiety levels using both standard and alternative communication methods such as social networks and digital communication platforms to prevent social isolation (Bannerjee, 2020).

In a meta-analysis of the existing research works, Salari et al. (2020) measured the prevalence of stress, anxiety and depression in adult samples during the pandemic. They found the prevalence of stress in five studies (total sample size of 9074) as 29.6%, the prevalence of anxiety in 17 studies (sample size of 63,439) as 31.9% and depression in 14 studies (sample size of 44,531) as 33.7% This evidence suggests that the pandemic had in various ways amplified anxiety, anger, confusion and stress to significant levels (Brookes et al., 2020).

Different cohorts of society appear to be afflicted to different degrees by declines in mental health. In recent studies, the prevalence of anxiety and depression and stress during the pandemic is shown to be higher in women than in men (Liu et al., 2020). In Australia, over the last two years there has been a rising flood of all age ranges contacting mental health clinics, recording around a 140% increase over 2021, with women particularly seeking treatment for burnout and chronic stress. Neuroscientists claim women suffer more than men because their brains are wired slightly differently. Women, particularly those who have it all, are more susceptible as they are used to being in control and their neurobiology drives them to solve all problems and keep things moving both at work and home. The pandemic, out of their control, throws up large-scale uncertainty which impacts on their hormones and stress levels.

Another group where the levels of anxiety, depression and stress are significantly higher is the 21–40 age group where, for example in Australia, the mental health of millennials and Gen Z has been badly damaged by the pandemic. Data from major insurer Allianz (28-09-22) show that between 2019 and 2021 there was a 17% increase in psychological injury claims from millennials (26–41 years) and a 27.8 increase from Gen Z (10–25 years). Allianz predicts that by 2030 the relic effects of mental health issues will account for half of workplace injuries as mental health takes longer to treat and requires longer time off work than physical injury. The main reason for this seems to be that this age group is concerned over future consequences and economic challenges caused by the pandemic, as they are key active working forces in society and are therefore mostly affected by redundancies and business closures (Huang & Zhao, 2020). Some researchers have argued that a greater anxiety among young people may be due to their greater access to information through social media, which can also cause stress (Cheng et al., 2014).

Another positive correlation arising from research lies between higher education levels and higher levels of anxiety and depression levels (Wang et al., 2020a, 2020b). A Chinese study revealed higher prevalence of mental stress was associated with those with higher levels of education possessing high self-awareness of their own health (Zhang & Ma, 2020). In addition, anxiety levels are significantly higher in people with at least one family member, relative or a friend with Covid (Cao et al., 2020; Moghanibashi-Mansourieh, 2020). Other revealed associations occur between medical history and increased anxiety and depression caused by the Covid spread where those who have a history of medical problems and also suffering from poor health may feel more vulnerable to a new disease with increased psychiatric distress levels (Mazza et al., 2020).

The psychological effects of the contagion are not limited to the fear of contracting the virus but from effects derived from separation from loved ones, loss of freedom and movement, uncertainty about the trajectory of the disease and the feeling of helplessness (Cao et al., 2020). These latter aspects can lead to dramatic consequences, such as the rise of suicidal behaviours among people who lived/live in the most affected areas (Kawohl & Nordt, 2020; Mamun & Griffiths, 2020). In the light of these consequences, a careful evaluation of the potential benefits of quarantine/lockdown should have occurred taking into account the high psychological, social and economic costs (Mazza et al., 2020). This cost–benefit issue will be covered in depth in discussion of ethical and moral implications of national government actions in Chap. 10.

In a meta-analysis of adults in the UK, Fancourt et al. (2021) aimed to explore the trajectories of anxiety and depression over the first 20 weeks after lockdown was announced in England end March 2020, with data from over 70,000 adults. Being a woman or younger, having lower educational attainment, lower income, or pre-existing mental health conditions and living alone or with children were all risk factors for higher levels of anxiety and depression during the early part of lockdown. Some of these impacts reduced as lockdown continued, although these differences were still evident 20 weeks after the start of lockdown.

These data suggest that the highest levels of depression and anxiety occurred in the early stages of lockdown but declined fairly rapidly, possibly because individuals adapted to circumstances. The findings emphasise the importance of supporting individuals in the lead-up to future lockdowns to try to reduce distress and highlight that groups already at risk for poor mental health before the pandemic have remained at high risk throughout lockdown and its aftermath.

Dawel et al. (2020) investigated the effects of Covid on mental health and wellbeing of a representative sample from the Australian population also at the early phase of the pandemic. Depression, anxiety and psychological wellbeing were measured with well-validated scales. Pandemic-induced impairments in work and social functioning were strongly associated with elevated depression and anxiety symptoms, as well as decreased psychological wellbeing. The Dawel et al. (2020) study also found well-established risk factors for poorer mental health among younger age groups particularly females and having a pre-existing mental health condition was associated with increased risk within the pandemic context, but catching Covid did not appear to create anxiety. Governments should consider additional measures to monitor and support these at-risk groups.

Overall the Australian Dawel study highlights that pandemics may cause serious problems for community mental health in the early phase of disease, similarly to the UK Fancourt results noted above. They are also consistent with another UK-based study where citizens were more concerned about how societal changes will impact their psychological and financial wellbeing, than becoming unwell with the virus (Holmes et al., 2020). This finding is also consistent with emergent work indicating that loneliness is playing a central role in the observed mental health impacts of the Covid pandemic (Palgi et al., 2020). Catching the virus seems to be the least of the worrying problems!

In June 2020, 40.9% of 5412 US adults in a nationally representative survey study reported having experienced, attributed to Covid, adverse mental or behavioural health symptoms, including those of an anxiety or depressive disorder (30.9%), a trauma- and stressor-related disorder (26.3%), having started or increased substance use (e.g. alcohol, legal or illegal drugs, or prescriptions drugs that are taken in a way not recommended by a doctor) to cope with stress or emotions related to Covid (13.3%) and having seriously considered suicide (10.7%) (Czeisler et al., 2020, 2021). In the USA, data recently released by the Centres for Disease Control and Prevention (2021) report that in 2020 the proportion of mental health-related emergency department visits among adolescents rose 31% compared with the previous year.

Since then, a study of the electronic health records of nearly 70 million patients from 54 healthcare organisations in the USA found that 18.1% of patients hospitalised for Covid were diagnosed with a psychiatric condition in the 14 to 90 days following Covid diagnosis, including 5.8% who received first-time psychiatric diagnosis (Mahase, 2020). By comparison, less than half the percentage (2.8%) of individuals from a matched cohort of hospitalised influenza patients were diagnosed with a psychiatric condition in the same interval.

In 2021, American workers across the board saw heightened rates of burnout, and according to APA's 2021 Work and Wellbeing Survey of 1501 US adult workers, 79% of employees had experienced work-related stress in the month before the survey. Nearly 60% employees reported negative impacts of work-related stress, including lack of interest, motivation, or energy (26%) and lack of effort at work (19%). Meanwhile, 36% reported cognitive weariness, 32% reported emotional exhaustion, and an astounding 44% reported physical fatigue, a 38% increase since 2019. Income affected the prevalence of both anxiety and depressive disorder symptoms which were nearly double among those with a household income of less than $25,000 versus $200,000 or more (30.8% versus 17.0%, respectively), consistent with prepandemic evidence that low household income was associated with increased incidence of mood disorders (Sareen et al., 2011) Wealth may also be a factor, as having less than $5000 in savings was associated with increased odds of depression during the pandemic compared to those with at least $5000 in savings (Ettman et al., 2020).

Essential workers in the USA also experienced worse adverse mental and behavioural health compared to other employed respondents, with more than twice the prevalence of having started or increased substance use (24.7% versus 10.5%, respectively) and nearly 3 times the prevalence of serious suicidal ideation (21.7% versus 7.8%, respectively) (Czeisler et al., 2020). Some occupations are more vulnerable than others to the effects of burnout, with teachers and healthcare workers uniquely prone to high rates of burnout, as was the case even before the pandemic. It's been so much harder to keep up with demands during a pandemic in caretaking professions. Healthcare personnel may face increased psychological distress related to caring for patients with Covid and operating with limited resources that may directly influence patient survival and their own risk for infection. These conditions may be associated with symptoms of depressive or anxiety disorder, insomnia, plus guilt and moral injury in resource-limited settings. Poor mental health and sleep disturbance may be detrimental for the healthcare personnel and their patients, as positive screenings for sleep disorders and anxiety or depression have been associated with increased incidence of adverse safety outcomes by 83% and 63%, respectively (Weaver et al., 2018). Similarly, law enforcement personnel with diagnosed or undiagnosed sleep disorders also had higher odds of serious errors, including making an error or safety violation and uncontrolled anger towards suspects.

Unpaid caregivers for adults are often overlooked as an at-risk population, yet in the USA there was a near-threefold increased prevalence of symptoms of anxiety or depressive disorder and ninefold increased prevalence of suicidal ideation among unpaid caregivers than among non-caregivers (Czeisler et al., 2020). As expected, adverse mental health symptoms were highly prevalent among those with a diagnosed psychiatric disorder in the USA. Most notably, suicidal ideation was present in approximately one quarter of those with anxiety disorder and depressive disorder and nearly half of those with PTSD (Czeisler et al., 2020)

Deleterious Coping Strategies

Early evidence of deleterious financial (and health) coping strategies includes a 54% increase in national sales of alcohol immediately following stay-at-home orders in the USA, with online sales increased 262% from 2019, corresponding to a 14% increase in frequency of alcohol consumption and 41% increase in frequency of heavy drinking for women (Lund et al., 2019; Pollard et al., 2020). There has also been an acute increase in opioid-related overdoses, an acceleration of an epidemic that was already worsening before the pandemic (American Medical Association, 2020).

Simultaneously, firearm purchases have soared during the pandemic, with 17 million new firearm purchases as of the end of October according to estimates from Small Arms Analytics (Beckett, 2020) more than any full year on record. Beyond concerns related to early findings of increased firearm violence and anticipated increased gun murder in the USA, increased prevalence of guns and first-time gun owners may be associated with increased suicides, as more than 60% of US gun deaths are suicides (Schleimer et al., 2020).

While the American Psychological Association's (APA) 2021 data suggest persistent workplace stress has contributed to reduced efficacy and exhaustion, there is also increased cynicism American too, another classic sign of burnout, based around issues like the politicisation of masks and vaccines and feelings of lack of support from the government and workplaces have caused workers especially those in public-facing jobs to become cynical about their jobs. This kind of cynicism is powerful because it undermines the people's feelings about the value of their work, which could have helped motivate them during hard times.

Impact of Covid Among Children and Young People

While much media attention has been focussed on adult self-indulgent calls for freedom and protest marches where they could let off steam and rail against the government on various issues, young people's problems have fallen through the cracks. The Australian National Children's Health and Wellbeing Strategy (2021) indicated that in Australia, half of all adult mental health challenges arise before the age of 14 and many within this age group have been through various impacts of the pandemic which does not augur well for the future mental health of some of them. More than 50% of children currently experiencing mental health problems are not receiving any professional support.

While the past two years in Australia have been taxing for adults, it has been even tougher for young people. Their lives have been disrupted and panicked by extensive bush fires, massive heat waves, flash floods, mouse plagues, climate warming threats, bullying, both physical and online and discussion of suicide and self-harm on some nasty mass media. Into this mix comes a global pandemic with governments and health officials preaching overwhelming hospitalisation and mortality rates from initial unreliable modelling, with long periods of schooling missed with the corollary of lost peer friendship and companionship. Additionally, more children have been exposed to the rising tide of domestic violence that was engendered by weeks of close proximity in lockdown. Without the experience to know that these things come and go in a periodic fashion, the last few years have shunted them through one catastrophe to another, sometimes simultaneously.

Young peoples' mental health appears to be rapidly deteriorating. In mid-2021, Dooley et al. (2022) using a global sample charted the impact of the pandemic on mental health in children. Even after one year, 25% of the global sample experienced elevated depression, while 20% had elevated anxiety. These were double the prepandemic figures. Young people are designed to be social bonding with peers, and exploring the 'world', game to take risks and embrace life; living should be a sequence of first and gradual independence. The pandemic has produced the opposite scenario for many, with cancelled life steps, isolation and the dread of uncertainty. There is no proper database available for presecondary children to act as a guide for potential future problems from a pandemic and its restrictions. But a recent study (Goldfeld et al., 2022) has provided some startling insights suggesting that many children will face a generational defining disruption from Covid, not from the disease itself which has been generally mild, but from under three broad categories of deficits:

- Child-level factors (poorer mental health, poorer child health and development, poorer academic achievement),
- Family-level factors that affect children (poorer parent mental health, reduced family income and job losses, increased household stress, increased abuse and neglect, poorer maternal and newborn health) and
- Service-level factors that affect children (school closures, reduced access to health care, increased use of technology for learning, connection and health care).

These mental and health impacts show up worldwide almost from the start of the pandemic so immediately devastating has it been.

Goldfeld et al. (2022) also noted 20–46% children who experienced a second lockdown registered high levels of mental health issues. Demand for help from Kids Helpline surged by 4.6% per month with a 5.7% increase in help seeking for suicidal ideation and self-harm. They did less exercise with 81 min per day less time outdoors but screen time rose by 55 min per day. Vital milestone health checks were missed, and 31% of unwell children avoided accessing care as parents feared family exposure to the virus. 46% parents reported an impact on their own mental health which undoubtedly would have some impact on home life. Due to increased stress and isolation for families and reduced access to support (child welfare visits; child protection services), the expectation is that there will have been increased levels of family violence and child maltreatment. There is continuing and increasing demand for youth mental health services which cannot be met from an overwhelmed and under-resourced professional workforce. In Australia, a recent report from the Australian Psychological Society (February 2022) revealed that around 30% of psychologists were turning away new patients and waiting times had blown out. de Figueiredo et al. (2021) produced a similar range of impacts in a comprehensive literature review of the effects of Covid on children and adolescents internationally.

The snapshot offered by Goldfield et al. (2022) and de Figueiredo et al. (2021) structured into Fig. 8.1 reveals that the indirect impacts of Covid will likely have broad, long-lasting implications for children, and it is children already experiencing adversity that lose out the most, with the potential for wider health inequities.

In China, an evaluation of 1036 quarantined children and adolescents in an 6–15 age range, revealed 112 presented depression, 196 anxiety and 68 both (Chen et al., 2020a, 2020b). Similarly in India, a high prevalence of psychological distress was evident with quarantined children and adolescents experiencing helplessness (66.11%), worry (68.59%) and fear (61.98%), compared to non-quarantined children (Saurabh & Ranjan, 2020). Moreover, it was also reported in China that children and adolescents aged 3–18 years presented symptoms of inattention, clinging, worry and irritability during this pandemic (Jiao et al., 2020).

Children and young adults are particularly at risk of developing anxious symptoms in the early stages of the pandemic (Orgilés et al., 2020). The research involved a sample of 1143 parents of Italian and Spanish children aged

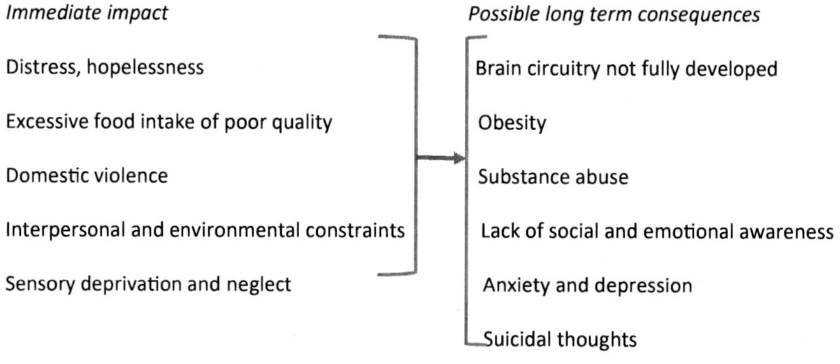

Fig. 8.1 Summary of major immediate and long-term concerns for children and adolescents

3–18. In general, parents observed emotional and behavioural changes in their children during the quarantine: symptoms related to difficulty concentrating (76.6%), boredom (52%), irritability (39%), restlessness (38.8%), nervousness (38%), sense of loneliness (31.3%), uneasiness (30.4%) and worries (30.1%). Chinese data on a sample of college students at the time as the epidemic spread in China showed that anxiety levels were lower where there was family economic and social stability and cohabitation with parents (Cao et al., 2020), but having infected relatives or acquaintances leads to a worsening in anxiety symptoms. The economic problems and the slowdown in academic activities in the EU are related to anxious symptoms in youth (Alvarez et al., 2020).

Children's mental health crises are on the rise in the USA. From March 2020 to October 2020, mental health-related emergency department visits increased 24% for children ages 5–11 and 31% for those ages 12–17 compared with 2019 emergency department visits (Leeb et al., 2020). In a 2020 survey of 1000 US parents around the country facilitated by the Ann & Robert H. Lurie Children's Hospital of Chicago (Lurie Children's Blog), 71% of parents said the pandemic had taken a toll on their child's mental health, and 69% said the pandemic was the worst thing to happen to their child. A US national survey of 3,300 high schoolers conducted in spring 2020 by the APA found close to a third of students felt unhappy and depressed much more than usual (American Psychological Association (APA) 2020 *Trends Report*).

Large-Scale Multinational Studies of Young People

Lockdown conditions due to the pandemic have affected the mental health of youth in Egypt, Ghana, India, Pakistan and the Philippines according to Shaikh et al. (2021). Philippines had the highest mean score in all three domains followed by Egypt, Pakistan, India and then Ghana. There was a significant association of female gender with stress, educational status with depression and anxiety with stress. Students tended to have the highest levels of anxiety, and close friends/family infected with Covid was found to be associated with depression and stress scores. The most common student coping strategy for the Philippines was suicide (a bit of paradoxical coping!!); for Pakistan was religion (Islam); and for Egypt, India and Ghana was acceptance. The highest scores observed in all three domains of stress, anxiety and depression were associated with avoidant coping (i.e. not facing up to the issues and using denial).

A global meta-analysis (Panchal et al., 2021) of 61 research articles comprising over 54,000 children and adolescents (mean age = 11.3 years, 49.7% female) revealed anxiety and depression symptoms were common as well as irritability and anger. Significant risk factors for anxiety were children with special needs and presence of mental disorders before the lockdown, alongside excessive unhelpful media exposure. Important protective factor for anxiety and depression was good parent–child communication and relationships. Another meta-analysis (Bussières, 2021) identified 28 empirical studies worldwide with prospective or retrospective longitudinal data that were included in their quantitative synthesis and produced similar results to Panchal et al. (op cit.). Covid lockdown measures were associated with negative general mental health outcomes among children. Moreover, results did not differ between children from the general population and those from clinical populations such as children with epilepsy, oncology, neurodevelopmental disorders or obesity. Both studies found that children's mental health was less negatively impacted during the early part of the pandemic than at later stages where problems and issues built up.

A third major systematic meta-analysis (Panda et al., 2021) of 22,996 children/adolescents from a total of 15 studies attempted to provide an accurate picture of psychiatric/behavioural problems for the benefit of health and educational authorities to plan appropriate mitigating measures. Between 30 and 40% of children were found to be suffering from one or more symptoms of anxiety, depression, irritability and inattention. At least 22.5% of children had a significant fear of Covid, and 35.2% and 21.3% of children, respectively, had boredom and sleep disturbance. Similarly, 52.3% and 27.4% of caregivers developed anxiety and depression, respectively, while being in isolation with children and this can so easily be modelled by the children. Children with pre-existing behavioural problems like autism and attention deficit hyperactivity disorder had a high probability of their behavioural symptoms worsening. Anxiety, depression, irritability, boredom, inattention and fear of Covid are predominant as psychological problems were made worse during the pandemic.

During the current ongoing Covid pandemic, psychological problems like anxiety, depression, irritability, mood swings, inattention and sleep disturbance appear to be fairly common among quarantined children. UNICEF in its first State of the World's Children Report (2022) notes that the impact of Covid will be a very visible tip of the iceberg in children's mental health outcome and will have continuing disastrous results long after the pandemic has passed. It reports there is a staggering number of young people with mental health problem worldwide with around 89 million boys and 77 million girls aged 10–19 affected. Suicide is the fifth major cause of death in this age group, with the highest prevalence rates in Europe, the Middle East, N. America and N. Africa. Fears about the disease itself added to the dislocation it's caused to education, home life and friendship groups, has also added to the burden of existing issues such as poverty, domestic violence, displaced and homeless persons/families.

Suicide

In Australia, much against an intuitive belief that Covid and the restrictions it has brought would have fired mental health cases among young people through the roof, a paradox of falling death by suicide rate has actually occurred. The decline in suicide rates for youth suicide in 2020 showed a 6.2%

decrease from the previous year. But this did not continue as the pandemic surged in 2021 bringing with it a surge in mental health problems as registered in Lifeline's 2021 records. The Australian Institute of Health and Welfare Report (2021) noted that from May 2020 to February 2021, the weekly volume of mental health-related prescriptions rose above the previous year. There has been a rapid increase in demand for the Australian national Kids Helpline too, with common reasons for contact including mental health (4.6% monthly increase) and suicidal ideation or self-harm (5.7% monthly increase) (Batchelor et al., 2021). Additionally, some children with existing mental health disorders have experienced an exacerbation of symptoms (Evans et al., 2020). Mental health difficulties significantly increased for children who experienced a second lockdown (20–46% in high range; 2–13% in very high range) compared with a normative sample (De Young et al., 2021).

Parent mental distress tripled from 8% before the pandemic to 24% during the pandemic (Broadway et al., 2020), with Lifeline Australia reported its highest volume of calls in its 58-year history in the first week of August 2021, while much of Australia was in lockdown. Mental health needs are rarely prioritised during pandemics, with limited access to trained mental health professionals. In Australia, the benefit of the Australian Government's increase in funding to suicide prevention organisations has paid off as there are more supportive person-to-person 'chats' and interventions being conducted heading off many suicidal intentions. Studies from both the USA and the UK report a substantial decrease in child abuse notifications as school staff account for approximately 21% of child protection referrals. This is because school closures are also combined with an overall decrease in social work home visits and primary care visits, leaving children vulnerable.

Adolescence as a Critical Period

It has been known for several decades that during early childhood and into adolescence, the central nervous system is vulnerable to stressful challenges at the time of critical periods of neural development triggering short and long-term physiological, cognitive and behavioural damage with social isolation in pre-adulthood as a major risk factor for depression in adult life (Danese et al., 2009). Longitudinal studies have significantly correlated the presence of psycho-social stressors such as social isolation during childhood and adolescence with high levels of C-reactive protein (an inflammatory biomarker) later in life (Lacey et al., 2014). Adolescence has also been shown in past studies to be a stress-sensitive developmental window relative to fear regulation with chronic stress impacting the amygdala-prefrontal cortex connectivity and activity, impairing, for instance, the extinction of fear memory so earlier fear experiences can be easily activated and replayed (Tottenham & Galvan, 2016).

These issues raise serious questions about the harmful effects on the developing brain in the context of the pandemic during adolescence. In addition, there is major developmental transition between childhood and adulthood brain circuits that involves maturation in frontal cortical neural systems and in social and affective circuitry that occurs in response to social experiences (e.g. relationships and interactions that a person experiences with others, including that from the same age), socio-economic status and culture (Foulkes & Blakemore, 2018). This transition and learning can be interfered with if social and emotional experiences are restricted.

Adolescence is also the well-known peak age of onset for the most common psychiatric disorders such as attention deficit/hyperactivity disorder, anxiety, depressive mood and schizophrenia (Kessler et al., 2005); it is also a time of high risk for substance abuse and suicidal behaviour. The peak onset of mental illness during the teenage years can also be impacted by the surges of sex hormones.

During adolescent development, the central nervous system undergoes an intense process in the formation and maintenance of synaptic connections and finalisation of myelinisation of nerve networks which guide intellectual, social and emotional behaviour into adulthood modes. From this perspective, the adolescence period is critical for logical thinking and deep learning about the social environment including the comprehension of other people's emotions, intentions and beliefs. For most teenagers, school is one of the most important social environments and one in which peers increasingly affect adolescents' self-concept, wellbeing and behaviour. Social touch is important to human development especially during childhood and adolescence. Even when virtual relationships are established, they cannot cater to all physical needs for contact in the context of quarantine. This poses some questions that only the future can answer. Could social isolation and adversities that inhibited some cognitive, emotional and social learning experiences during the pandemic result in future inability to develop and maintain relational experiences and result in decreased neuronal and synaptic growth in the brain? What will be the effects of this long-term switch to 'virtual contact' on human interactions? During pre-adulthood, adverse experiences can induce long-term impacts on brain development as well as promote mental and behavioural disturbances through neurochemical and physiological mechanisms (De Bellis & Zisk, 2014). The sum of the effects can be devastating, and detection might be several years later.

Psychological and Social Impact of Covid on Healthcare Workers *(HCW)*

Healthcare workers (*HCWs*) at all levels are a segment of population particularly affected by stress (Lai et al., 2020) and are at risk of developing symptoms common in catastrophic situations, such as post-traumatic stress disorder, burnout syndrome, physical and emotional exhaustion, depersonalisation, and dissociation (Grassi & Magnani, 2000; Øyane et al., 2013). However, a pandemic presents different peculiarities compared to a one-off catastrophic event, for instance, the stigmatising attitudes in particular towards health professionals, who are in daily contact with the risk of infection (Brooks et al., 2020). During SARS, up to 50% of healthcare professionals suffered from acute psychological stress, exhaustion and post-traumatic stress, caused by the fear of contagion of their family members and the prolonged social isolation (Maunder et al., 2006). Covid is not likely to be different and even worse due its geographical spread and lengthy period of impact.

Studies from previous infectious disease outbreaks such as SARS and MERS revealed long-term and persistent psychopathological consequences among healthcare workers who reported lack of workplace support and resources leading to acute distress (Tam et al., 2004). SARS and MERS experiences crucially compromised healthcare professionals' wellbeing a warning red flag for the current situation. After SARS, health professionals reported that clear directiveness and support from the supervisors, adequate training, precautionary measures, social, religious and familiar support were the most effective coping strategies (Maunder et al., 2006). During the SARS emergency, personality traits of optimism, resilience and altruism reduced psychological distress among healthcare workers (Lee et al., 2007). After MERS, medical staff reported that strict protective measures, the presence of a cohesive team, positive attitudes in the workplace and the recognition of their efforts by the hospital helped them to face the situation (Khalid et al., 2016). These clear positive approaches did not seem to filter through to this Covid pandemic.

Italian frontline *HCWs* for example have experienced savage increases in workload in a context of uncertainty and powerlessness and are more vulnerable to the infection due to their direct contact with patients, which also increases in turn their concerning about infecting their families and colleagues (Liu et al., 2020). By the end of April 2020, about 12,000 doctors and nurses were infected by Covid, and 228 doctors and 26 nurses had died (Fusaroli et al., 2020; Manzoni & Milillo, 2020).

In line with these results, Rossi et al. (2020) evaluated mental health outcomes among *HCW* in Italy during the pandemic, confirming a high increase in mental health issues, particularly among young women and frontline workers, with women more likely to be affect by anxiety, depression and distress. A relationship was found by Liang et al. (2020) in China between age and depressive symptoms associated with the pandemic where younger medical staff (< 30 years) reported higher self-rated depression scores and more concern about infecting their families than older staff, while those > 50 years of age reported increased stress due to patient death, the prolonged work hours and the lack of personal protective equipment. Other early studies as Covid spread across Asia were consistent too revealing HCW in India who were overworked suffered high levels of psychophysical stress (Mohindra et al., 2020), and data from Lai et al. (2020) in China on 1257 HCW who assisted patients in Covid wards and other understaffed wards showed high percentages of depression (50%), anxiety (44.6%), insomnia (34%) and distress (71.5%). Also, the constant fear of contagion leads to obsessive thoughts (Brooks et al.,

2020), increasing the progressive closure of the person and reducing social relationships.

A study by Giusti et al. (2020) sought to assess the prevalence of burnout and psychopathological conditions in three hundred and thirty North Italian health professionals and identify socio-demographic, work-related and psychological predictors of burnout, employing an online anonymous survey. The results revealed a startling amount of health disruption as they worked obviously highly worried within a Covid health context. Two hundred and thirty-five health professionals (71.2%) had scores of anxiety above the clinical cut-off, 88 (26.8%) had clinical levels of depression, 103 (31.3%) of anxiety, 113 (34.3%) of stress and 121 (36.7%) of post-traumatic stress. Regarding burnout, 107 (35.7%) had moderate and 105 (31.9%) severe levels of emotional exhaustion; 46 (14.0%) had moderate and 40 (12.1%) severe levels of depersonalisation; 132 (40.1%) had moderate and 113 (34.3%) severe levels of reduced personal accomplishment. Predictors of burnout were work hours, psychological co-morbidities, fear of infection and perceived level of support by friends. Predictors of both emotional exhaustion and depersonalisation were female gender, being a nurse, working in the hospital, being in contact with Covid patients.

Pappa et al. (2020) investigated with meta-analysis the prevalence of depression, anxiety and insomnia among healthcare workers across a number of countries. Thirteen studies were included in the analysis with a combined total of 33,062 participants. Anxiety was assessed in 12 studies, with a pooled prevalence of 23·2% and depression 22·8% in ten studies. A subgroup analysis revealed gender and occupational differences with female medical staff exhibiting higher rates of affective symptoms compared to male and medical staff, respectively. Finally, insomnia prevalence was estimated at 38·9% across five studies.

In Singapore, a study by Tan et al. (2020) on the psychological impact of the Covid pandemic on healthcare workers there produced interesting findings that it was the non-medical healthcare personnel at higher risk for psychological distress during the outbreak compared to other medical staff.

Doctors in the frontline are also suffering from a high level of work stress and emotional stress working with Covid. A longitudinal survey (Roberts et al., 2021) of 5400 frontline doctors' mental health and experiences of Covid in the UK and Ireland found that 44% were experiencing psychological stress. Doctors reported '*feeling like COVID cannon fodder*' let down by government and NHS Trusts that were not supportive of frontline medical staff in an overwhelmed system. This UK study led to a working party of medical staff/experts creating a Covid-19 Clinical Cohort (CoCCo) model of well-being emphasising what doctors needed, such as places to sleep and rest, hot meals, good communication between sections, compassionate peer support and access to psychological support. The British Psychological Society Psychologist February 2022 provides details on qualitative feedback on doctors experiences.

An Australian study (Quigley et al., 2021) shows that HCWs were at nearly 3 times the risk of infection compared to the general population. Of concern, this nearly tripling of risk occurred during a period of low community prevalence suggesting failures at multiple hazard levels including PPE policies within the work environment. Even in a country with relatively good control of Covid, *HCWs* are at greater risk of infection than the general community with substantial effects on workforce capacity by the quarantine of numerous HCWs during an outbreak. The study identified at least 36 outbreaks in healthcare facilities and at least 536 *HCW* infections in the 6 months up to 8 July 2020 in Australia. The burden of Covid extended beyond the individual *HCW* and resulted in the closure of two hospitals, and in most cases, quarantine of many *HCW* contacts.

The occurrence of hospital outbreaks highlights the high-risk setting that hospitals present in a pandemic. Australia faced the second and third waves of Covid after the Quigley et al. (2021) study period, with multiple hospital outbreaks. In other countries, Covid infections have been estimated at greater than 150,000 in *HCW* in Europe alone by June 2020 (Bandyopadhyay et al., 2020), with over 620 HCW deaths (European Public Service Union, 09-19-2020). The United States of America has seen over 19,000 HCW infections with close to 400 HCW deaths in the same time period. These sort of numbers now extending through a three-year pandemic illustrate the gross impact that the pandemic has had not only on *HCW* but also the hospital systems and other actual or potential patients who have detrimentally missed out on normally provided care.

In another Australian study (Dobson et al., 2021), despite low levels of Covid contact, moderate to high levels of psychological distress were reported with HCWs showed significant symptoms of moderate–severe level depression (21%), anxiety (20%) and post-traumatic stress disorder (29%), associated with burnout and resilience levels.

New research from Edith Cowan University (2021) has shed light on the emotional strain Australian doctors, nurses and paramedics have faced throughout the pandemic. A survey of almost 600 frontline healthcare staff during Australia's first wave in 2020 revealed a workforce less willing to work than before, with concerns ranging from availability of personal protective equipment, family members' worries and risk of contracting the virus. Back during Australia's first wave of community transmission, one-third of participants reported at least one symptom of burnout (35%), 30% had symptoms of depression and 16% disclosed absenteeism. It's reasonable to suggest these figures would be even higher now. Potentially, factors such as burnout and depression are likely to impact on the quality of patient care, three quarters of respondents said they had wrestled even with their obligation to work and the risk of infecting themselves and their families, with 42% reporting they were less willing to work than they had been prior to the outbreak.

Moral distress is also a concerning problem discerned in the Edith Cowan 2021 study as healthcare workers were being forced not only to their physical limits during the pandemic but also to confront significant moral challenges, such as the fair allocation of limited resources, restrictions such as isolation and quarantine and being held responsible for patients' care despite personal risk. When healthcare workers compromise their core values, they can feel shame, guilt and even isolation, and unresolved moral distress can result in depression and other mental, emotional and spiritual health struggles. The nursing profession, in particular, is experiencing a high staff exodus, largely due to burnout, exhaustion and accumulated unresolved moral distress. Despite the number of workers being less willing to work during the pandemic, only a quarter (26%) claimed their workplace had issued communications addressing staff members' obligation to work during Australia's first wave.

Given the relative novelty of this crisis, no valid published studies have collected data on interventions to improve psychological health and overall wellness for *HCWs* who face Covid-specific challenges. There appears to be no methodological sound repeated measures *before and after* study to determine whether wellness or stress changed significantly within the same individuals due to the intervention.

The review of *HCW* literature has revealed consistent reports of stress, anxiety, moral distress and depressive symptoms as a result of Covid with multiple studies confirming significant anxiety regarding patient care in addition to the possibility of infecting own families. Primary concerns of all levels of *HCWs* revealed in studies above during 2020 and into 2022 were the availability of personal protective equipment, of paramount importance to help all HCW feel more protected from infection, which may lessen fear of infecting loved ones. In addition, distress related to Covid among *HCWs* also extends beyond occupational exposure risk, with further impacts that also affect the general public preoccupation with the pandemic, involving its uncertain future course with variants arising, socio-economic and lifestyle upset, exposure to unwelcome negative media offerings and the limitation of social supports. This emphasises the importance of making supports flexible and available to *HCWs*, as they bear both workplace and general public impositions.

Healthcare employers need to be able to recognise early symptoms of psychological trauma in their workers. This will help them develop appropriate measures to intervene and help alleviate conditions such as severe depression, post-traumatic stress disorder and substance abuse, or prevent them from developing in the first place. Psychological resilience appears to be a valuable mediator of the stress response to trauma (Kaplan et al., 2017). High levels of psychological resilience are protective against the development of mental illness, and this was reflected in this study (Kaplan et al., 2017). There need to be serious consideration given to introducing resilience training as a preventative treatment for the reduction of mental health outcomes among first responders, particularly *HCWs* in anticipation of further public health emergencies.

There is also a strong relationship between individual coping mechanisms and moral distress, so nurses need to understand some appropriate coping strategies, which might include, positive reframing and growth (e.g. showing appreciation for the staff who helped during critical times instead of complaining about staffing shortage or being grateful for having the ability to care for patients during a pandemic), active coping (e.g. facing problems and seeking solutions like professional help), mutual social support, permissible ventilation of emotion, meditation, humour and mental and behavioural disengagement to remove the stressor. Meditation spaces can be created to provide the staff with an opportunity to disconnect from morally challenging situations and relax in a quiet place. Peer support from colleagues or managers could help nurses cope and ventilate their feelings. Group-based counselling or virtual peer support sessions to feel connected despite social distancing guidelines could reduce moral distress and burnout during Covid. Some co-workers initiated successful virtual sessions for physical activities like workouts and yoga. Getting recognition from co-workers and leadership even for small achievements also helped improve staff morale. Daily huddles at the beginning of shifts can provide a safe space for all healthcare professionals to discuss any clinical or non-clinical concerns, which were forgotten over time with the increasing workload.

To summarise, the evidence is clear from studies across many nations that HCWs at all levels have a high risk of working in conditions that cause burnout, PTSD, psychical and mental problems and moral distress. Medical staff need to utilise effective individual and/or group coping strategies, while managers, employers and organisations need to provide safe working environments and access to mental health care and other additional support to ensure the wellbeing of medical staff.

Domestic Violence (DV)

The psycho-social effects of the pandemic extend to the inside of our homes, where many people find themselves in sudden forced proximity with their immediate family. People subject to quarantine or self-isolation are at risk of anxiety, confusion and anger (Brooks et al., 2020), trying to contain emotional tendencies that can be explosive when multiple household members simultaneously endure each other for weeks or months on end. Indeed, some studies suggest that this forced proximity and subsequent tension is a major risk factor for aggression (Greenaway et al., 2015) and domestic violence (Owen, 2020).

The pandemic provided '*perfect storm conditions*' for DV abusers, where family members spent an unusual amount of time together in confined spaces, often unsuitable for the purpose itself. This context of enforced living together in a time of stress, with it's increased financial difficulties, loss of employment and childcare pressures, fed into the mix of conditions that lead to abuse or amplified existing abuse. Perpetrators of violence and abuse in the home pretty much had the person they were abusing present 24/7, who was unable to get support, and whom they could monitor all the time. Domestic abuse victims both adults and children have in effect been imprisoned with their abusers during the pandemic who also can be adults and other children. This situation has emerged in the UK where a 33% increase was recorded in 2020 in domestic violence reports as the unprecedented lockdown restrictions forced women to isolate with their abusers (Marie Stopes Report, 2020).

Additional interesting findings show a negative correlation between periods of systemic closure such as during the first UK Covid national lockdown in 2020 and a decline in the number of referrals to a primary care linked DVA support programme simply because people were imprisoned were unable to get out of the house. But at the same time, Panovska-Griffiths et al. (2022) noted a reduction in referrals contrasted with the reported increases in domestic violence reports in the UK as calls to the 24-h national domestic violence helpline managed by Refuge in England surged by 60% during 2020 compared to equivalent period in the previous year. At this time, France also showed a 30% increase in helpline reports of domestic violence, while 50% increased call centre help was recorded in Brazil during 2020. These sets of data are in line with the application of the term '*pandemic paradox*' where DV help calls increase as referrals decrease. DV has been termed a '*shadow epidemic*' carried out under the cover of the Covid pandemic.

There was also a surge in Australia in the reporting DV from women as they emerged from the various lockdowns. The Australian Institute of Criminology (Boxall et al., 2020) found in a survey of 15,000 women that one in 12 experienced physical violence from their live-in partner in the first three months of the pandemic, when most Australians were locked down. More than one in five women experienced emotionally abusive and controlling behaviour from their live-in partners. Half of the women who experienced violence or coercive control from a current or former live-in partner before the pandemic indicated the violence increased in the first three months of the pandemic. For those who had experienced violence and abuse in an intimate partnership during lockdowns, two-thirds reported an escalation in prior violence or abuse, while a minority others experienced violence for the first time.

A study of 362 domestic violence providers surveyed by the Queensland University of Technology in mid-2020 (Carrington et al., 2020) revealed that almost two-thirds, 62%, reported the pandemic restrictions had increased the number of clients wanting help for domestic violence. An overwhelming 82% of domestic violence workers said perpetrators had used isolation to control their victims with increased surveillance and monitoring, cutting the victim off from friends and family. Coercion, control and domination over somebody else are the crux of what domestic and family violence is all about. All those things are intended to take control over that other person and restrict their autonomy. Nearly half, 43%, of the domestic violence workers said abusers used the pandemic environment to control victims by making threats to the safety of the women and their children. There is no acceptable level of violence, and there is evidence that bystanders can be very effective in reducing DV and coercive control by becoming more aware of what they are witnessing and hearing. Griffith University has developed an app with Telstra that provides bystanders with the resources to evaluate what is transpiring and access to a list of support services.

Elder Abuse

Equally concerning data about the effects of the pandemic on older people are beginning to emerge too, with reports of elder abuse increasing around the world. In the UK, the charity Hourglass, which is dedicated to elder abuse, recorded about a 30% increase in calls from older people reporting abuse during lockdown, whereas a survey in the USA of 897 older people sheltering at home during the pandemic found that the prevalence of elder abuse was approximately one of five—an 83.6% increase compared with prevalence estimates before the pandemic (Chang & Levy, 2021). This data is especially alarming when you consider that elder abuse is systematically under-reported: one estimate suggests that only one of every 24 cases is reported.

The pandemic has resulted in an escalation of elder abuse as several generations ended up in close proximity in one dwelling during periods of lockdown or isolation. This contributed to more arguments, disagreement and annoyance as intergenerational differences arose. The Australian Elder Abuse Prevention Unit Report (2021) shows that its helpline received 31.8% more reports of abuse during the pandemic in 2020–2021. The helpline received 2022 abuse notification calls over the period, the highest yearly total recorded since data collection began 20 years ago. In 80% of cases, the perpetrator was a person in a close or intimate relationship with the victim, and in two-thirds of cases the victim and perpetrator were living together. Psychological abuse was most commonly reported in 72.9% of calls, followed by financial and social abuse at 62.6% and 28%, respectively. The most common forms of psychological abuse were pressuring, shouting and degrading victims. Of the financial abuse reported, 32.9% of calls included undue influence and demands followed by misuse of an executive power of attorney at 18.6%.

Uniting Care's Australian wellbeing services have indicated it was common for around 60% of victims to experience numerous types of abuse at once. There was a broad range of contributing factors to the horrendous issue, such as ageism, and expectations about wealth transfer. The problems were compounded by a lack of public awareness in the cocooned environment and limited support programmes. People were reporting that perpetrators were often adult children or grandchildren that had moved into the home because of the financial impact of the pandemic and had become frustrated as house price and rent hikes prevented them moving on with the elderly seen as unwilling to help.

Online Medical, Psychological and Psychotherapy Support

As a consequence of the restrictions on patients/clients going out, many health and social support professionals have moved to provide medical and psychological support online. This has raised awareness among such professionals of the potentials of the online services, exploring where and how best to deploy particular method/devices (phone chat, video-audio consultation, Facebook, etc.) in order to use them effectively in relation to specific purposes identified by the professional. Saladino et al. (2020) identify new perspectives of online intervention are congruent with and avoid the deliberately erected public health mandate barriers against virus transmission. A variety of online techniques permit effective medical consultations and counselling for prolonged stress effects manifesting as anxiety, depression and the inability to manage traumatic and negative emotions.

In particular, the use of already available resources like digitised cognitive behavioural therapy (*CBT*) that is provided in some heath systems can be rapidly extended. Such digitised *CBT* should include components of mindfulness, and emotion regulation and coping skills tailored to address Covid-related stressors (Lopes & Jaspal, 2020). This is vital to ameliorate the potential negative impact of Covid of the increase in common mental health problems such as depression and anxiety but also less common psychiatric conditions such paranoia and hallucinations (Perrin et al., 2020; Pietrabissa et al., 2015). Ensuring that therapies are effective across cultures and socio-economic backgrounds will be crucial to the world's recovery from Covid. But in practice, there is actually a major problem in obtaining psychological help due to a dearth of psychologists to meet escalating demand. For example, a survey by the Australian Psychological Society (24 Feb 2022) reveals that 33% of psychologists in Australia turn new clients away up from 1% prepandemic. In the Australian Capital Territory, 50% are turned away and in Tasmania 86% had wait lists. In S. Australia even those accepted waited an average of 76 days to be seen. Most increases in clients were children. On average, psychologists worked 17 h unpaid each work. The outcome can only be increasing mental health issues building up for the future.

In the current pandemic situation, online services provide several advantages:

- Help many people quickly in a short period of time,
- Reduce the risk of contagion and the strong anxiety felt by both professional and patient, who feel uncomfortable in traditional face-to-face methods due to the pandemic (Békés & Aafjes-van Doorn, 2020),
- Decrease waiting for the consultation, because it takes place at home or at the workplace, even after hours saving time and expense,

- Remove necessity of travel for those who use it, avoiding difficulties related to mobility for some, and even rental costs for the office for those who provide the service,
- Facilitate access to people who struggle to find support close in a closed social environment,
- Help people who have less confidence in face-to-face consultations/ psychotherapy as online takes place in one's comfort zone and facilitate the expression of problems and feelings.

Online services are flexible using different mediums with, for example, a phone chat to establish a first assessment of a person who feels uncomfortable in using a visual set up initially. Online consultation tends to reduce the hierarchical dominant-dominated relationship between professional and client facilitating a greater sense of freedom to express oneself and less concern about judgement. Online also enables professional and patient to record the sessions via chat and in video mode with the informed consent of the participants. Evidence from the brave new world of digital and remote service provision on a limited basis during the pandemic suggests a useful tool to develop for future use in appropriate general health circumstances and leads to the proposition that the pandemic might be a turning point for medical and mental healthcare provision.

Activities to Manage and Ease Stress

In the face of a global pandemic, avoiding stress is simply not an option. Fortuitously, the past twenty years of research on coping and stress suggest that it's not the type or amount of stress that determines its impact. Rather, developing positive mind-sets and realistic situation appraisals about stress can alter its impact (Crum et al., 2020). There are steps to take to help handle stress in a positive way and keep it from making yourself debilitated:

1. *Acknowledge the stress.* Start dealing with stress by acknowledging that you are currently experiencing it. Recognise signs of your body's response to stress, such as difficulty sleeping, increased alcohol and other substance use, being easily angered, feeling depressed and having low energy. Without acknowledgement, you will not alleviate it.
2. *Identify the source(s).* Write a to-do list of the things that cause you stress. Set priorities—by working out which problems you can solve now and which can wait or are beyond your control for the moment. From your list start with the little ones, keep calm, think of possible solutions and take action. Solving small problems will give you confidence to tackle the big ones and help you feel less stressed. Note what you have accomplished at the end of the day, not what you have been unable to do.

3. *Set limits* so things become more manageable. When it comes work and family, consider what you can really do. There are only so many hours in the day. Don't be afraid to say NO to requests for your time and energy if they are putting you into overload. Write out a plan for each day building in relaxation, dog walking, or meeting friends time, etc.
4. *Relaxation and breathing*. These exercises usually involve the following:

   (a) Find a quiet place and sit or lie comfortably. After breathing in (deep breaths), count to four; then breathe out gently and count to four again before taking another breath in and repeat 6 times. If you're feeling really stressed, taking a few deep breaths makes you breathe slower and helps your muscles relax before starting the exercise. Repeat several times a day as convenient.
   (b) Stretch. Stretching can also help relax your muscles and make you feel less tense.
   (c) Massage tense muscles. Having someone massage the muscles in the back of your neck and upper back can help you feel less tense.
   (d) Take the time to relax to do the things that you really want to do. Perhaps listening to music, playing a musical instrument, reading a book, painting, patchwork, taking the dog for a long walk, or going to a movie, etc. Think of this as an order from your doctor, so you won't feel guilty!

5. *Meditation and mindfulness and self-care practice*. Sometimes doing nothing, especially at the beginning, is the best way to understand and handle the top stressors. While this advice may seem counter-intuitive, sometimes the best thing to do is nothing, which covers what superficially appears to be going on in meditation. Meditation refers to a group of techniques including mindfulness which may be practised for many reasons, such as to increase calmness and physical relaxation, to improve psychological balance, to cope with illness, or to enhance overall wellness. Combining data from 23 studies, Bartlett et al. (2019) found statistically strong beneficial effects for ameliorating stress, anxiety, psychological distress, and for improving wellbeing and sleep. Most types of meditation have four elements in common:

   (a) A quiet location with as few distractions as possible. This can be particularly helpful for beginners.
   (b) A specific, comfortable posture. Depending on the type being practised, meditation can be done while sitting, lying down, standing, or walking.
   (c) Focussing one's attention is an essential part of meditation. For example, the meditator may focus on a mantra (a specially chosen word or set of words), an object, a picture, country scene or the sensations of the breath. Having an open attitude during meditation

means letting distractions come and go naturally without judging them.

To meditate is a bit paradoxical, as it is an exercise of 'non-doing'. Generally speaking, the work is to become an observer of one's inner world, exerting minimal effort and adopting a stance of non-judgement.

Mindfulness is a type of meditation which involves developing self-awareness, deep breathing, doing one thing at a time, observing a healthy diet and taking adequate rest; you deliberately focus on something usually on being intensely aware of what you're sensing and feeling in the moment, without interpretation or judgement. Mindfulness has been found effective for stress management (Owens, 2020). Some stress coping programmes may combine meditation, yoga, t'ai chi, or other gentle exercises.

6. *Exercise.* This is an excellent way to manage stressful life events. Do it regularly, even just a daily gentle walk can help boost mood and reduce stress. Level of intensity and duration don't matter but ensure the activity is enjoyable, non-competitive and personally satisfying. Just ten minutes of daily physical activity can be enough to reset your mental and emotional state. Endorphins are produced during exercise which are morphine-like substances providing painkilling effects and promote a sense of euphoria removing anxiety and depression. To reduce stress by exercise on the most stressful days, you can try slow and soothing exercise such as gentle, restorative yoga and flowing t'ai chi to manage stress.
7. *Improving health status*. This will help in managing stress.
   (a) Getting enough sleep helps you recover from the stresses of the day. Being well-rested helps you think better so that you are prepared to handle problems as they come up. Most adults need 7–9 h of sleep a night to feel rested.
   (b) Eat right. Fuel up with fruits, vegetables, beans and whole grains. Don't be fooled by the jolt you get from caffeine or high-sugar snack foods. It wears off quickly, and you could wind up feeling more tired than you did before.
   (c) Don't deal with stress in unhealthy ways like using alcohol, drugs, smoking or overeating.
8. *Social support*. Coping with stress can be helped by social support from individuals and/or community (Chap. 6). Stay in touch with friends, family and community or religious organisations. Talking about your problems with friends or family members can sometimes help you feel better. They might also help you see your problems in a new way and suggest solutions that you hadn't thought of. Seek help from a qualified healthcare provider if you are overwhelmed, feel you cannot cope, have suicidal thoughts or are using drugs or alcohol to cope. They may suggest

counselling to help you learn better ways to deal with stress. Your doctor may also prescribe medicines, such as antidepressants or sleep aids. Help others. Volunteering in your community can help you make new friends and feel better about yourself.

9. *Positive thinking and a positive self-concept.*

The use of negative statements about oneself even in terms of thinking stimulates self-defeating behaviour lowers resilience and self-esteem. This sort of faulty thinking generates stress. Therefore, the focus must be on positive thinking. In maintaining negative self-talk such as '*What's the point*', '*It's another of those days*', '*I don't think I can manage to teach the children at home*', we set a ceiling for our performance, and by anticipating a poor performance, this creates the self-fulfilling prophecy; we perform poorly and perpetuate a failure picture of ourselves. All this amplifies our negative self-concept even further. As Shakespeare once wrote in Measure for Measure, '*our doubts are traitors making us lose the good we might oft win by fearing to attempt*'. Feeling negative, incompetent and inferior is then supplemented by the stresses and strains of actually not coping with life's events and changes. A positive self-concept person will, in meeting a stressful situation, be resilient enough to say, '*It is a difficult situation but I know I will manage it, so best foot forward*'. After having some success, they will reward themselves by positive self-talk to reinforce the behaviour, such as '*I did that reasonably well*'. This limits and manages the stress. So think positively and promote positive feelings about yourself, and there will be much less stress in your life (Burns, 1993 Chaps. 3, 4 and 5 contain exercises for improving positive thinking, self-concept enhancement and stress management).

Several books that provide extended discussion stress and how to manage it with exercises are

Burns (1993) *Managing People in Changing Times*. Allen and Unwin: Sydney.
Burns (2003) *Unwind: 10 Ways to Manage Stress*. Revised 2nd Edition. Allen and Unwin: Sydney.

The review of research above reveals that multifaceted threats of Covid to which all age groups are exposed collaborate for future unpredictable damages particularly in the mental health areas and may heighten pre-existing difficulties and problems for the future. Health authorities and government need to be alert to a long-term public health issue of mental stress with the need for prolonged governmental support and not as something whose outcome is short-lived once Covid is conquered. In the young, mental stress impacts critical central nervous system processes that transport young people through adolescence to adulthood in terms of thinking skills and socio-emotional control, damaging ability to form and retain mutually satisfying social relationships. It has potential consequences of unemployment on their future long-term employment prospects and finances. The main danger is that it leaves a legacy of stress, anxiety and depression, and for few, psychoticism that can replay as PTSD.

A major problem is that there is insufficient school and clinical psychologists to deal with the crisis in most nations. Addressing those needs may not be a realistic solution until the workforce grows. Before the pandemic, only 1% of psychologists in Australia were unable to accept new patients. In mid-2022 around 30% have closed their books. Not only has demand increased during the pandemic but training places for clinical psychologists are sparse with very valid applicants turned away. One university had 700 applicants from qualified psychologist to undertake the post-grad clinical course but only 21 places. But taking over and working well in Australia is a focussed preventative approach by government funding organisations (e.g. Lifeline in Australia) which field the initial help requests and provide counselling. It is this sort of provision that has remarkably helped to reduce the suicide numbers despite increasing distress from Covid impacts as recorded from the increased calls for help. Some school teachers are also providing children with basic social and emotional skills to help students cope with stress and anxiety in real time.

Given a similar shortage of experts in the USA, psychologists in some districts are training teachers in equipping kids with coping skills and resilience in the classroom that can prevent strain on school psychologists while also improving students' ability to learn and relate to others. Such in-service courses incorporate pandemic-relevant topics like awareness of anxiety, trauma and warning signs of suicide into their classes as well as teaching students emotional intelligence skills. One-on-one therapy won't be available for every child who's struggling, so a multipronged approach to help build the capacity of teachers and staff to support young people who are critical to the future of society in the classroom setting is essential. Increasing access to mental health services in the community is becoming important policy goals to minimise pandemic-related impacts on mental health and wellbeing.

In general, the reopening of economies and societies generally has thankfully been fund to lead to a rapid rebound in personal wellbeing. Thus, the priority should be to return to normal as far as possible and as quickly as possible to restore familiar routines, interactions and behaviours. With the rise in new coronavirus variants as well as other global health issues, this is not the last time that a pandemic, epidemic or national emergency could prompt strict mandated behavioural controls. Therefore, systems must evolve to reflect the growing body of research and evidence about the harms of heavy-handed restrictions on peoples' health, their social, psychological and economic wellbeing and life expectancy.

References

Adams, J. G., & Walls, R. M. (2020). Supporting the health care workforce during the COVID-19 global epidemic. *JAMA, 323*, 1439–1440. https://doi.org/10.1001/jama.2020.3972

Alvarez, F., Argente, D., & Lippi, F. (2020). A simple planning problem for Covid-19 lockdown. *Covid Economics, 14*, 1–33. https://doi.org/10.3386/w26981

Allianz Insurance Company. (2022, 28 September). *The workplace wave: the next wave of the pandemic disrupting workplace mental health* . Retrieved 30 October 2022 from https://www.allianz.com.au ›media › news › the-workplace

American Medical Association. (2020). Retrieved 30 October 2020 from http://www.asapnys.org/wp-content/uploads/2020/07/Issue-brief_-Reports-of-increases-in-opioid-related-overdose-and-other-concerns-during-COVID-pandemic.pdf

American Psychological Association (APA). *2020 trends report*. Retrieved 30 October 2020 from https://www.apa.org/monitor/2022/01/special-childrens-mental-health

American Psychological Association (APA). (2021). *Work and well-being survey 2021.* Retrieved 30 October 2020 from https://www.apa.org/pubs/reports/work-well-being/compounding-pressure-2021

Australian Elder Abuse Prevention Unit Report. (2021). Retrieved 4 January 2022 from https://eapu.com.au/research-elder/

Australian Institute of Health and Welfare. (2021). *Australia's Welfare 2021 Report*. Retrieved 4 January 2022 from https://www.aihw.gov.au/news-media/media-releases/2021-1/september/aihw-releases-2021-report-card-on-the-wellbeing.

Australian Institute of Family Studies. (2022, August). Elder helpline. *Elder abuse in Australia Report*. Retrieved 28 September 2022 from https://aifs.gov.au/projects/elder-abuse-research.

Australian National Health and Wellbeing Strategy. (2021). Department of Health and Aged Care. Canberra.

Australian Psychological Society. (2022). Media Release: 24 February 2022. *Unpaid, underfunded and overworked: Psychologists on the brink*. Retrieved 28 September 2022 from https://psychology.org.au/about-us/news-and-media/media-releases/2022/unpaid,-underfunded-and-overworked-psychologists

Bandyopadhyay, S., Baticulon, R. E., Kadhum, M., et al. (2020). Infection and mortality of healthcare workers worldwide from COVID-19: A systematic review. *BMJ Global Health, 5*, e003097. https://doi.org/10.1136/bmjgh-2020-003097

Banerjee, D. (2020). The COVID-19 outbreak: Crucial role the psychiatrists can play. *Asian Journal of Psychiatry, 50*, 102014. https://doi.org/10.1016/j.ajp.2020.102014

Bartlett, L., Martin, A., Neil, A. L., et al. (2019). A systematic review and meta-analysis of workplace mindfulness training randomized controlled trials. *Journal of Occupational Health Psychology, 24*, 108–126. https://doi.org/10.1037/ocp0000146

Batchelor, S., Stoyanov, S., Pirkis, J., & Kõlves, K. (2021). Use of kids helpline by children and young people in Australia during the COVID-19 pandemic. *Journal of Adolescent Health, 68*, 1067–1074. https://doi.org/10.1016/j.jadohealth.2021.03.015

Beckett, L. (2020). Americans have bought record 17m guns in year of unrest, analysis finds. *The Guardian*. Retrieved 15 December 2020 from https://www.theguardian.com/us-news/2020/oct/29/coronavirus-pandemic-americans-gun-sales
Békés, V., & Aafjes-van Doorn, K. (2020). Psychotherapists' attitudes toward online therapy during the COVID-19 pandemic. *Journal of Psychotherapy Integration, 30*, 238–247. https://doi.org/10.1037/int0000214
Bowling, A. (1987). Mortality after bereavement: A review of the literature on survival periods and factors affecting survival. *Social Science and Medicine, 23*, 117–124. https://doi.org/10.1016/0277-9536(87)90244-9
Boxall, H., Morgan, A., & Brown, R. (2020). The prevalence of domestic violence among women during the COVID-19 pandemic. *Statistical Bulletin no. 28. Canberra: Australian Institute of Criminology*. https://doi.org/10.52922/sb04718
Broadway, J. et al. (2020). Behind closed doors: The surge in mental distress in paents. *Melbourne Institute Research Insights*, Article 21.
British Psychological Society. (2022). *The psychologist February 2022. Feedback on doctors experiences*. Retrieved 23 March 2022 from https://www.tninyurl.com/46khfe98
Brooks, S. K., Webster, R. K., Smith, L. E., et al. (2020). The psychological impact of quarantine and how to reduce it: Rapid review of the evidence. *Lancet, 395*, 912–920. https://doi.org/10.1016/S0140-6736(20)30460-8
Bueno-Notivol, J., et al. (2021). Prevalence of depression during the COVID-19 outbreak: a meta-analysis of community-based studies. *International Journal of Clinical and Health Psychology, 21*, 100–196. https://doi.org/10.1016/j.ijchp.2020.07.007
Burns, R. (1982). *Self concept development and education*. Holt Rinehart and Winston.
Burns, R. (1993). *Managing people in changing times*. Allen and Unwin.
Burns, R. (2003). *Unwind: 10 ways to manage stress* (Revised 2nd edn). Allen and Unwin
Bussières, E. L. (2021). Consequences of the COVID-19 pandemic on children's mental health: A meta-analysis. *Frontiers Psychiatry*. https://doi.org/10.3389/fpsyt.2021.691659
Cao, W., Fang, Z., Hou, G., et al. (2020). The psychological impact of the COVID-19 epidemic on college students in China. *Psychiatry Research, 287*, 112934. https://doi.org/10.1016/j.psychres.2020.112934
Carrington, K., Morley, C., Warren, et al. (2020). *Impact of COVID on domestic and family violence workforce and clients*: Research Report QUT Centre for Justice, QUT, Brisbane, Australia. Retrieved 16 January 2021 from https://research.qut.edu.au/centre-for-justice/wp-content/uploads/sites/304/2020/11/Research-Report-Series-November-2020-COVID.pdf
Centers for Disease Control and Prevention. (2021). United States, January–June 2021. Supplement. 71 No. 3 April 1, 2022. *Adolescent behaviors and experiences survey*. https://doi.org/10.15585/mmwr.su7103a3external
Chang, E. S., & Levy, B. R. (2021). High prevalence of elder abuse during the COVID-19 pandemic: Risk and resilience factors. *The American Journal of Geriatric Psychiatry, 29*, 1152–1159. https://doi.org/10.1016/j.jagp.2021.01.007
Chen, F., Zheng, D., Liu, J., et al. (2020a). Depression and anxiety among adolescents during COVID-19: A cross-sectional study. *Brain, Behavior, and Immunity, 88*, 36–38. https://doi.org/10.1016/j.bbi.2020.05.061.S0889-1591(20)30891-6

Chen, Q., Liang, M., Li, Y., et al. (2020b). Mental health care for medical staff in China during the COVID-19 outbreak. *The Lancet Psychiatry, 7*, e15–e16. https://doi.org/10.1016/S2215-0366(20)30078-X

Cheng, C., Jun, H., & Liang, B. (2014). Psychological health diathesis assessment system: A nationwide survey of resilient trait scale for Chinese adults. *Studies of Psychology and Behavior, 12*, 735–742. https://doi.org/10.1136/gpsych-2020-100213

Cox, T. (1981). *Stress*. MacMillan.

Crum, A., Jamieson, J., Akinola, M., et al. (2020). Optimizing stress: An integrated intervention for regulating stress responses. *Emotion, 20*, 120–125. https://doi.org/10.1037/emo0000670

Czeisler, M., Howard, M., & Rajaratnam, S. (2021). Mental health during the COVID-19 pandemic: Challenges, populations at risk, implications, and opportunities. *American Journal of Health Promotion, 35*, 301–311. https://doi.org/10.1177/0890117120983982b

Czeisler, M., Lane, R. I., Petrosky, E., et al. (2020). Mental health, substance use, and suicidal ideation during the COVID-19 pandemic—United States. *Morbidity and Mortality Weekly Report, 69*, 1049–1057. https://doi.org/10.1016/j.jpsychires.2021.05.080

Danese, A., Moffitt, T. E., Harrington, H., et al. (2009). Adverse childhood experiences and adult risk factors for age-related disease: Depression, inflammation, and clustering of metabolic risk markers. *Archives of Pediatrics and Adolescent Medicine, 163*, 1135–1143. https://doi.org/10.1001/archpediatrics.2009.214

Dawal, A., Shou, Y., Smithson, M., et al. (2020). The effect off COVID-19 on health and well being in a representative sample of Australian adults. *Font Psychiatry, 11*, 579985. https://doi.org/10.3589/fpsyt.2020.619331

De Bellis, M. D., & Zisk, A. (2014). The biological effects of childhood trauma. *Child and Adolescent Psychiatric Clinics of North America, 23*, 185–222. https://doi.org/10.1016/j.chc.2014.01.002.vii

de Figueiredo, C. S., Sandre, P. C., Portugal, L., et al. (2021). COVID-19 pandemic impact on children and adolescents' mental health: Biological, environmental, and social factors. *Progress in Neuro-Psychopharmacology & Biological Psychiatry., 106*, 110–171. https://doi.org/10.1016/j.pnpbp.2020.110171

De Young, A., Paterson, R., March, S., et al. (2021). *COVID-19 unmasked. Report 2: Impact of the second wave in Australia on the mental health of young children and parents*. Queensland Centre for Perinatal and Infant Mental Health, Children's Health Queensland Hospital and Health Service. Retrieved 8 January 2022 from https://www.childrens.health.qld.gov.au/wp-content/uploads/PDF/COVID-19/COVID19-Unmasked-Survey-Progress-Report-02.pdf

Dobson, H., Malpas, C., Burrel, A., et al. (2021). Burn out and psychological stress among Australian HCW during the Covid-19 pandemic. *Australasian Psychiatry, 29*, 26–30. https://doi.org/10.1177/1039856220965045

Dooley, D., Rhodes, H., & Bandealy, A. (2022). Pandemic recovery for children—beyond reopening schools. *JAMA Pediatrics, 176*, 347–348. https://doi.org/10.1001/jamapediatrics.2021.3227

Edith Cowan University Report. (2021). *Australian healthcare workers facing burnout, less willing to work since COVID outbreak*. Retrieved 6 January 2022 from https://www.ecu.edu.au/newsroom/articles/research/australian-healthcare-workers-facing-burnout-less-willing-to-work-since-covid-outbreak

Elder Helpline. (2022). *Elder Abuse Prevention Unit Report 2022.* Retrieved 1 November 2022 from https://eapu.com.au/research-elder/

Ettman, C. K., Abdalla, S. M., Cohen, G. H., et al. (2020). Prevalence of depression symptoms in US adults before and during the COVID-19 pandemic. *JAMA Network Open, 3*(9), e2019686. https://doi.org/10.1001/jamanetworkopen.2020.19686

European Public Service Union. (2020). *Press Release, Brussels, 9 October 2020.* Retrieved 20 July 2021 from https://www.epsu.org/article/european-mobilization-health-and-care-workers

Evans, S., Mikocka-Walus, A., Klas, A., et al. (2020). From "it has stopped our lives" to "spending more time together has strengthened bonds": The varied experiences of Australian families during COVID-19. *Frontiers in Psychology, 11*, 588667. https://doi.org/10.3389/fpsyg.2020.58866

Fancourt, D., Steptoe, A., & Bu, F. (2021). Trajectories of anxiety and depressive symptoms during enforced isolation due to COVID-19 in England: A longitudinal observational study. *The Lancet Psychiatry, 8*, 141–149. https://doi.org/10.1016/S2215-0366(20)30482-X

Fegert, J. M., Vitiello, B., Plener, P. L., & Clemens, V. (2020). Challenges and burden of the coronavirus 2019 (COVID-19) pandemic for child and adolescent mental health: A narrative review to highlight clinical and research needs in the acute phase and the long return to normality. *Child and Adolescent Psychiatry and Mental Health, 14*, 20. https://doi.org/10.1186/s13034-020-00329-3

Foulkes, L., & Blakemore, S. J. (2018). Studying individual differences in human adolescent brain development. *Nature Neuroscience, 21*, 315–323. https://doi.org/10.1038/s41593-018-0078-4

Freudenberger, H. (1974). Staff burnout. *Journal of Social Issue, 30*, 159–165. https://doi.org/10.1111/j.1540-4560.1974.tb00706.x

Fusaroli, P., Balena, S., & Lisotti, A. (2020). On the death of 100 + Italian doctors from COVID-19. *PubMed, 48*(5), 803–804. https://doi.org/10.1007/s15010-020-01436-1

Giusti, E. M., Pedroli, E., D'Aniello, G. E., et al. (2020). The psychological impact of the COVID-19 outbreak on health professionals: A cross-sectional study. *Frontiers in Psychology, 11*, 1684. https://doi.org/10.3389/fpsyg.2020.01684

Goldfeld, S., O'Connor, E., Sung, V., et al. (2022). Potential indirect impacts of the COVID-19 pandemic on children: A narrative review using a community child health lens. *Medical Journal of Australia, 216*, 364–372. https://doi.org/10.5694/mja2.51368

Grassi, L., & Magnani, K. (2000). Psychiatric morbidity and burnout in the medical profession: An Italian study of general practitioners and hospital physicians. *Psychotherapy and Psychosomatics, 69*, 329–334. https://doi.org/10.1159/000012416

Greenaway, K., Jetten, J., & van Bunderen, L. (2015). The dark side of inclusion: Undesired acceptance increases aggression. *Group Process Intergroup Relations, 18*(2), 173–189. https://doi.org/10.1177/1368430214536063

Holmes, E. A., O'Connor, R. C., et al. (2020). Multidisciplinary research priorities for the COVID-19 pandemic: A call for action for mental health science. *The Lancet Psychiatry, 7*, 547–560. https://doi.org/10.1016/S2215-0366(20)30168-1

Holmes, T., & Rahe, T. (1967). The social readjustment rating scale. *Journal of Psychosomatic Research, 11*, 213. https://doi.org/10.1016/0022-3999(67)90010-4

Huang, Y., & Zhao, N. (2020). Generalized anxiety disorder, depressive symptoms and sleep quality during COVID-19 outbreak in China: a web-based cross-sectional survey. *Psychiatry Research, 288*. https://doi.org/10.1016/j.psychres.2020.112954

Jakovljevic, M., Bjedov, S., Jaksic, N., & Jakovljevic, I. (2020). Covid-19 pandemic and public and global mental health from the perspective of global health security. *Psychiatria Danubina, 32*(1), 6–14. https://doi.org/10.24869/psyd.2020.6

Jiao, W., Wang, L., & Liu, J. et al. (2020). Behavioural and emotional disorders in children during Covid-19. *The Journal of Pediatrics, 221*, 264–266. https://doi.org/10.1016/j.jpeds.2020.0.013

Kaplan, J., Bergman, A., Christopher, M., et al. (2017). Role of resilience in mindfulness training for first responders. *Mindfulness, 8*, 1373–1380. https://doi.org/10.1007/S12671-017-0713-2

Kawohl, W., & Nordt, C. (2020). COVID-19, unemployment, and suicide. *The Lancet Psychiatry, 7*, 389–390. https://doi.org/10.1016/s2215-0366(20)30141-3

Kessler, R. C., Berglund, P., Demler, O., & Walters, E. E. (2005). Lifetime prevalence and age-of-onset distributions of DSM-IV disorders in the national comorbidity survey replication. *Archives of General Psychiatry, 62*(6), 593–602. https://doi.org/10.1001/archpsyc.62.6.593

Khalid, I., Khalid, T. J., Qabajah, M. R., et al. (2016). Healthcare workers emotions, perceived stressors and coping strategies during a MERS-CoV outbreak. *Clinical and Medicine Research, 14*, 7–14. https://doi.org/10.3121/cmr.2016.1303

Lacey, R., Kumari, M., & Bontley, M. (2014). Social isolation in childhood and adult inflammation. *Psychonueroendocrinology, 5*, 85–94.

Lai, J., Ma, S., Wang, Y., et al. (2020). Factors associated with mental health outcomes among health care workers exposed to coronavirus disease 2019. *JAMA Network Open, 3*, e203976. https://doi.org/10.1001/jamanetworkopen.2020.3976

Lee, A. et al. (2007). Stress and psycholoical distress among SARS survivors. *Canadian Journal of Psychiatry, 52*, 233–240.

Lee, S., & Ward, K. (2020). *Stress and parenting during the coronavirus pandemic*. Retrieved 23 November 2021 from https://www.parentingincontext.org/uploads/8/1/3/1/81318622/research_brief_stress_and_parenting_during_the_coronavirus_pandemic_final.pdf

Leeb, R. T., Price, S., Sliwa, S., et al. (2020). COVID-19 trends among school-aged children—United States, March 1–September 19, 2020. *MMWR Morbidity Mortal Weekly Report, 69*(45), 1410–1415. https://doi.org/10.15585/mmwr.mm6939e2

Liang, Y., Chen, M., Zheng, X., & Liu, J. (2020). Screening for Chinese medical staff mental health by SDS and SAS during the outbreak of COVID-19. *Journal of Psychosomatic Research, 133*, 1101–1102. https://doi.org/10.1016/j.jpsychores.2020.110102

Liberati, E., Richards, N., Willars, J., et al. (2021). A qualitative study of experiences of NHS mental healthcare workers during the Covid-19 pandemic. *BMC Psychiatry, 21*, 250. https://doi.org/10.1186/s12888-021-03261-8

Liu, C. H., Zhang, E., Wong, G. T. F., et al. (2020). Factors associated with depression, anxiety, and PTSD symptomatology during the COVID-19 pandemic: Clinical implications for U.S. young adult mental health. *Psychiatry Research, 290*, 113172. https://doi.org/10.1016/j.psychres.2020.113172

Lopes, B., & Jaspal, R. (2020). Understanding the mental health burden of COVID-19 in the United Kingdom. *Psychological Trauma: Theory, Research, Practice, and Policy., 12*, 465–467. https://doi.org/10.1037/tra0000632

Lopes, B., Bortolon, C., & Jaspal, R. (2020). Paranoia, hallucinations and compulsive buying during the early phase of COVID-19 in the United Kingdom: A preliminary experimental study. *Psychiatry Research, 293*, 13455. https://doi.org/10.1016/j.psychres.2020.113455

Lund, C., Docrat, S., Abdulmalik, J., et al. (2019). Household economic costs associated with mental, neurological and substance use disorders: A cross-sectional survey in six low- and middle-income countries. *Bjpsych Open*, *5*(3), e34. https://doi.org/10.1192/bjo.2019.20

Lurie Children's Blog. (2021). *Children's mental health during the COVID-19 pandemic*. Retrieved 12 July 2021 from https://www.luriechildrens.org/en/blog/childrens-mental-health-pandemic-statistics/

Mahase, E. (2020). Covid-19: Nearly 20% of patients receive psychiatric diagnosis within three months of COVID. *BJM, 371*. https://doi.org/10.1136/bmj.m4386

Mamun, M. A., & Griffiths, M. D. (2020). First COVID-19 suicide case in Bangladesh due to fear of COVID-19 and xenophobia: Possible suicide prevention strategies. *Asian Journal of Psychiatry, 51*. https://doi.org/10.1016/j.ajp.2020.102073

Manzoni, P., & Mililllo, C. (2020). Covid-19 mortality in Italian doctors. *Journal of Infection, 81*. https://doi.org/10.1016/j.jinf.2020.05.034

Marie Stopes Report. (2020). *33% rise in domestic violence reports under COVID-19 lockdown*. Retrieved 06 June 2021 from https://www.msichoices.org.uk/news/33-rise-in-domestic-violence-reports-under-covid-19-lockdown/

Maunder, R. G., Lancee, W. J., Balderson, K. E., et al. (2006). Long-term psychological and occupational effects of providing hospital healthcare during SARS outbreak. *Emerging Infectious Diseases, 12*, 1924–1932. https://doi.org/10.3201/eid1212.060584

Mazza, C., Ricci, E., Biondi, S., et al. (2020). Nationwide survey of psychological distress among italian people during the COVID-19 pandemic: Immediate psychological responses and associated factors. *International Journal of Environmental Research Public Health, 17*. https://doi.org/10.3390/ijerph17093165

Moghanibashi-Mansourieh, A. (2020). Assessing the anxiety level of Iranian general population during COVID-19 outbreak. *Asian Journal of Psychiatry, 51*, 102076. https://doi.org/10.1016/j.ajp.2020.102076

Mohindra, R. R. R., Suri, V., Bhalla, A., & Singh, S. M. (2020). Issues relevant to mental health promotion in frontline health care providers managing quarantined/isolated COVID-19 patients. *Asian Journal Psychiatry, 51*. https://doi.org/10.1016/j.ajp.2020.102084

Neria, Y., & Sullivan, G. M. (2011). Understanding the mental health effects of indirect exposure to mass trauma through the media. *JAMA, 306*(12), 1374–1375. https://doi.org/10.1001/jama.2011.1358

Orgilés, M., Morales, A., Delvecchio, E., et al. (2020). Immediate psychological effects of the COVID-19 quarantine in youth from Italy and Spain. *PsyArXiv* 1–13. https://doi.org/10.1017/s0033291720001841

Owen, L. (2020). 5 ways the corona virus is hitting women in Asia. *BBC News*. Retrieved 13 January 2021 from https://www.bbc.com/news/world-asia51705199

Owens, R. (2020). *Meditation*. Retrieved 9 April 2021 from https://insighttimer.com › lamarod › guided-meditations

Øyane, N. P. S., Elisabeth, M., Torbjörn, A., & Bjørn, B. (2013). Associations between night work and anxiety, depression, insomnia, sleepiness and fatigue in a sample of Norwegian nurses. *PLoS One* e70228. https://doi.org/10.1371/journal.pone.0070228

Palgi, Y., Shrira, A., Ring, L., et al. (2020). The loneliness pandemic: Loneliness and other concomitants of depression, anxiety and their comorbidity during the COVID-19 outbreak. *Journal of Affective Disorders, 275*, 109–111. https://doi.org/10.1016/j.jad.2020.06.036

Panchal, U. S., de Pablo, G., Franco, M., et al. (2021). The impact of COVID-19 lockdown on child and adolescent mental health: Systematic review. *European Child and Adolescent Psychiatry, 18*, 1–27. https://doi.org/10.1007/s00787-021-01856-w

Panda, K., Gupta, J., Chowdhury, S., et al. (2021). Psychological and behavioral impact of lockdown and quarantine measures for COVID-19 pandemic on children, adolescents and caregivers: A systematic review and meta-analysis. *Journal of Tropical Pediatrics, 67*(1). https://doi.org/10.1093/tropej/fmaa122.

Panovska-Griffiths, J., Szilassy, E., Johnson, M., et al. (2022). Impact of the first national COVID-19 lockdown on referral of women experiencing domestic violence and abuse in England and Wales. *BMC Public Health, 22*, 504. https://doi.org/10.1186/s12889-022-12825-6

Pappa, S., Ntella, V., Giannakas, T., et al. (2020). Prevalence of depression, anxiety, and insomnia among healthcare workers during the COVID-19 pandemic: A systematic review and meta-analysis. *Journal Brain, Behavior, and Immunity, 88*, 901–907. https://doi.org/10.1016/j.bbi.2020.05.026

Perrin, P., Rybarczyk, B., Pierce, B., et al. (2020). Rapid telepsychology deployment during the COVID-19 pandemic: A special issue commentary and lessons from primary care psychology training. *Clinical Psychologist, 76*, 1173–1185. https://doi.org/10.1002/jclp.22969

Pietrabissa, G., Manzoni, A., et al. (2015). Facebook use as access facilitator for consulting psychology. *Australian Psychologist, 50*, 299–303. https://doi.org/10.1111/ap.12139

Pollard, M. S., Tucker, J. S., & Green, H. D. (2020). Changes in adult alcohol use and consequences during the COVID-19 pandemic in the US. *JAMA Network Open, 3*, e2022942. https://doi.org/10.1001/jamanetworkopen.2020.22942

Quigley, A. L., Stone, H., Nguyen, P. Y., et al. (2021). Estimating the burden of COVID-19 on the Australian healthcare workers and health system during the first six months of the pandemic. *International Journal of Nursing Studies, 114*, 103811. https://doi.org/10.1016/j.ijnurstu

Rajaratnam, S. M., Barger, L. K., Lockley, S. W., et al. (2011). Sleep disorders, health, and safety in police officers. *JAMA, 306*(23), 2567–2578. https://doi.org/10.1001/jama.2011.1851

Roberts, T., Daniels, J., Hulme, W., et al. (2021). Psychological distress during the acceleration phase of the COVID-19 pandemic: A survey of doctors practising in emergency medicine, anaesthesia and intensive care medicine in the UK and Ireland. *Emergency Medicine Journal, 38*, 450–459. https://doi.org/10.1136/emermed-2020-210438

Rossi, R., Socci, B., Pacitti, F., et al. (2020). Mental health outcomes among frontline and second-line health care workers during the coronavirus disease 2019 (COVID-19) pandemic in Italy. *JAMA Network Open, 3*(5), e2010185. https://doi.org/10.3389/fpsyt.2020.00790

Rubin, G. J., & Wessely, S. (2020). The psychological effects of quarantining a city. *BMJ, 28*(368), m313. https://doi.org/10.1136/bmj.m313

Saladino, V., Algeri, D., Auriemmam, V., et al. (2020). The psychological and social impact of Covid-19: new perspectives of well-being. *Frontiers in Psychology, 11*, 577684. https://doi.org/10.3389/fpsyg.2020.577684

Salari, N., Hosseinian-Far, A., Jalali, R., et al. (2020). Prevalence of stress, anxiety, depression among the general population during the COVID-19 pandemic: A systematic review and meta-analysis. *Globalization and Health, 16*(1), 57. https://doi.org/10.1186/s12992-020-00589-w

Sareen, J., Afifi, T. O., McMillan, K. A., & Asmundson, G. J. (2011). Relationship between household income and mental disorders: Findings from a population-based longitudinal study. *Archives of General Psychiatry, 68*(4), 419–427. https://doi.org/10.1001/archgenpsychiatry.2011.15

Saurabh, K., & Ranjan, S. (2020). Compliance and psychological impact of quarantine in children and adolescents due to Covid-19 pandemic. *Indian Journal of Pediatrics, 87*, 532–536. https://doi.org/10.1007/s12098-020-03347-3

Schimmenti, A., Starcevic, V., Giardina, A., et al. (2020). Multidimensional assessment of COVID-19-related fears (MAC-RF): A theory-based instrument for the assessment of clinically relevant fears during pandemics. *Frontiers in Psychiatry, 11*, 748. https://doi.org/10.3389/fpsyt.2020.00748

Schleimer, J. P., McCort, C. D., Pear, V. A., et al. (2020). Firearm purchasing and firearm violence in the first months of the coronavirus pandemic in the United States. medR xiv. https://doi.org/10.1101/2020.07.02.20145508

Selye, H. (1976). *The stress of life* (Revised). McGraw-Hill.

Shaikh, A., Peprah, E., Mohamed, R. H., et al. (2021). COVID-19 and mental health: A multi-country study—the effects of lockdown on the mental health of young adults. *Middle East Current Psychiatry, 28*(1), 51. https://doi.org/10.1186/s43045-021-00116-6

Tam, C. W. C., Pang, E. P. F., Lam, L. C. W., et al. (2004). Severe acute respiratory syndrome (SARS) in Hongkong in 2003: Stress and psychological impact among frontline healthcare workers. *Psychological Medicine, 34*, 1197–1204. https://doi.org/10.1017/S0033291704002247

Tan, B. Y., Chew, N. W. S., Lee, G. K. H., et al. (2020). Psychological impact of the COVID-19 pandemic on health care workers in Singapore. *Annals of Internal Medicine*, M20–M1083. https://doi.org/10.7326/M20-1083

The Guardian Newspaper. (2021). Our key findings about US healthcare worker deaths in the pandemic's first year. Retrieved 24 January 22 from https://www.theguardian.com/us-news/ng-interactive/2020/dec/22/lost-on-the-frontline-our-findings-to-date

The Australian Government's National Children's Mental Health and Wellbeing Strategy. (2021). Retrieved 17 February 2022 from https://www.mentalhealthcommission.gov.au/getmedia/5b7112be-6402-4b23-919d-8fb9b6027506/National-Children%E2%80%99s-Mental-Health-and-Wellbeing-Strategy-%E2%80%93-Report.

Tottenham, N., & Galvan, A. (2016). Stress and the adolescent brain: Amygdala-prefrontal cortex circuitry and ventral striatum as developmental targets. *Neuroscience and Biobehavioral Reviews, 70*, 217–227. https://doi.org/10.1016/j.neubiorev.2016.07.030

UNICEF State of World's Children Report. (2022). Retrieved 3 November 2022 from https://data.unicef.org/resources/sowc-2022/

Wang, G., Zhang, Y., Zhao, J., et al. (2020a). Mitigate the effects of home confinement on children during the COVID-19 outbreak. *Lancet, 395*, 945–947. https://doi.org/10.1016/S0140-6736(20)30547-X

Wang, Y., Di, Y., Ye, J., et al. (2020b). Study on the public psychological states and its related factors during the outbreak of coronavirus disease 2019 (COVID-19) in some regions of China. *Psychology, Health & Medicine, 30*, 1–10. https://doi.org/10.1080/13548506.2020.1746817

Weaver, M. D., Vetter, C., Rajaratnam, S. M., et al. (2018). Sleep disorders, depression and anxiety are associated with adverse safety outcomes in healthcare workers: A prospective cohort study. *Journal of Sleep Research, 27*, e12722. https://doi.org/10.1111/jsr.12722.

World Health Organization. (2020). Coronavirus disease 2019 (COVID-19) Situation Report—116. Retrieved 28 February 2021 from https://www.who.int/docs/default-source/coronaviruse/situation-reports/2

Zhang, Y., & Ma, Z. F. (2020). Impact of the COVID-19 pandemic on mental health and quality of life among local residents in Liaoning Province, China: A cross-sectional study. *International Journal of Environmental Research and Public Health, 17*(7), 2381. https://doi.org/10.3390/ijerph17072381

Zhou, S.-J., Zhang, L.-G., Wang, L.-L., et al. (2020). Prevalence and socio-demographic correlates of psychological health problems in Chinese adolescents during the outbreak of COVID-19. *European Child and Adolescent Psychiatry, 29*(6), 1–10. https://doi.org/10.1007/s00787-020-01541-4

CHAPTER 9

Managing Grief and Death

Abstract The most devastating effect of the pandemic has been the sudden unexpected increase in deaths, mourning and loss inflicted around the world, particularly among the elderly, generating considerable grief. Early grief models suggested a sequential process of 'grief work' is critical to resolution/recovery. New grief models are now identifying patterns and relations of complex idiosyncratic grief experience and do not support former popular notions that grieving is necessarily associated with depression, anxiety and PTSD. Two concerning forms of grief, Prolonged Grief Disorder (PGD) and Complicated Grief (CG), are identified and elaborated. The extraordinary circumstances of deaths during Covid pandemic have been challenging for the deceased's families and have evoked novel approaches to relatives' grieving processes and managing funerals within restrictions of lockdown, assembly and movement. Examples and evidence of successful grief counselling are detailed.

Keywords Grief disorders · Death · Bereavement · Mourning · Grief counselling · The aged

Introduction

Grief and death are an inevitable part of life and unfortunately have been and continue to be the tragic end of many Covid cases. Current worldwide figures indicate around 6,300,000 reported deaths caused by the new coronavirus so far, around one in ten of the total world cases to date and averaging now about 10 K per day. Estimates suggest each death affects around nine close relatives and friends which means the bereaved and grieving are almost as large

© The Author(s), under exclusive license to Springer Nature Singapore Pte Ltd. 2023

R. B. Burns, *The Human Impact of the COVID-19 Pandemic*,
https://doi.org/10.1007/978-981-99-1710-5_9

a number as that of the total cases! After nearly three years, over 1 million US citizens have died and in India 500,000, Brazil 700,000, UK 210,000 and Australia 16,000. (Our World in Data undated weekly) These are astonishing figures that have become so horrendously apparent in most countries with the daily presentations in news media of the previous day's death toll and case death (mortality) rate. These death rates are far in excess of normal levels due to the pandemic. Excess mortality is a term used in epidemiology and public health that refers to the number of deaths from all causes during a crisis above and beyond what we would have expected to see under 'normal' conditions. Globally, this is about 14% more but varies tremendously depending on quality and quantity of healthcare availability and geographical situation such as close living arrangements in apartments of cities in Europe and Asia compared to New Zealand and Australia where the isolated island nature enables lockdown of each country from outside, significantly lowering excess death rates. The global figures mean that in all countries families, friends and hospital staff are meeting grief, death and even guilt, particularly ICU and Ventilation ward nurses, who endure a their own perceived sense of failure on a daily basis.

In many Western nations, mortality figures have been more devastating because a large percentage have been persons in aged care homes where varying levels of inadequate service have been offered due to staff shortages (infected or close contacts), staff still working when infected and slow vaccination rates. In Australia for example, the first two months of 2022 produced nearly 800 aged care Covid deaths, although authorities knew aged care was struggling before the epidemic with under-resourcing and depleted staffing, and over 600 aged care homes still had Covid infections through mid-to-late 2022. Australians might have thought the elderly would have been prioritised for booster shots but by late July 2022, during the new reset without mandates around 40% still had not had their second booster. This is part of the ethical dilemma of balancing opening up the country for the general population and accepting increasing mortality among the more vulnerable, mainly immune compromised, disabled and aged. In late 2022 a fourth wave rapidly expanded around the world and the agedwere still the main bait. While most of the community is able to live with Covid, vulnerable older people in aged care are dying from it. The answer is really for the state governments to recommend more strongly and promote measures in the wider community that will rapidly decelerate the growth of Covid such as mask wearing and other protective behaviours. People need to realise that although Covid spreading might not feel a serious issue to them now, taking preventive measures protects older people.

Grief

Grief can be a roller coaster. Early grief theories each postulated a stage sequence through the grieving process (e.g. Engel, 1962; Kubler-Ross, 1969). These models have been strongly criticised for suggesting that all individuals must move through these stages and implied that failure to complete any of these stages would result in a variety of complications. Stage theories did have a seductive appeal, bringing a sense of order to a complex process and seemed to offer the desired end point, the emotional promised land of 'recovery' and 'closure'. However, they failed to capture the complexity, diversity and idiosyncratic quality of each individual's grieving experience by not addressing the multiplicity of physical, psychological, social and spiritual needs experienced by bereaved people, their families and intimate networks. Each experience is so different, moderated by very specific interaction of factors providing multiple trajectories through grief. Specific factors that create the individuality include personality, anticipatory processes, closeness of the bereaved to the loss, suddenness of loss, impact of loss, guilt feelings, availability of empathic support (understanding and talking through) and practical support (organising funeral and other bureaucratic requirements), etc.

So instead of a series of fixed stages, the grieving process is better conceptualised as a roller coaster, with ups and downs, highs and lows, twists and turns relating to the individual's situation and feelings, not a straight line from A to B. In the beginning, the ride may be rougher, and lows deeper and longer, but as time elapses the difficult periods should become less intense and shorter. There will also be times when the anniversary of the death, of birthdays and visits to old neighbourhoods will evoke sadness, yearning and temporary awareness of the loss again. Grief is probably best conceived as a 'period of learning'; how to live in a world minus a loved one. The learning is to restore a meaningful life. At a basic level, every bereaved person has to relearn every small habit that incorporated 'we' to just 'me' and relearn how to connect with relatives and friends still around.

The normal grieving period is about 6 months, and this period is used as the cut off to classify those who have continuing *Prolonged Grief Disorder (PGD)* or *Complicated Grief (CG)*, two psychologically recognised syndromes (see later this chapter). Even years after a loss, especially at special events such as a family wedding or the birth of a child, a strong sense of grief may still be revived.

Symptoms of Grief

While loss affects people in different ways, many experience the following symptoms when grieving:

Shock and disbelief. Right after a loss, it can be hard to accept what happened. Some people feel numb, have trouble believing that the loss happened or even deny the truth. If someone they loved has died, for example, they may keep expecting them to show up, even though they know they're gone.

Sadness. Profound sadness is probably the most universally experienced symptom of grief, with feelings of emptiness, despair, yearning or deep loneliness and periods of crying.

Guilt. Some people may regret or feel guilty about things they did or didn't say or do. They can also feel guilty about certain feelings (relieved when a person died after a long, difficult illness, for example). They may even feel guilty for not doing more to prevent their loss, even if it was completely out of their hands.

Fear. A significant loss can trigger a host of worries and fears. If it's a spouse/ partner, they may feel anxious, helpless or insecure about the future. They may even have panic attacks. The death of a loved one can trigger fears about their own mortality, of facing life without that person, or the responsibilities now to be faced alone.

Anger. Even if the loss was nobody's fault, there may be anger and resentment. They may be angry with themselves, God, the doctors or even the person who died for abandoning them. This is because they may feel the need to blame someone for the injustice that was done to them.

We often think of grief as a strictly emotional process, but grief often involves physical problems, such as fatigue, nausea, weight loss or gain, aches and pains and insomnia. Put simply, grief is the natural and normal reaction to loss, the price we pay for love and caring, and a natural consequence of forming emotional bonds to people, projects and possessions. All that we value we will someday lose. As Freud once famously declared in his essay *Beyond the Pleasure Principle* (1920) that the death drive (or instinct) is the drive towards death and destruction, so that '*the aim of all life is death*'. For many, the desire to 'make sense' and 'find meaning' in the wake of loss is central. Neimeyer and Sands (2011) have emphasised that the reconstruction of meaning represents the critical issue in grief and must be approached in a positive way where possible despite emotional and physical pain. Of course help and support and advice are always required and ways found to provide these, just as a toddler learning to walk needs the security and comfort of an adult hand for encouragement to move on. These sort of crises always require some measure of personal adjustments and external adaptations if resolution is to be successful. Unresolved grief and guilt can lead to psychiatric illness. Sometimes delayed grief occurs as a result of denial in order to support the morale of others such as one's children and can suddenly erupt as a torrent of emotional expression in reaction to some minor event.

More Recent Approaches to Grief Trajectories

There is also a growing awareness that losses can provide the possibility of positive life-enhancing 'post-traumatic growth' as one copes with the lessons of loss and resilience. How we adapt to these patterns shapes who we become.

For example, a study of spousal bereavement identified the most common trajectories of adjustment to loss (Bonanno et al., 2002) and made the compelling finding that resilience is actually the most common trait and that chronic and delayed grief reactions are less common than thought. Five different distinct trajectories covered the outcome patterns of most participants: (1) common grief or recovery (11%); (2) stable low distress or resilience (46%); (3) depression followed by improvement (10%); (4) chronic grief (16%) and (5) chronic depression (8%) (Bonanno et al., 2004).

In Bonanno's 2004 research, for those not normally depressed before the loss, level of dependency on the deceased was an important predictor of grief reactions and those who experienced the highest levels of distress were those with high levels of personal dependency prior to the death of their spouse. A lack of expectation of loss or lack of psychological preparation for the loss also contributed strongly to increased distress. There is no single set of stages or tasks in adapting to loss, but instead distinct paths through bereavement, which calls for a closer understanding of both the individual's personality and their usual way of behaving and coping.

Two of the most comprehensive and influential grief theories are the *Dual-Process Model* of Stroebe and Schut (1999) and the *Task-Based Model* developed by Worden (2008). These models serve both counsellors and clients by offering frameworks that guide interventions and enhance clients' self-awareness and self-efficacy. The *Dual Process Model of Grief* developed from a cognitive stress perspective describes grief as a process of oscillation between two contrasting modes of functioning. In the 'loss orientation', the griever engages in emotion-focussed coping, exploring and expressing the range of emotional responses associated with the loss. At other times, in the 'restoration orientation', the griever engages with problem-focussed coping and particularly focussing on the many external adjustments required by the loss, including attention to ongoing life demands. The model suggests that the focus of coping may differ from one moment to another, from one individual to another, and from one cultural group to another.

Worden's (2008) *Task-Based Model* suggests that grieving should be considered as an active process that involves engagement with four tasks: (1) to accept the reality of the loss; (2) to process the pain of grief; (3) to adjust to a world without the deceased and (4) to find an enduring connection with the deceased in the midst of embarking on a new life. Worden also identifies seven determining factors that are critical to appreciate in order to understand the bereaved person's experience. These include (1) who the person who died was; (2) the nature of the attachment to the deceased; (3) how the person died; (4) historical antecedents; (5) personality variables; (6) social mediators and

(7) concurrent stressors. Those who counsel bereaved people must recognise the unique reactions, needs and challenges, the risk and protective factors that individuals and their families cope with and base their support and counselling tailored to an individual's needs at the time. Grief counselling after Covid must recognise and appreciate the idiosyncratic nature of the grief experience.

Loss Can Cause Disease and Mortality Among the Bereaved Too

The life events which are consistently rated as most unpleasant and requiring most adjustment appear to be those involving a personal loss, particularly of a close individual, such as a spouse. Some research workers in this area believe that a generalised sense of loss (actual, potential or imagined) and bereavement are significant factors in the onset of disease. They contend that loss and bereavement can give rise to an emotional response of hopelessness and helplessness which results in the individual literally 'giving up'. When this happens, the individual can no longer cope, psychologically and biologically, with environmental demands. If the individual has a predisposition to disease, then being in this psychological state makes the disease more likely to occur because the body is made less capable of dealing effectively with the processes which give rise to the disease.

Many studies have shown that the recently bereaved are much more likely to develop physical and psychological symptoms, including that the bereaved have a higher mortality rate within the six months following the death of a spouse (Parkes, 1983). It would appear that those who show a strong initial grief reaction and who are able to express their emotions are able to make the best physiological and psychological adjustments. In contrast, there appears to be a less satisfactory outcome for the bereaved person who has had an over-reliant relationship with the deceased, who has limited social support and experiencing other stressors. These individuals often experience recurrent pangs of depression and are most at risk for their susceptibility to other diseases.

As with many psycho-social stressors, there is increasing evidence in the way that one copes with bereavement is more critical in determining vulnerability than the actual occurrence of loss. It is the meaning of the loss, not loss per se that appears more likely to determine susceptibility to illness. This explains why counselling programmes for those close to experiencing bereavement cope better when bereavement occurs (Parkes, 1983). Anticipatory grieving does not remove grief after death but mitigates possible adverse reactions later.

The process of recovery from grief is a process of reconstruction as it is necessary to develop new roles, new behaviours and new relationships as the survivor must live without a former crucial relationship: a widow or widower, a child without one parent or parent without one child. The period of adjustment may never be complete but generally lasts up to 6 months. Gradually with the decline and lightening of mood, decisions and actions are more feasible and an active process of commencing life again begins, although perhaps in a modified form. Therefore, professional care and support should not end with the death of a patient. Predominantly causes of death are coronary thrombosis and other degenerative heart diseases with most the result of continued stress and lack of self-care. Every effort should be made to ensure the support is available to the bereaved person who needs someone to listen when they want to talk and someone who will support them emotionally and practically as appropriate. This demands an informal rather than a formal professional response.

Spontaneous Strategies for Mourning Under Covid Restrictions

The extraordinary circumstances of deaths during Covid pandemic have been challenging for the deceased's families and have been affecting relatives' grieving process (Simon et al., 2020), especially for people who lost a relative at the hospital. In the Covid situation, most of the processes that psychologists know as helpful for patients and families dealing with a death in the hospital, like family involvement, physical presence, clear information, and preparation, have been negated. Many Covid deaths have been solitary, without traditional rituals, often unexpectedly fast, without clear information or preparation and with limited or interrupted communication. Imposed public health safety measures and restrictions often prevented physical closeness; families could not stay close to the loved one in the last moments of life (Sun et al., 2020).

Moreover, some people have been forced to stay at home after the loss to prevent the spread of the virus, reducing the possibility of support from their social network (Carr et al., 2020). Also, traditional funeral ceremonies which usually have an important role in the grieving and recovery process, as they foster emotion expression, social support and give meaning to the loss, have been banned or limited. The complexity and simultaneity of these stressful issues and restrictions have had to be faced all over the world, making the grieving process extremely challenging for families; therefore, the possibility of processing the loss of the deceased has been at risk (Sun et al., 2020). Furthermore, the support usually provided by healthcare professionals has also been limited by Covid safety restrictions. In such a unique scenario, some spontaneous strategies have emerged to deal with this extraordinary grief situation enabling families to process the loss of a relative during the pandemic in a variety of ways.

In a recent study by Borghi and Menichetti (2021), families reported 2–3 days after the loss of a loved one in hospital the main strategies that they developed as their devised way to cope with the bereavement. These strategies were combined into the following six behaviours: finding alternative rituals; normalising the loss; addressing faith and hope; highlighting the positives of isolation; supporting others in need and communicating the bad news. Such strategies are reported below in more detail.

Creating Alternative Rituals for Grieving

Physical distance and isolation could lead to a detached experience, transforming the loss into a 'shadow death', not completely real, and therefore not processed. But Borghi and Menichetti (2021) discovered this did not happen with bereaved families and showed that those lonely funerals and limited social rituals were not perceived or experienced as only partial funerals. Similar to what happened with the Ebola disease outbreaks (IASC Reference Group, 2015), families found new ways to say the last goodbye and to celebrate the dead; they created new rituals to ease pain.

Undertakers had a key role to facilitate this process. For example, families often asked them to drive by the family home on their way to the crematorium/cemetery. This way, the last goodbye from those unable to attend due to number restrictions could take place at the window, with a word, song or prayer. In other cases, the undertaker was asked to place special items in/on the coffin or to take a picture of the prepared body. Furthermore, when at least one family member was able to physically attend the funeral, the last goodbye sometimes became a digital experience with a shared video or broadcast of the funeral to family and friends. Prayers also became a shared digital experience: e.g. prayers were said together with the hospital priest on a video call. Overall, technologies, phone calls, video calls and messages had a key role to help families feel present and involved, not segregated or alone. Moreover, the idea of an anticipated future visit to the grave sooner or later was something that gave a timeframe to the context.

Normalising or Rationalising a Loss in the Covid Context

When the Covid victim was already sick and/or old, the thought of a quick death often alleviated the sufferance, as death was seen as the natural course of events. '*He/she was very old or had a terminal illness, sooner or later this had to happen*' was a recurrent thought/statement among relatives that 'normalised' a death brought forward under extraordinary circumstances. Furthermore, especially families already expecting the loss used the period before the death as an opportunity to express their love. This limited regrets and facilitated acceptance, leading to 'peaceful' grief, with death sometimes seen as a relief from very painful conditions.

Religious and Existential Anchors

Addressing faith or hopes, with thoughts like '*it was destiny*' or '*he is with his wife now*', helped to come to terms with the death. Faith and spirituality represent a strong inner anchorage for families in some cultures searching for meanings in an unpredictable and uncontrollable situation as the pandemic. This reframed a stressful situation into a larger, more benevolent meaningful system within a faith context. While spiritual resources like attending church or talking to their local religious leader were often limited, many families relied on an inner faith as a way to positively cope with the loss.

More Time to Process the Loss

Besides its many downsides, the safety measures and confinement restrictions offered some advantages: for example, families had more time to process the bad news, because they did not need to come back to normality immediately. This extension of both time and space facilitated some aspects of the mourning process, such as reflecting on the loss and emotions processing, with a small group. At the same time, the practicalities required by the extraordinary situation of the pandemic (e.g. bureaucracy requirements, coroner's duties legalities with wills, etc.) enabled an oscillation between facing painful reality and focussing on necessary actions.

Supporting Others, Supporting the Self

In the context of the pandemic, one death could be part of a larger crisis scenario in which stressors piled up; there could be more than one sick relative within an infected family, who may have been hospitalised or also dead because of coronavirus. Some people struggled to contain the spreading of the virus among the whole family when in lockdown. This resulted in feelings of anxiety and distress, but also of helpfulness. Focussing on other family members' physical or psychological health had been found to help all members feel valuable, fostering their sense of helpfulness, mutual support and self-confidence. This also occurs in the larger community as they pull together and support each other.

Delivering the Bad News

Relatives and close family members often had to deliver the bad news to others. This could be a difficult task to accomplish in the first days after the loss. However, it seemed to help bereaved individuals uncover the silence surrounding the death and start to process it as they talked. Indeed, choosing the words can become a constructive activity of meaning-making in the mourning process. Especially in the confused and disruptive Covid circumstances, delivering the bad news helped families translating experiences into meaningful narrations to embrace the reality. Social media can be useful in letting others know about your loss and reaching out for support. However, it can also attract Internet trolls who post inappropriate, insensitive or even abusive messages. To spare yourself additional pain and heartache at this time, you may want to limit your social media use to closed groups rather than public postings that can be commented on by anyone.

In summary, the spontaneous strategies used by family members in Borghi and Menichetti (2021) study to cope with the losses may represent a precious resource, providing first indications of bereavement processes that seem to work in restrictive situations preventing further psychological distress. Such strategies represent new and creative ways to activate and to organise substitutive rituals and actions for grieving, involving concrete actions which give meaning to the loss, helping a positive adjustment and may be helpful irrespective of the specific cultural and religious backgrounds of family members.

Prolonged Grief Disorder (PGD) and Complicated Grief (CG): Same or Different?

The Covid bereavement situation has given rise to two serious grieving disorders; *Prolonged Grief Disorder (PGD)* and *Complicated Grief (CG).* The totality of the upsurge of bereavement grief due to Covid is quite inconceivably unimaginable when we consider each of those 6,600,000 deaths (so far) and their social circles and families, all of whom have been touched by loss. While grief is a normal reaction to loss, some bereaved people develop Prolonged and Complicated Grief reactions, including high levels of grief and an unprecedented need for increased access to psychological support, in considering the aftermath of the pandemic. The restrictions in place because of the virus have led to relatives and friends having a very different experience of the death of their loved ones. This can make their grief journey very different, particularly if they are isolated grieving from their usual supports.

There exists a general consensus that *Prolonged Grief Disorder* (*PGD*) represents a distinct mental disorder worthy of diagnosis and treatment. Nevertheless, confusion remains over whether different names and proposed symptom criteria for PGD identify the same or a different diagnostic entity named *Complicated Grief* (*CG*). Are these two substantively different or merely semantically different names? The Yale Bereavement Study (Maciejewski et al., 2016) attempted to answer this question. Data were derived from a longitudinal community-based study of bereaved individuals funded by the US National Institute of Mental Health, designed explicitly to evaluate diagnostic criteria for *CG*. The results for the *CG* test had only limited agreement with those for PGD, leading the researchers to conclude that *PGD* and *CG* are different disorders although perhaps close relatives.

Semantic differences between *PGD* and *CG* also hinge on the response to the central question: '*is all grief normal*?'. For PGD, the answer is: '*no, not all grief is normal; in particular prolonged, unresolved, intense grief is not normal*'. From the *PGD* perspective, all symptoms of grief immediately after bereavement are normal; for *PGD*, the pathology is in the severity and prolongation, not in the symptoms per se. So *PGD* is characterised by *normal* symptoms of grief that remain too intense for too long. There are complications (mental disorders) in bereavement aside from grief that merit clinical attention, e.g. bereavement-related depression or trauma, that interfere with otherwise normal grief processes, and these lie in the ambit of *CG* (Zisook et al., 2012). For *CG*, the pathology is attributed to factors other than grief.

Prolonged Grief Disorder (PGD)

We will discuss *PGD* first and *CG* in the next section. Millions of families around the world have been faced in this Covid outbreak with the sudden death of loved ones, as well as eventual likelihood of death of those in ventilation and *ICU* wards.

Over the past two decades, there has been increasing awareness and conclusive research demonstrating that *PGD* involving intense, prolonged symptoms of grief, coupled with some form of functional impairment beyond 6 months post-loss, constitutes a distinct mental disorder (Prigerson et al., 2009). Numerous studies have demonstrated that symptoms of grief are distinct from symptoms of depression and anxiety disorder and post-traumatic stress disorder (Prigerson et al., 1996; and that PGD is associated with significant suffering and enduring functional impairments (Boelen et al., 2007).

This disorder was recently added to the Diagnostic and Statistical Manual of Mental Disorders (*DSM*) and International Statistical Classification of Diseases and Related Health Problems (*ICD*) in response to ongoing worldwide mass deaths due to Covid. All this combines into unwelcome upsetting experiences of bereavement stress with accepted cultural and religious processes constrained and diminished to meet health mandates. Those with the condition experience bereavement difficulties which persist or grow, rather than diminishing over time, and can remain indefinitely without treatment.

The most recent diagnostic criteria for PGD require the death to have occurred at least 12 months before diagnosis with thinking dominated by yearning or preoccupation with thoughts or memories of the deceased. *PGD* is associated with elevated risk for suicidal ideas, and data from clinical research settings suggest anywhere from 20 to 50% of treatment-seeking individuals endorse suicidal ideation (Frumkin, 2021). Moreover, PGD reactions are uniquely associated with general health impairments including cancer and health problems as well as alcohol and substance use disorders.

Risk factors for development of *PGD* include pre-existing psychiatric conditions, nature of the death, inadequate social support, female gender, older age and lower socio-economic status. *PGD* prevalence is also higher among individuals with a history of a mood disorder (e.g. bipolar disorder, major depression) as well as those who experienced childhood adversity. Furthermore, depression that is present in early bereavement may increase risk of developing *PGD*. Those bereaved by sudden losses as in Covid are also more likely to develop *PGD* conditions.

Pre-Covid prevalence of *PGD* estimates sit at around 10–20%. However, some initial estimates of *PGD*'s prevalence during the pandemic within Chinese populations place this figure much higher where the first mass of deaths and funeral rituals occurred within strict restraints because of the inability to say goodbye in the expected manner and guilt feelings that the deceased was not being honoured with the normal cultural ceremony, but in undignified haste. Using online versions of the *International Prolonged Grief Disorder Scale* and the *Traumatic Grief Inventory Self-Report*, researchers Tang and Xiang (2021) assessed grief in 422 Chinese participants who had recently lost a loved one to Covid. From this, they were able to arrive at a higher estimate of between 29 and 38% of participants experiencing symptoms of *PGD*.

In the USA, Simon et al. (2020) estimate that PGD characterised by ≥ 6 months of intense longing and preoccupation with the deceased, and by emotional pain, loneliness, difficulty reengaging in life, avoidance, and feeling life is meaningless, had a 10% prepandemic prevalence among bereaved individuals (Lundorff et al., 2017). With each Covid death leaving an estimated nine family members bereaved (Verdery et al., 2020), and a cumulative death toll across the USA of more than 1 million by mid-November 2022, there could be as many as 9 million bereaved Americans, leading to an estimated prevalence of 100,000 Americans with *PGD* due to Covid.

Several assessment measures, including self-report and clinician-rated questionnaires, can be used to assess specific grief symptoms and to track progress in treatment over time. Evidence-based approaches, including cognitive behavioural therapy (*CBT*), exist for treating *PGD* symptoms in a short-term framework. Future research and clinical work should focus on improving the understanding of the potential role of pharmacological treatments.

Complicated Grief

While the bereavement process can become troublesome, prolonged and develop into *PGD*, with people stuck indefinitely in grieving, preventing them from processing the death and moving on with life, *CG* may eventually arise.

CG is a chronic, impairing form of grief, involving other mental disorders like depression, anxiety and post-traumatic stress disorder for example, and other conditions that may follow the death of a loved one (Dell'Osso et al. 2012). *CG* has its historical roots in the concept of depression as a bereavement-related complication and now encompasses other problems (Boelen et al., 2005; Horowitz et al., 1997).

The prevalence of *CG* in the general population ranges from 2 to about 7% (Middleton et al., 1996), but estimates increase steeply in older adults grieving spouse loss, people grieving for unexpected/violent deaths, bereaved people exposed to natural or human-made disasters, or other traumatic events (Kristensen et al., 2012). Most of the recent data on natural disaster *CG* come from earthquakes, tsunamis and hurricanes. Prevalence estimates of *CG* among bereaved survivors evaluated up to 18 months after these types of disasters range from 9 to 80%, with the loss of a child or a spouse both being associated with *CG* symptoms. It is only now that study can be made of *CG* in a pandemic context.

Many of the deaths occured in the *ICU* environment which was a traumatic experience for both patients and relatives: people are rolled in, often unable to communicate, hooked up to machines, ventilated or intubated. During the pandemic, patients entered the *ER*, after the development of an acute respiratory distress syndrome, were taken into the *ICU*, and never came back. As noted above, to keep them isolated, visits were strictly controlled, and critical events, including death, happen quickly, with no chance for relatives to be informed timely and to say goodbye. The situation would prove to be extremely traumatic.

Prevalence estimates of *CG* in relatives of *ICU* decedents are quite variable, ranging from 5 to 52% as evaluated on average six months after the death (Downar et al., 2014; Probst et al., 2016). In a study conducted among 50 family members of ICU inpatients, 46% of those whose relative died presented with both *CG* and *PTSD* after six months (Anderson et al., 2008). In a larger study involving 282 relatives of *ICU* decedents, the prevalence of *CG* at six months was as high as 52.1%, and CG symptoms were associated with the presence of depressive symptoms at three months.

A review by Gesi et al. (2020) of *CG* underlines that female sex is a risk factor for *CG* among bereaved people of ICU decedents. Given that the vast majority of deaths due to Covid is among older males, a special clinical attention to widows is needed. The evidence suggests that the more the bereaved person develops PTSD-related symptoms, the higher the risk of concurrent *CG*. Important risk factors for *CG* with ICU death are the same as those indicated for *PGD* in that family members may be unable to say goodbye to their loved one with this separation from the decedent which appears to contribute to yearning, anger and bitterness over the death, ultimately leading to *CG* (Kentish-Barnes, 2010). In addition, the bereaved often blame themselves for not having tried harder to see their loved one while in hospital and for not taking care of their relative's comfort and dignity during the hospital stay, and feel guilty about not being present at the time of death, although witnessing the death has been shown to raise the risk of *CG* in one previous study on bereavement after ICU stay (Kentish-Barnes, 2010). Again, better grief outcomes are highlighted by research as deriving from greater levels of social support (Kentish-Barnes, 2010), but different from mass short time period disasters, the pandemic is a long-lasting disaster associated with social distancing which prevents much face-to-face counselling.

The Covid pandemic has brought unprecedented circumstances that public funerals are virtually banned in many countries due to restrictions against gatherings and to cemeteries' overloading. But even limited rituals as noted above allowed mourners achieve better outcomes in later grief (Gamino et al., 2000). From this perspective, being prevented from being allowed to be involved in any funeral arrangements and rituals might prevent Covid mourners from gaining awareness of the reality of the death and eliminating a significant occasion of social support from other mourners.

If every death leaves up to nine people grieving, and that the prevalence of *CG* is estimated at approximately 10% to 20% of bereaved people (Middleton et al., 1996), the number of cases of *CG* following Covid deaths may virtually reach the number of overall Covid deaths. The chance of lowering the psychological impact of bereaved people during the current pandemic is small due to restrictions. One concrete option is to safeguard the connectedness between relatives and Covid inpatients and to improve the communication between medical staff and relatives as much as possible. Secondly, as living alone after the death has been found to be associated with the presence of CG symptoms, it could be crucial to provide bereaved relatives with effective social support again difficult under Covid restriction although some other family member could live in temporarily.

Symptoms of CG

During the first few months after a loss, many signs and symptoms of normal grief are the same as those of *CG*. However, while normal grief symptoms gradually start to fade over time, those of *CG* linger or get worse. *CG* is like being in an ongoing, heightened state of mourning that keeps you from healing. *CG* can affect you physically, mentally and socially as complications are added to the grief. These complications can be common and explain why it is termed Complicated Grief and why it is distinct from *PGD* (long-term severe grief without any other major complications) and often include a number of the following:

- Depression, guilt/self-blame,
- Anxiety, including *PTSD*,
- Significant sleep disturbances,
- Increased risk of physical illness, such as heart disease, cancer or high blood pressure,
- Long-term difficulty with daily living, relationships or work activities; have serious trouble carrying out normal routines,
- Extended isolation from others and withdrawal from social activities; emotional numbness or detachment.

Other complications may include

- Intense sorrow, pain and rumination over the loss of your loved one with a focus on little else but your loved one's death,
- Extreme focus on reminders of the loved one or excessive avoidance of reminders,
- Intense and persistent longing/pining for the deceased,
- Bitterness about your loss; problems accepting the death,
- Inability to enjoy life or think back on positive experiences with your loved one,

- Believe that you did something wrong or could have prevented the death,
- In an attempt to escape or cope, detrimental levels of alcohol or drug use, poor diet, lack of activity, self-harm or overworking may be seen.

Study of both *PGD* and *CG* is still in their infancy, and more research is needed to establish prevalence, and how restriction factors associated with Covid may be making them more prevalent, such as fear of infection or disrupted mourning practices, and whether this will differ markedly between cultures who have different attitudes, beliefs and practices towards bereavement. Little is known but given the potentially high prevalence of both brought on by the pandemic, combined with the sheer number of people requiring lengthy support since these disorders are long-lasting and for some people will even outlast the current pandemic, continued attention should be paid to psychotherapeutic support over the long term and more research into best counselling practice and delivery methods to aid mitigation.

Mortality After Covid

Discharge from hospital does not appear to be the light at the end of the tunnel for full recovery for many patients. In an important groundbreaking study by Mainous et al. (2021), analysis of electronic health records for 13,638 patients, including Covid positive and a comparison group of Covid negative patients, who were followed for 12 months post-discharge in one health system was conducted. Both Covid positive patients and Covid negative patients were *PCR* validated. Covid positive patients were classified as severe if they were hospitalised within the first 30 days of the date of their initial positive test. The 12-month risk of mortality was assessed as well as separate subgroup analyses were conducted for (a) patients aged 65 and older and (b) those < 65 years.

In the discharged Covid patient cohort, 2686 died within 12 months. The vast majority of deaths (79.5%) were for causes other than respiratory or cardiovascular conditions. Only 20.5% of the post-acute Covid deaths were for respiratory or cardiovascular causes which implicates other serious organ damage and physiological stress from Covid as significant for the other 80%. Even among younger patients aged < 65 years, the pattern was similar. This suggests that the Covid patients had experienced on overall decline in their health status that left them vulnerable. Patients aged 65 and older with severe Covid were at an increased 12-month mortality risk. The results indicate that patients with a Covid hospitalisation were at significantly increased risk for immediate future mortality, with a significantly increased risk compared to those with no Covid infection.

Mainous et al. (2021) provide evidence that the increased risk of death from Covid is not limited to the initial episode of Covid. In fact, the risk of 12-month mortality among adults over 65 who are hospitalised with Covid is increased by 233% over those who are Covid negative, i.e. more than twice as likely to die over the following year than those who remain uninfected. The benefits of preventing Covid go beyond flattening the curve to prevent overwhelming the health system with hospitalised patients but extend to an increased 12-month mortality risk for conditions other than Covid directly. Prevention of prior significant Covid infection is the most effective way to decrease the risk of death following discharge. In a time when nearly all Covid hospitalisations are preventable with high population vaccination rates and small outbreak area lockdowns, this study points to an important and under-investigated consequence of Covid, and those discharged need regular and thorough medical surveillance perhaps for at least two years.

Anticipatory Grief Counselling

When a death event is possible or known about in advance such as in terminal illness or on ventilation in a Covid ward, anticipatory grief counselling facilitates the alleviation of the eventual impact. This anticipatory process enables those involved to cope by discussing the event before it occurs enabling affected persons to work through it in advance. This mobilises psychological strength, lowers anxiety, guilt and grief, developing a readiness for a less psychologically painful reaction.

Most nursing staff can feel grief at the impending and final loss of a patient with whom they have formed a bond. They may feel guilt and failure too. The professional attitude is that nurses should not express such emotional needs, particularly when on duty; yet nurses are human and often bottle up their feelings, letting go only when alone. To defend too strongly against stress, grief and anxiety may create barriers to the development of warm, caring interpersonal relationships with clients.

The best way to help those bereaved and other colleagues cope with grief and loss is 'acceptant' listening, willing to listen and accept what they say, allowing expression of the emotion. It is easy for staff members to take other staff members for granted, forgetting that they too are human and have needs which they are often trying to suppress. There must be some opportunity provided for even staff to obtain emotionally open support, for emotional interactions with patients are far more easily coped with when staff are also able to communicate openly and supportively with each other about such emotions.

Re-grief After Covid-19; Social Support and Loneliness in Grief

Re-grief is part of the grieving process but occurs as a sudden and unexpected wave of emotion that can hit at any time. Triggers or reminders of the person who died cause re-grief. Re-grief includes vividly remembering the loss or experiencing the pain again as if it happened just yesterday. Evidence suggests individuals can experience re-grief, with feelings from a past bereavement returning following a trigger experience, which for many already previously bereaved is the Covid pandemic. Times of mass death like this may evoke a re-grief response triggering thoughts and feelings previously related to the past bereavement, leading people to imagine a scenario where they or someone else they care about dies. This may be exacerbated by news reports and official advice of ways to reduce risk of death. This reigniting of grief elicits a range of negative mental distress behaviours, such as anxiety, depression, isolation, substance use or self-harm.

Social support can help during these times; however, the rules of social distancing and close contact isolation during Covid did limit direct physical contact support from friends and family. These restrictions to physical connectedness are likely to be detrimental although the use of Internet visual/oral communication of the Zoom type and telehealth has helped to mitigate for some. Those who have been bereaved often feel better understood by others who have also experienced a loss. But the re-grieving person may not cry out to others to establish any support and try to keep it hidden as a supposed stigma. As a society, we need to find ways to encourage and reach out to those grieving.

Cacciatore et al. (2021) explore what good grief support is after traumatic grief. Social support is beneficial to feeling, particularly when faced with stressful life challenges. It improves mental, physical and emotional health outcomes and has been studied extensively within varying disciplines over the last 40 years with similar results. Conversely, poor social support and loneliness are a social determinant of poor health outcomes and can adversely affect physical, emotional and mental wellbeing. Social support is therefore especially important in traumatic grief. However, from the perspective of those being helped, the ways in which grieving individuals interpret and define social support are not well understood, and little is known about what specific behaviours are perceived as helpful. Cacciatore et al. (2021) found just over one-third of the sample rated the level of social support they received post-loss as excellent or good, with 38% rating it as poor or very poor. Specific actors who provided good or excellent social support in more than 50% of the sample included animals, support groups, counsellors or therapists and friends, while the percentage was below 50% for family, faith leaders, colleagues and community members.

There are four categories of social support defined in the literature that have been widely used over the past four decades. Structures and processes of social support, broadly speaking, include (1) informational, (2) instrumental, (3) appraisal and (4) emotional. Many grieving persons have needs related to loss that traverse all four categories of social support such as funeral planning, financial aid, trauma and crisis care and emotional experiences related to the loss. Different groups may benefit more from some types of support than from others, depending on their needs and circumstances.

Cacciatore et al. (2021) findings suggest that emotional support is the most desired type of support following traumatic loss and for supporting bereaved individuals within and beyond the context of the Covid-19 pandemic. Specifically, emotional support in grief can be defined as being present and holding space for the griever, more specifically focussed on listening and allowing grief without judgement, platitudes or an agenda. This means being available for the griever, spending time and centring on griever's needs and not imposing a time limit on grief. Acts of emotional concern can be expressed by remembering (asking about, sharing memories of and speaking the name of) the person who died, acknowledging important dates and engaging in emotionally sensitive communication. It is not simply the amount of contact with family and friends that equates to good social support, but also the quality of the connection, with the presence of emotional support and expression of caring being highly valued.

Research on bereavement suggests that loneliness and inadequate social support are common giving rise to concerns about the risks to emotional, mental and physical health for grievers. This situation has been worsened considerably by the Covid pandemic with a significant increase in loneliness during the pandemic and links to increases in depression, suicidality and other mental health concerns. Restrictions on social activities have been associated with higher rates of loneliness, and measures such as quarantine, while reducing the spread of the illness, have been associated with a number of adverse psychological effects. Authors of many studies on loneliness and Covid have called for increased attention to addressing loneliness and related mental health concerns that are unfolding along with the health crisis plus downstream consequences.

Some studies show that both the quantity and quality of social support may influence wellbeing for grievers. Bereaved people who have more frequent contact with family and friends tend to report better quality of life, whether this support comes through technology (email and the Internet) or in-person. However, the number of contacts in a person's social network does not always predict wellbeing, pointing to the importance of the quality of relationships.

Pitman et al. (2020) identified thwarted belongingness, withdrawal from others, lack of connection and loneliness as significant risk factors for suicidality in *PGD*. Strong social support for those dealing with intense grief may not accelerate recovery, but it may improve the capacity to cope. Typically, much of the responsibility for grief support falls on family and friends. Yet, bereaved people often report insufficient support from these sources. While each person has unique needs, those who have lost a spouse at an early age or a child often need more support than family or friends are typically able to give and may benefit the most from grief counselling or support groups. Additionally, while the death of a loved one sometimes strengthens family relationships, often these relationships are strained, as family members may also be grieving, adding to the psychological distress of the bereaved; additionally, much of the support offered in early grief diminishes quickly while the need for support continues.

A breakdown in social relationships after a loss is not uncommon and loneliness, particularly salient during the Covid pandemic, may exaggerate that effect for grievers increasing the risk for poor outcomes. Despite findings that perceived social support mitigates risk in bereaved individuals, a dearth of qualitative research exists in understanding the specifics of this supportive care. Very limited knowledge exists about the effects of grief support groups or grief counselling. Medical professionals, too, often have little training in dealing with the grief of their patients. Overall, many providers who are present at the time of death are unable to provide sufficient crisis or long-term support to bereaved individuals.

Was 'Heaven' Ever an Ethical Issue?

In early 2022, the end of restrictions and the road to freedom in most nations was exemplified as a metaphorical '*heaven*' for most people on TV as passengers were seen to rip off masks on US planes; as jubilation was witnessed at the lifting of the dancing and singing bans; as extasy from joyous long-awaited reunions between relatives and friends rang through airports as borders opened. Everyone was desperate to get out, visit restaurants, enjoy picnics, take part in sports, renew social connections and celebrate as life became heaven on earth again.

But the '*heaven*' awaiting those in aged care and with disability was of a different kind, a life ending experience for many despite the warnings from advocates of these groups, ignored in the strongly emerging popular demands that mandated restrictions had to end. But the ethics of this two faced drama was not a majority focus or thought through. In many Western nations, mortality figures have been more devastating because a large percentage have been persons in aged care homes where varying levels of poor service have been offered due to staff shortages (infected or close contacts), staff still working when infected and slow vaccination rates.

The figures globally are astounding for old age care homes deaths from Covid. Canadian Institute of Health Information (2020) shows that deaths in aged care homes made up 42% of all Covid deaths reported across the OECD. In Australia, 28% of all deaths from the coronavirus at that time were from residential aged care. Germany reported that 34% of all Covid deaths were in such care homes, the Netherlands 15%, a figure that has since increased significantly. The USA reported 31%, the UK 27%, Italy 32%, France 48% and Spain 66%. The highest of all was Canada, where deaths in aged care homes represented 81% of the comparatively large national total of deaths due to Covid. These Canadian Institute of Health Information (May 2020) figures probably under-report the extent of such corona deaths. There was a failure to include care home deaths where Covid was not explicitly diagnosed in many countries, including the UK and the USA. This was often due to a lack of testing, particularly where the old person also had a prior known co-morbidity.

In Australia, the first two months of 2022 produced nearly 800 aged care Covid deaths, although authorities knew aged care was struggling before the epidemic with under-resourcing and inadequate staffing, and over 600 aged care homes still had Covid infections through August 2022. Australians might have thought the elderly would have been prioritised for booster shots but by late July 2022, during the new reset without mandates around 40% still had not had their second booster. This is part of the ethical dilemma of balancing opening up the country for the general population and accepting increasing mortality among the more vulnerable mainly immune compromised, disabled and aged. The road to Covid salvation became littered by the bodies of the aged who died from Covid, and we all have accepted this and bear some guilt by not putting far greater pressure on governments. Despite warnings, politicians went ahead and most of us eagerly jumped on-board. It may be uncomfortable for the public to accept that in the decision to open up, increased deaths and risk for those most vulnerable to Covid were inevitable; death was an unspoken part of the bargain.

While most of the community is able to live with Covid, vulnerable older people in aged care are still dying from it. The impact overall has been disproportionately felt by older people. The Federal Health Department has broken down the cumulative number of Covid deaths in Australia by age group, and it shows by July 2022 almost 97% were aged 65 years or older with half not having received the approved number of boosters. The answer is real for the state governments to promote measures vigorously in the wider community that will rapidly decelerate the growth of Covid such as mask wearing, disinfecting hands and other protective behaviours. People need to realise that although Covid spreading might not feel a serious issue to them, taking preventive measures protects older people. Currently, in this pandemic, people die every day from Covid and we seem to be OK with that compared to the onset of the pandemic when people globally were aghast at the thought of a single Covid case, let alone a death!

It was a hard decision by public health officials in many Western nations but suggests aged care and disability care individuals have been sacrificed by deliberate action to favour economy over some citizens' lives. Public opinion globally apart from China has quietly moved towards an acceptance norm of influenza, which claims thousands of lives each year and is heading that way with more acceptance of Covid aged care deaths. As noted in other parts of this text (particularly Chap. 10), Covid has exposed the facts that governments make ethical choices regularly (ABC Net News 3 April 2022).

Public messages about Covid-related deaths need to be handled sensitively. Sometimes it may be perceived that some deaths seem to be more important than others; a young person is highlighted, but if you're old or you've got an underlying condition, it seems to matter less and bound up in a general problem of aged care deficiencies and statistics rather than a focus on the person. That can add to bereaved relatives' feelings of helplessness, and we really need to capture the people behind the statistics.

Activities to Support Resolution of Grief

Physical activity particularly with others as a support 'medicine' for grief.

Physical activity can provide significant benefit to those who have been bereaved, and this is particularly found in outdoor activities. The importance of outdoor physical activity has been recognised during the Covid 'lock-down'. It is one of the few legal reasons for which people are allowed to leave their home. Being physically active particularly with others can reduce grief outcomes, including levels of depression, anxiety, loneliness and post-traumatic stress disorder. It can also build social support and a sense of belonging. Depending on age and physical condition try things, you can do with others such as walking, cycling, park runs, tennis, golf, bridge, choir and volunteering.

A Set of Resources
The *BPS Covid-19 Bereavement group* have designed an invaluable set of resources to support people before, during and after the Covid crisis. They are for people in different population groups and ages, for the public and professionals working with grieving people. So far they have produced a range of booklets on supporting each other through death and grief, managing death and grief in care homes and coping with the death of a colleague and are well worth accessing.

Psychologists health and social care professionals have a role in helping communities and the government to plan for a social recognition of lasting Covid grief ensuring that any response is inclusive and that everyone can have access to the best quality evidence-based support they need to readjust to their lives without their loved ones as this will undoubtedly impact on the grief journeys of many people and ultimately on their psychological health and wellbeing.

Valuable texts for more detailed discussion of the topics in this chapter are

Gross (2018). *The Psychology of Grief.* Taylor and Francis: London.
O'Connor (2022). *The Grieving Brain. The Surprising Science of How We Learn from Love and Loss.* HarperOne: NY.
Worden (2008). *Grief Counselling and Grief Therapy.* Springer: NY.

References

ABC News. (2022, April 3). Retrieved 3 April 2022 from https://www.abc.net.au/news/2022-04-30/qld-covid19-coronavirus-data-cases-tolerate-deaths-australia/101024646

ABC News. (2022, 30 April). Retrieved 03 April 2022 from https://www.abc.net.au/news/2022-04-30/covid-cases-vaccines-hospitalisations-daily-statistics-australia/101028736

American Psychiatric Association. (2022, March). *Diagnostic and statistical manual of mental disorders*. (DSM; latest ed DSM-5-TR). Retrieved 16 May 2022 from https://www.psychiatry.org. dsm.

Anderson, W. G., et al. (2008). Posttraumatic stress and complicated grief in family members of patients in the intensive care unit. *Journal of General Internal Medicine, 23*, 1871–1876. https://doi.org/10.1007/s11606-008-0770-2

Boelen, P. A., & Prigerson, H. G. (2007). The influence of symptoms of prolonged grief disorder, depression, and anxiety on quality of life among bereaved adults. *European Archives of Psychiatry and Clinical Neuroscience, 257*(8), 444–452. https://doi.org/10.1007/s00406-007-0744-0

Boelen, P. A., & van den Bout, J. (2005). Complicated grief, depression, and anxiety as distinct postloss syndromes: A confirmatory factor analysis study. *American Journal of Psychiatry, 162*, 2175–2177. https://doi.org/10.1176/appi.ajp.162.11.2175

Bonanno, G. A., Wortman, C. B., Lehman, D. R., et. al. (2002). Resilience to loss and chronic grief: A prospective study from preloss to 18-months postloss. *Journal of Personality and Social Psychology, 83*, 1150–1164. https://doi.org/10.1037//0022-3514.83.5.1150

Bonanno, G. A., Wortman, C. B., Nesse, R. M., et al. (2004). Prospective patterns of resilience and maladjustment during widowhood. *Psychology and Aging, 19*(2), 260–271. https://doi.org/10.1037/0882-7974.19.2.260

Bright, J., Au, H., Bailey, H., et al. (2020). Coronavirus coverage by state-backed English-language news sources. *Oxford internet institute data memo*. Retrieved 28 August 2021 from https://comprop.oii.ox.ac.uk/wp-content/uploads/sites/93/2020/04/Coronavirus-Coverage-by-State-Backed-English-Language-News-Sources.pdf

British Psychological Society Covid Bereavement Group. Retrieved 11 December 2021 from https://www.bps.org.uk/covid-19-coordinating-group. Also https://www.bps.org.uk/coronavirus-resources

Cacciatore, J., Thieleman, K., Fretts, R., Jackson, L. B., et al. (2021). What is good grief support? Exploring the actors and actions in social support after traumatic grief. *PLoS ONE, 16*(5), e0252324. https://doi.org/10.1371/journal.pone.0252324

Canadian Institute of Health Information. (2020, May). Retrieved 15 November 2021 from https://www.cihi.ca/en/long-term-care-and-covid-19-international-comparisons

Carr, D., Boerner, K., & Moorman, S. (2020). Bereavement in the time of coronavirus: Unprecedented challenges demand novel interventions. *Journal of Aging & Social Policy, 32*, 425–431. https://doi.org/10.1080/08959420.2020.1764320

Dell'osso, L., & Pini, S. (2012). What did we learn from research on comorbidity in psychiatry? Advantages and limitations in the forthcoming DSM-V era. *Clinical Practice and Epidemiology in Mental Health, 8*, 180–184. https://doi.org/10.2174/1745017901208010180

Downar, J., Barua, R., & Sinuff, T. (2014). The desirability of an intensive care unit (ICU) clinician-led bereavement screening and support program for family members of ICU decedents (ICU Bereave). *Journal of Critical Care, 29*(311), e9-311.e16. https://doi.org/10.1016/j.jcrc.2013.11.024

Engel, G. L. (1962). *Psychological development in health and disease*. W. B. Saunders.

Frumkin, H. (2021). COVID-19, the built environment, and health. *Environmental Health Perspectives, 129*(7), 75001. https://doi.org/10.1289/EHP8888

Gamino, L. A., Easterling, L. W., & Sewell, K. W. (2000). Grief adjustment as influenced by funeral participation and occurrence of adverse funeral events. *OMEGA—Journal of Death and Dying, 41*, 79–92. https://doi.org/10.2190/QMV2-3NT5-BKD5-6AAV

Gesi, C., Carmassi, C., Cerveri, G., et al. (2020). Complicated grief: What to expect after the coronavirus pandemic. *Frontiers in Psychiatry, 11*, 489. https://doi.org/10.3389/fpsyt.2020.00489

Horowitz, M. J., Siegel, B., Holen, A., et al. (1997). Diagnostic criteria for complicated grief disorder. *American Journal of Psychiatry, 154*(7), 04–10. https://doi.org/10.1176/ajp.154.7.904

IASC Reference Group on Mental Health and Psychosocial Support in Emergency Settings. (2015). *Mental health and psychosocial support in Ebola virus disease outbreaks: A guide for public health programme planners*. Retrieved 18 August 2021 from https://www.mhinnovation.net/sites/default/files/downloads/resource/ebola_guide_for_planners.pdf

Kentish-Barnes, N., Chaize, M., Seegers, V., & Jaber, S. (2010). Complicated grief after death of a relative in ICU. *European Respiratory Journal, 45*, 1341–1352. https://doi.org/10.1016/j.jad.2010.11.032

Kübler-Ross, E. (1969). *On death and dying*. Macmillan.

Lundorff, M., Holmgren, H., Zachariae, R., et al. (2017). Prevalence of prolonged grief disorder in adult bereavement: a systematic review and meta-analysis. *Journal of Affective Disorder, 212*, 138–149. https://doi.org/10.1016/j.jad.2017.01.030

Maciejewski, P. K., Maercker, A., Boelen, P. A., & Prigerson, H. G. (2016). "Prolonged grief disorder" and "persistent complex bereavement disorder", but not "complicated grief", are one and the same diagnostic entity: An analysis of data from the Yale bereavement study. *World Psychiatry, 15*, 266–275. https://doi.org/10.1002/wps.20348

Mainous, A. G., Rooks, B. J., Wu, V., & Orlando, F. A. (2021). COVID-19 post-acute sequelae among adults: 12 month mortality risk. *Frontiers in Medicine (lausanne), 1*(8), 778434. https://doi.org/10.3389/fmed.2021.778434

Neimeyer, R. A, & Sands, D. C. (2011). Meaning reconstruction in bereavement: from principles to practice. In R.A. Neimeyer, D.L. Harris, H.R. Winokuer, & G.F. Thornton (Eds.), *Grief and bereavement in contemporary society: bridging research and practice* (pp. 9–22). Routledge.

Our World in Data. *Continually updated*. Online at https://ourworldindata.org/grapher/weekly-covid-deaths

Parkes, C. M., & Weiss, R. S. (1983). *Recovery from bereavement*. Basic Books.

Pitman, A. L., King, M., Marston, L., et al. (2020). The association of loneliness after sudden bereavement with risk of suicide attempt: A nationwide survey of bereaved adults. *Social Psychiatry and Psychiatric Epidemiology, 55*(8), 1081–1092. https://doi.org/10.1007/s00127-020-01921-w

Prigerson, H. G., Bierhals, A. J., Kasl, S. V., et al. (1996). Complicated grief as a disorder distinct from bereavement-related depression and anxiety: A replication study. *American Journal of Psychiatry, 153*(11), 1484–1486. https://doi.org/10.1176/ajp.153.11.1484

Prigerson, H. G., Horowitz, M. J., Jacobs, S. C., et al. (2009). Prolonged grief disorder: Psychometric validation of criteria proposed for DSM-V and ICD-11. *PLoS Medicine, 6*, e1000121. https://doi.org/10.1371/journal.pmed.1000121

Probst, D. R, Gustin, J. L., Goodman, L. F., et al. (2016). ICU versus non-ICU hospital death: Family member complicated grief, posttraumatic stress, and depressive symptoms. *Journal of Palliative Medicine, 19*, 387–393. https://doi.org/10.1089/jpm.2015.0120

Simon, N. M., Saxe, G. N., & Marmar, C. R. (2020). Mental health disorders related to COVID-19 related deaths. *JAMA, 12.* https://doi.org/10.1001/jama.2020.19632

Sun, Y., Bao, Y., & Lu, L. (2020). Addressing mental health care for the bereaved during the COVID-19 pandemic. *Psychiatry and Clinical Neurosciences, 74*, 406–407. https://doi.org/10.1111/pcn.13008

Tang, S., & Xiang, Z. (2021). Who suffered most after deaths due to COVID-19? Prevalence and correlates of prolonged grief disorder in COVID-19 related bereaved adults. *Global Health, 17*, 19. https://doi.org/10.1186/s12992-021-00669-5

Verdery, A. M., Smith-Greenaway, E., Margolis, R., & Daw, J. (2020). Tracking the reach of COVID-19 kin loss with a bereavement multiplier applied to the United States. *Proceedings of the National Academy of Sciences u.s.a., 117*(30), 17695–17701. https://doi.org/10.1073/pnas.2007476117

WHO Coronavirus Dashboard. Continually updated online at https://covid19.who.int/table

WHO. (2022). International classification of diseases (ICD) (11th Revised edn). Retrieved 15 October 2922 from https://icd.who.int/en

Worden, J. W. (2008). *Grief counseling and grief therapy: A handbook for the mental health practitioner* (4th ed.). Springer.

Zisook, S., Pies, R., & Corruble, E. (2012). When is grief a disease? *Lancet, 379*(9826), 1590. https://doi.org/10.1016/S0140-6736(12)60679-5

CHAPTER 10

An Ethical Dilemma: Freedom Versus Authority

Power tends to corrupt, and absolute power corrupts absolutely
Lord Acton, 1887

Abstract This chapter investigates the dilemmas facing governments in balancing freedom with authority when issuing public health mandates. There has been considerable criticism globally that governments and public health officials have indulged in over-reach with mandated quarantine, vaccination and lockdowns. Ethical principles promoted in the Nuffield Council of Ethics report, viz. gravity of threat, treatment is safe and effective relative to alternatives, and coercion is proportionate to risk, are discussed in relation to the restrictions and mandates imposed as part of the attempts to curb Covid infections. Additional biomedical ethical concepts of beneficence, non-maleficence, autonomy and justice are also considered in relation to the freedom versus authority dilemma of democracies. Research on the cost–benefit analysis of lockdowns, movement restrictions and other controls suggest that such restrictions produced limited benefit at great cost. Moral failures over unequal global distribution of vaccines between nations, the apparent vulnerability of minority groups within countries and the moral distress experienced by many healthcare staff with limited appropriate equipment and facilities even in some developed countries are raised.

Keywords Freedom · Totalitarianism · Over-reach · Bioethics · Cost–benefit analysis · Moral distress

© The Author(s), under exclusive license to Springer Nature Singapore Pte Ltd. 2023

R. B. Burns, *The Human Impact of the COVID-19 Pandemic*,
https://doi.org/10.1007/978-981-99-1710-5_10

Respect for the Law

We have already drawn attention to the twin viruses of (a) the pandemic and (b) misinformation/conspiracy theories in the opening chapters. Another viral spin off is a worrying '*creeping authoritarianism*'. The line in the sand between authority and freedom has always been a confronting uncompromising issue in democratic government decision making. Naturally at the beginning of the pandemic, rapid tough action was required as no one really knew what they were dealing with. At least there is now growing acceptance that suppressing the virus and living with it, supported by high vaccination rates and sensible levels of individual responsibility, is really the only way forward rather than some idealistic battle to annihilate it as was seemingly attempted earlier by some governments and still is by China reaping street riots.

The hype, panic and hysteria generated by the pandemic stop people from thinking rationally. They then tend to do and say silly things. This goes for both the false information mob as well as national governments which have become, to many citizens, dysfunctional nanny states, too frequently, and for far too long. Free speech seemed at times unacceptable when discussing some Covid issues. Pregnant women have been arrested at home for disagreeing online about the mandated restrictions, and a basketball star was threatened by the Victorian Electoral Commission for an anti-government tweet about the pandemic, whereas extreme views arguing for blanket vaccine mandates, extended lockdowns, school closures and continuing harsh border controls were not silenced and evidence for the validity of these actions was silenced unable to be raised in rational debate.

The tilt towards authoritarianism happened nearly all over the world to varying degrees. For example, in Australia there was a secret but damning move from democracy to authoritarianism during the first year of Covid, when the initial threat of the pandemic was drear and difficult to prognosticate, as the then Prime Minister Morrison appointed himself to five additional portfolios in secret including health, finance, treasury, home affairs and industry, science and resources. His concern apparently was what would happen if certain ministers were unable to fulfil their duties including their responsibility to make regulations like Public Health Orders and Immigration movements necessary to control the virus and protect the people. He became the only backup for these five ministerial posts with presidential powers potentially a very damaging insidious weakening in what was a very open democracy, particularly able to impose extreme measures within the Bio-Security Act. Only members of the National Security Committee and the Governor General knew that the prime minister now had authority that amounted to effective power of martial law. While there was no illegality in the delegation of ministerial power to the prime minister, there remain significant matters of principle, practice, convention and propriety involved that undercut democracy, and he has now been censured by parliament. In Victoria and Queensland, one can even portray Premiers and their Chief Medical Officers as exemplars of people seduced by power, hiding behind the mantra '*we will keep you safe*', while Witty and Fauci in the UK and US, respectively, manoeuvred into sitting on top of rapidly expanding empires like the CDC in the US.

All these actions and many more generate '*moral injury*' a perception of state sanctioned injustice which goes against the moral order of society leading to bewilderment, anxiety, vulnerability and anger among the population. It is viewed as a betrayal by someone who holds legitimate authority of what is morally correct. Many Covid power grab examples reveal an almost literary replica of tragedy for those seduced by power as evoked in Faust and the Game of Thrones as those attempting to do good somehow becoming 'bad' and dictator-like. Power brings respect and fame, so why would not you grab it. But as Lord Acton wisely wrote (1887), '***Power tends to corrupt, and absolute power corrupts absolutely***'. Nearly all great persons in history were eventually 'bad', an issue avoided in history classrooms where power is celebrated.

Baring a few occupations, like aged care and medical/health staff who all deal with the vulnerable, the rest of the populations in most countries had been initially promised that vaccination would be voluntary as is the case with any other medical procedure. Choosing or not choosing a medical treatment or procedure is generally a patient's right even when the reasons for choosing or not choosing a particular option seem irrational, are unknown or even non-existent. These rejected medical advices about treatment often relate to non-transmittable conditions such as various sorts of cancers, cornea transplants and hip operations which have serious implications for the patient although only of some nuisance value for carers. This highly contagious Covid virus which is continuing to mutate raises a different argument about balance where some consideration must be afforded to the problem of transmission not only to close relatives and friends but also work colleagues and through them the general community, remembering the Omicron *Rtt,* and subsequent variants are high on this index. Therefore, arguments for vaccination should be directed sensitively towards vaccination of hesitant persons like pregnant ladies and those whose experiences with previous vaccination episodes have been somewhat disconcerting, for whom the right to refuse treatment must always remain available and understandable.

However, there are situations where mandated vaccinations for continuing in certain occupations/professions should exist; these are generally made under public health regulations which offer very limited options to refuse, and '*personal choice*' is not a reason permitted. Should any person not wish to receive the required vaccination schedule and use their right to reject treatment, then they must accept personal responsibility for their choice and also accept there is no inherent right to be able to attend a particular place of work, entertainment venue or sporting event, or high risk setting as the unvaccinated have found out. In supporting this belief in freedom of personal choice, there must be clear explanation, recognition and acceptance of consequent implications.

The Anti-Discrimination Act in Australia does allow employers to impose '*genuine occupational requirements*', which in this setting is a full set of vaccinations and to do things which may appear to be discriminatory if it's reasonably necessary to protect public health or the health and safety of other workers or visitors/clients in the work context, as employers also have legal obligations under industrial law to provide a safe working environment. Queensland have fined all teachers who refused to get vaccinated as well as standing them down without pay when they originally refused to be vaccinated on the grounds of ensuring a safe working environment for students and vaccinated teachers. It is accepted generally that there must be rules for ordered life in democratic society. Total freedom is anarchy. Imagine being able to make a personal choice over whether to stop at a red light or to steal another person's property simply because you want it. Freedom involves responsibility and can only extend as far as not impinging on another's freedom.

Despite attempting to maintain as much freedom as possible in a pandemic, governments have an onerous duty to preserve the safety and health status of as many of its citizens as possible just as they can impose massive safety restrictions in all sorts of other grave situations such as outbreak of warfare, terrorist acts and climate emergencies. But when governments extend mandated restrictions on a close relative doing a check visit to the grandparents, block the state border to prevent you returning to your own home or prevent you from sitting on a park bench to have a sandwich, then democracy and freedom for some actually become seriously impaired on a proportionate basis to the danger involved, especially when as one Australian premier implied a stark division in society when stating, '*there is going to be a vaccinated economy and you get to participate in that if you are vaccinated*'. This situation has risen because for two years 2020 to mid 2022, health officials have been shutting down society at the stroke of a pen on a public health order cheered on by epidemiologists and senior politicians seeking to firm their positions for the next electoral victory.

There were 31 pages of rules and regulations of Public Health Directives created by public health bureaucrats just for entering into the State of Queensland that bypassed review by the elected Queensland Parliament. There was an obvious lack of equity, fairness and even handedness, in the examples noted in the next section that then leads too easily towards contempt for the law and to those who administer it in an unthinking, inhuman way. This is not scorn of authority, because that is the treacherous path to anarchy. This is simply recognising the fact that the democratic legitimacy of laws has been eroded over the last two years with many governments at all levels functioning largely at the behest of unelected health officials. It took nearly 20 months before a state premier made an obvious statement and declared that as state premier he was the elected official and proceeded to open up the state despite some health officials pushing for a longer lockdown.

Over-reach Has Infected Protest Rallies and Amplified Concerns About the Ethics and Morality of Some Government Actions

What is not in doubt is that over the t hree years, 2020-22 using massive emergency powers democratic governments worldwide have basically suspended normal parliamentary decision making and review processes as they imposed rules, restrictions and coercive enforcement, using Public Health Orders. The law has come into disrespect because some politicians and bureaucrats appear to have employed disproportionate powers to manage the virus, often without any disclosed supporting medical evidence, sometimes very clearly unfairly in relation to individual exemption claims, and this has become the basis for many protestors attending rallies. Here are a few of the thousands of examples painting a vivid picture of government over-reach just in Australia, which appear heartless and lacking any sense of humanity, fairness or reasonableness, consequently motivating many anti-mandate rallies:

- In some Australian states, it became illegal for a lengthy time to dance, sing or drink alcohol while standing, looking like it was plagiarised from the Taliban handbook, in the absence of any real medical evidence.
- Some brothel clients were fined for not wearing appropriate protection in Sydney—face masks!
- In some states, it became illegal to go fishing by yourself—can an 'infected' fish transfer the virus when in close proximity to you?
- In Perth, two Melbourne men were imprisoned for daring to cross a state border to watch their favourite football team.
- A footballer moved to W. Australia from Victoria on a contract. He committed suicide 9 months later. His parents were granted permission to travel to W Australia but on arrival were told they had to serve an immediate 14 days in quarantine. The parents indicated they only wanted to do two things: legally identify their son and pack up his things and then leave immediately. The bureaucrats denied their request.
- A double-vaccinated son was refused entry to cross one border to care for his dying mother.
- One Premier banned two people in a loving relationship who lived apart from seeing each other as '*that's not care*' one of the rigid criteria for visiting another person.
- Two elderly ladies eating a sandwich on a park bench were hassled nastily by police to move on as they were not '*exercising*' one of the few criteria for being allowed outside.
- Tourism and hospitality venues were shut down in several states at the height of the Xmas and New Year season (2021) because one employee or customer had later tested positive, meaning all contacts including staff must isolate. Another example of overkill that brought financial ruin to many employees and some businesses.

There are many hundreds of these sort of stories, the most heartless being the plight of thousands of Queenslanders stuck on the NSW side of the state border and refused permission by Queensland to return to their homes with the border closed for close to 5 months! They became squatters in caravan sites, sleeping in their cars, in tents in paddocks and living on the good nature of the communities where they were stranded. A partial relaxation (November 2021) of the blocked border served no useful purpose for them as road crossing was still banned; they had to fly in, an obvious impossibility for those trapped in cars and caravans; that is go back to either Melbourne or Sydney airports (around 1400 and 800 km, respectively further south)!!

Luckily common sense returned with a pre-Xmas 2021 opening of road entry but only with *PCR* or *RATs* 72 h before arrival and five days after. This inundated testing and pathology laboratories preventing people managing the time line set, coupled with insufficient supply of *RAT* test kits. Another failure in planning that had to be drastically modified after denying many tourists their entry access for prebooked holidays unable to comply with testing requirements.

Rules seem to be made without sensible consideration in terms of risk assessment and degree of discretion allowed that could have been applied to the many Queenslanders trapped over the state border in New South Wales brutally denied access to their own state while fulfilling the then requirements of two vaccinations and regular testing. The stopping of their own citizens from returning across a state border and being trapped for many months leading to financial stress as jobs were lost, and savings eroded to maintain themselves in whatever accommodation they could find was absolutely disproportionate as well as being a malfeasance, to the risk these citizens posed if they had been allowed to return and undertake a short period of quarantine. This blockade occurred as the most vulnerable elderly persons, in aged care homes, were not afforded enough protection with aged care locations providing most of the deaths. It is one thing to quarrel with the content of a law but another when a law is applied arbitrarily, unevenly and unfairly benefitting some elites. No wonder legitimacy of the public health orders was increasingly damaged, especially as case after case of eminent persons both local and overseas, usually sports people or film stars including spouses and partners, were given special preferential exemptions to cross borders and quarantine minimally in rather exclusive houses and resorts, noted visually in the public arena of TV and internet for all to see.

During lockdown, while Australians overseas were stranded unable to return home, separated from family, the rich and famous jetted in and out. Hollywood stars like Julia Roberts and Matt Damon set up temporary home in Australia. Nicole Kidman and Dannii Minogue were allowed luxurious private quarantine, while other Australians lucky enough to get a flight back had to endure squalid small quarantine hotel rooms, many without proper access to fresh air for 14 days. Billionaire businessman Kerry Stokes and his wife, returning from the Colorado ski fields, were exempted from hotel quarantine on medical grounds. Like the UK 'Partygate', it all represents what many people believe, that it is one law for 'us' but a different law for 'them' as leaders who prescribe the strict lockdowns discriminate in who they apply the regulations to.

Sowing the Seeds of Totalitarianism

The fear is that the manner in which authorities sought to manage the pandemic might inadvertently lead onto the path towards undermining democracy. For example, in a major democratic society like the U.K., the Scientific Pandemic Influenza Group on Behaviour (SPI-B) which ***actually encouraged the use of fear to control people's behaviour*** and increase '*the perceived level of personal threat*' because the government felt '*a substantial number of people still do not feel sufficiently personally threatened*' during the Covid pandemic and have admitted its work was '*unethical*' and '*totalitarian*' (Rayner, 2021). Morgan (2021), a psychologist on the team, said: '*Clearly, using fear as a means of control is not ethical and smacks of totalitarianism*'. This admission supports repeated accusations that U.K. Ministers ramped up the threat from the pandemic to justify lockdowns and coerce the public into abiding by them, using the pandemic to drive through things that wouldn't happen otherwise.

The dilemma is perhaps understandable from state government perspectives. In Australia, there was a policy of '*Go Hard*' with lockdowns, quarantines and border restrictions to protect the citizens, then far too late, partially and gradually release the reins, portrayed as a reward for good behaviour (i.e. obedience) from a smiling motherly or fatherly Premier but at the same time create 'pariahs' of those in the minority who refuse to be jabbed by limiting their access to normal life, apparently to protect those who are jabbed (who have protected themselves proactively anyway).

Around the Western world, most of the measures have little to do with infection control and more to do with growing coercive control combined with relaxation to reinforce acceptable behaviour and negative reinforcement applied by banning access to certain desirable establishments; the sad misuse of a methodology clearly derived from Skinner's Behaviourist Psychology playbook. The willingness to acquiesce to government dictats has perhaps been conditioned by previous years of climate warming propaganda creating a constant state of anxiety, leading to an abandonment of scepticism with unquestioning acceptance of what 'experts' claim. Almost a wartime call to arms and collectivism with slogans like '*keeping us all safe*', '*we are all in this together*' and '*we'll all pull up our sleeves for the country*' was employed to mass motivate many countries in the face of the pandemic. On the other hand, politicians, epidemiologists, mass media and university researchers have failed to inform the general public of the initial untrusty pandemic modelling (see Chap. 11) which turned out to be as equally as untrustworthy as some of the climate warming models.

Some support for raising fear to increase adherence has been derived from a new survey scale *'Fear of Covid-19 Scale'* (Ahorsu et al., 2022) that has been used worldwide, translated into many languages and poses items to be checked like *'I cannot sleep because I am worried about getting coronavirus-19'*. Results commonly revealed that respondents who registered higher fear scores generally were ones who abided by and behaved in accordance with requirements. Thus, it could be argued that fear can be used ethically where it ensures increased protection from devastating consequences of not complying and protecting the general public, an example of the difficult ethical balance facing governments.

Coetzee (2021), the head of the South African Medical Association who first identified Omicron, indicated that the effect would be far less severe than Delta with most people only experiencing mild symptoms. This is now largely borne out by experience globally, but she became the target of pressure from politicians and scientists worldwide who wanted her to state that Omicron '*was more serious*' in another attempted fear strategy. This attempted fear campaign to rein in the general populace failed as she stuck to her guns to place Omicron in perspective and refused to be intimidated to hide the scientific truth. Scary tactics also have been used in public announcements in various Australian jurisdictions directed at millions of lay persons in the general public by Premiers and Chief Medical Officers claiming '*the virus is coming and everyone will get it*' or similar.

Until vaccination levels became almost maximally high, there was a concerted drive to weaponise behavioural psychology from altruism to manipulation. Nations took covert decisions to terrify the public to get compliance with rules, which raises extremely serious questions about the type of society we want Western democracies to be. There were considerable concerns that Western government policy was sowing the seeds of totalitarianism. The *Economist Intelligence Unit* 2021 *Democracy Index* noted an unprecedented withdrawal of civil liberties in democracies. Politicians world-wide needed reminding sChurchill claimed that democracy was *the worst form of government except for all the others*. While the emergency initially required temporary restrictions, we let our guard down. Even these restrictions should have been subject to parliamentary oversight and judicial eyes. Both were missing or deliberately avoided.

China tried to demonstrate that its system was superior by showing the disruption and pandemonium Covid restrictions cause to democracies, blithely ignoring the obvious that China's control over its people prevent issues of withdrawal of freedoms ever being an issue with the lockdowns of many millions over a three year period on and off manifesting barely a whimper until riots in November 2022. The Queensland government have refused to release the scientific evidence and cost–benefit analysis that informed its harsh decisions to close Queensland borders and impose lockdowns despite two Rights to Information requests from a major tourist group. It is only now that an end has come to vaccine mandates as a condition of employment in Australia and the UK where in the latter it had created a shortage of 140,000 healthcare workers.

Restrictive mandates had been imposed on the basis that the unvaccinated spread the disease. This rarely is the case now with well over 90% double vaccinated, variants of the virus are still infecting even many double- and triple-vaccinated people, although at a greatly reduced rate. Now with the dramatically less dangerous variants, only 1% of cases in Australia are in hospital, 0.1% in ICU and 0.04% dying. To gain perspective of the dramatic presentation of unnecessary fears and infections, in a normal year, around 400 persons die each day (around 150,000 annually) in Australia, mostly elderly and often from respiratory illnesses. Compare this with the national influenza report of 2019, the last year Australia really had any flu around, there was a hospitalisation rate of 10% similar to Delta, with 950 deaths, and a mortality rate of 0.03% that places it on a par with Omicron. If Australia and most other countries can live with flu epidemics that produce such data, then nations can live with these later Covid variants without mandates. Most nations have scrapped all restrictions, with the sick staying home, only the very sick go to hospital, while the rest get on with normal daily life with due regard for maintaining basic hygiene, pushing their economies and social lives back towards normal. The unvaccinated are putting no one at risk but themselves.

Kulldorff (2021) criticises that with lockdown, there was an untested policy that affected millions, with the denial and avoidance of any rigorous scientific debate and robust challenge to identify error, improve policy and save lives. Open and honest discourse is critical for science and public health. With lockdown, science was suppressed by politics and was translated from untested theory to unchallengeable orthodoxy, where dissenters faced personal attack. The authors of the *Great Barrington Declaration* 2020 *(GBD)* attempted to argue for focussed protection of those most at risk, rather than a blanket lockdown which inflicts so much harm on society. This strategy is similar to the current reset approaches adopted by many governments with the Omicron variant but probably 18 months too late. But the GBD writers were demonised as denialists at the time. It would be tragic if 400 years of scientific enlightenment established by Kepler, Galileo and Descartes ended up as one of the many casualties of this pandemic as a badly infected system.

Certainly, in future Covid must become one of the viruses we must be alert to, keeping our vaccinations up to date, knowing it will operate alongside flu and the common cold to cause some deaths, particularly among the elderly for whom there needs to be far greater concentration on their protection than is occurring presently. We need pragmatic not dramatic voices leading the way.

Some Legal Responses: The Tide Is Turning

The Human Rights Commissioner for Queensland opposed the Queensland government's new attempt to extend the Chief Health Officer's unprecedented powers in March 2022 to 31 October 2022. The Commissioner objected to the public health directive that restricted movement and gatherings, mandated quarantining, self-isolation and detention orders, as there was limited transparency in decision making, with medical evidence or research to support the directions not offered, especially as the initial urgency had passed and proportionality needs recalibrating as more is now known about the virus. The Commissioner's objections brought more balance to bear with transparent, accountable and human rights compatible legislation. This may have prevented the re-imposition of further excessive control.

The Victorian Ombudsman report of December 2021 into that state's border restrictions found that the bureaucrats operating the scheme failed to understand and take into account the genuine needs of some people to cross the border and was a cruel process in the way it operated. For example, in the report, one woman needed to travel to help her elderly mother to care for her intellectually disabled sister who had terminal cancer. She was required to jump through hoops providing inter alia evidence of her sister's cancer diagnosis, treatment and life expectancy, her birth and marriage certificates, drivers licence and a statutory declaration from her 86-year-old mother explaining why it was difficult for her to continue looking after the very sick daughter. The Ombudsman concluded that failure to exercise discretion fairly, not providing reasons for refusal, not offering right to review, all diminished public trust in and respect for law.

In South Australia, in late 2022 a case was heard to test the legitimacy of that state's emergency declarations, the proportionality of the government's response and the legal and medical bases for it all. The outcome fatally damaged the rationale for vaccine mandates and lockdowns nationally. The complainants wanted the emergency orders declared invalid so that they can return to work vaccinated or not. Legislations have been improperly sidelined with rules being imposed under emergency orders rather than legislation through parliament.

When the rule of law breaks down, respect for the laws does too. It is not surprising there is push back round the world at senselessly and unfairly applied restrictions. A line needs to be drawn sometimes when it comes to having to live under laws that operate in a morally inequitable fashion. To claim there is no line and all laws must be obeyed strikes at the heart of democracy and freedom. The success of the Boston tea party, the dismantling of apartheid and gaining women's suffrage name just a few events that have only been achieved by drawing a line. Compliance can so easily lead to tyranny as people become conditioned to obeying. This causes worry about whether countries will get back to 'normal freedoms' after the pandemic has been managed down to minimally endemic proportions.

The disease will be with us for a long time like the flu, but by late 2022 with a combination of high vaccination and booster rates and an aggressively contagious but much less severe variants, new policies to lower restrictions, more fairness and common sense rather than excessive interventions are evident. Although the rigid requirement for impossible number of virus tests to be carried out on cross-border and international travellers has recently been removed, it was evidence of a remnant of unwillingness to let go the reins sufficiently.

Freedom to and Freedom From

Feeding through all the issues is a clash between '*freedom to*' and '*freedom from*'. The former is strongly supported in democracies in relation to speech, religious observance, etc. It is bounded by responsibilities like not infringing the rights of others to enjoy the same freedoms and not advocating violence against others for what they believe, say or practice. Freedom is defined as liberty of conscience, thought, feeling and opinion, as John Stuart Mill the British philosopher stated '*liberty of tastes and pursuits ... doing as we like ... without impediment from our fellow creatures, so long as what we do does not harm them*'. (Mill, 1859). This moves the issue over to '*freedom from*' where all democratic societies curtail liberties as part of a social contract, to protect individuals from themselves and each other. Examples of the two sides:

- You have '*freedom to*' smoke, but are restricted to where you can smoke in order to provide '*freedom from*' the dangerous contents of smoke emissions on other peoples' health.
- You have *freedom to* drive on your own extensive property without a licence, be heavily intoxicated when you drive, ignore the necessity for seatbelts, vehicle registration and insurance, but venture onto public roads those freedoms cease as others have freedoms not to be injured or be unable to claim insurance damages.
- You have the *freedom to* vote in an election for the person of your choice and *freedom from* others mandating you vote a particular way.

Mandating and balancing certain rules for fair and sensible living like the above, which, with many other rules, are part and parcel of community living and without which society could quickly descend into self-destructive lawlessness is essential. We do this with freedom of speech and belief too. Freedom of speech has an important caveat, that everybody especially influencers and opinion leaders is responsible for the ideas and facts they put out into society. Get it wrong and there can be immense consequences. A person is entitled to hold views, opinions and beliefs that are, to the greater majority of the population, rather weird, scientific nonsense, irrational and even dangerous—*the freedom to*. But people have a right not to be verbally abused on the basis of their views on ethnicity, religion, sexuality, etc. or have violence urged against them—*the freedom from*. Agreeing to disagree has long been a hallmark of Western democracy. But *freedom from* the dissemination of false information that cannot be backed up by valid argument and that has the immediate potential to cause serious harm and even death to some if followed *is a genuine situation where some degree of control is necessary*. We should respect the legal and moral right of competent adults to refuse medical treatment. Yet many have often been seduced by fake news and dogmatic beliefs of others and are current victims of their own gullibility and possible future victims of the Covid virus.

The difficulty with the freedom rallies or convoys is that the '*freedom*' they chant is too empty, ill-defined and vacuous to be the basis of a valid manifesto. It seems to defy libertarianism as the participants actually demand government action to fix a whole range of things. The rallies and conveys have little respect for other peoples' freedoms (*freedom from*). The interference caused cancellation of an annual Lifeline bookfair in Canberra that raises funds to aid potential suicides and in Ottawa blocked main highways for several weeks needing police in riot gear attacked by gas canisters and smoke grenades as they cleared roads. One wonders what sort of freedom do they want because for some of them it is fuelled by a deep seated selfishness, psychological reactance and ultimately a sociopathic, megalomaniacal Machiavellian personality (sociopathy is a recognised anti-social personality disorder (*ASPD*)). Those with *ASPD* have no regard for others' rights or feelings, believe they should have their own way, lack empathy and remorse for wrongdoings and have the need to exploit and manipulate others for personal gain. In some participants' motivational drive, there may even be a degree of paranoia due to the belief that some dominant other(s) is controlling their life, nourishing an unrealistic distrust of others or of being persecuted an extreme level of external control end of the Locus of Control personality trait.

Societies do impose restrictions because rights are never absolute and responsibilities matter equally. In terms of vaccination success, there is no debate feasible now as the debate has been lost with most developed countries reaching over 90% double vaccination levels plus boosters and peak Omicron reached and passed. Rousseau's, 1762 statement that '*man is born free but everywhere he is in chains*' is a sound reflection of the current situation. The 'chains' are essentially those balances to freedom that nations employ to ensure stable democratic life, with the minimum of laws that permit maximum freedom without impinging on another's freedom. There are of course a number of nations where excessive and heavy 'chains' massively curtail basic freedoms where an imbalance of heavily restrictive laws imposes authoritarianism. The new normal must move back towards democratic society.

Ethics and Covid Regulations

When we're thinking about the ethics of a law or rule, there are lots of questions to ask. Is it fair and equitable? Is it proportionate to needs? Does it work? Who was consulted about it? Who made the decision? Can we understand it? Does it treat us like adults? Is it enforced appropriately? In the context of the initial onset of a pandemic, delivering inclusive, informed, nuanced and fair rules to such questions as these requires the crucial resource of time which was not at the disposal of anyone as the situation delivers rapid changes.

It means that leaders are thrust into hard decisions, and the rest of us must cope with living in a deeply imperfect moral world. The serious question for the future becomes whether the public will have become so inured to executive rule that governments feel confident in retaining some restrictions on our liberties and resist relinquishing many of their powers? QANTAS and Jetstar airline employees lost a High Court battle to save their jobs against the airlines' vaccination mandates, with the judge arguing that the airlines are simply seeking to comply with lawful public health orders. This implies if governments have ensured that the regulations and orders are watertight, there is little an aggrieved set of employees or public can do.

However, government policies have exhibited a heavy handed public policy 'duty of care' ostensibly to protect citizens from the virus and from those who refuse vaccination, extending the 'freedom from' argument beyond what many regard as fair and sensible limits. Thus, there is a challenge to our consciences to decide on a range of new behaviours in which a variety of positions could be argued such as:

- How far can our freedoms be rightly restricted in the name of the public interest and the greater good?
- Can refusal to receive newly developed Covid vaccines be morally acceptable?
- Are protest rallies against restrictions morally acceptable?
- Are protest rallies supporting fake news and conspiracy theories morally acceptable?
- Is it OK—or even obligatory—to 'dob' in mandate rule-breakers?
- Is it morally wrong to ignore social distancing rules and mask wearing?
- Is it acceptable to ignore tracing systems and not 'check-in'?
- Is it acceptable for those who do not follow various mandates be penalised?

Usually, responses to these ethically loaded questions are avoided by governments and health authorities by claiming they were *'just following the science'* of good public health management. But that is impossible as even where the scientific evidence is without question, issues of fairness, human rights, safety and freedom still impact political decision making as does the major issue of political positioning in the eyes of the electorate. But without a doubt, value judgements about fairness, human rights, safety and freedom have fed deeply into conversations about Covid rules. TV and newspaper reports that the rules have not applied equally to all on many occasions are only too common. Such issues as these have stimulated ethical thinking and discussion; *the pandemic may have been a benefit in encouraging more people to start thinking along ethical lines generally.*

While there are powerful ethical reasons supporting vaccine mandates, the shattering of people's life expectations nevertheless carries profound costs. Some people may be removed from careers they built their lives around. It's not a crime to have strange beliefs and odd values, so long as you still follow the relevant rules. But when a new regulation is imposed to prevent a person attending their workplace or right to leave the country or even local area, it raises personal disruption. Others may have lost the sense their future is able to be predicted, or that their lives are not in their control. We all have expectations and plans for our individual futures. Yet as the eighteenth-century philosopher Jeremy Bentham argued (1789), disruption is inherently ethically challenging because people build their lives around their expectations. We make decisions, investments and plans based on our expectations and adapt our preferences around them. When those expectations are violated, we can experience not only material losses, but losses to our autonomy and our perceived ability to navigate the world.

Ethics of COVID-19 Vaccination and Other Requirements

The major overlying issue is how far can and should governments proceed in the imposition of a range of heath mandates and whether sanctions should be levied on those who either disagree with them on ethical and moral grounds and refuse to obey or simply refuse to obey anyway. There does exist a large body of literature on the justification for the use of coercion in public health and infectious disease in particular. Mill, the nineteenth-century British philosopher, in his classical text *On Liberty* (1861) justified the utilitarian principle as the foundation of morals. This principle says actions are right in proportion as they tend to promote overall human happiness. Following Mill, the most prominent argument from bioethicists is that mandatory vaccination, including for Covid, can be ethically justified to prevent harm to others (Savulescu, 2021). The sole ground for the use of state coercion (and restriction of liberty) is when one individual risks seriously harming others. The Nuffield Council of Bioethics (2007) produced an influential report on public health ethics which has had strong influence globally on such matters. It provides clear unambiguous guidelines as to when coercion and mandatory vaccination might be justified leading the conclusion that there is a strong case for making any vaccination as universal as possible (i.e. compulsory) if four conditions are met:

1. There is a grave threat to public health.
2. There is high confidence that the vaccine is safe and effective; i.e. risks associated with vaccination are minimal.
3. Vaccination has a superior utility (cost/benefit) profile compared with other non-pharmaceutical alternatives.
4. The level of coercion is proportionate to the risk.

Each of these conditions involves value judgements. We will briefly explore the Nuffield Council of Bioethics (2007) criteria.

Gravity of Threat

Infection, hospitalisation, ventilation and mortality data are complex and difficult to compare with different testing rates, in ways of assigning deaths and collecting data differing from country to country. For example, Belgium counts deaths in care homes where there is only a suspicion that Covid was the cause (without the need for a positive test) and, until recently, the UK counted a death which followed any time from a Covid positive test as a Covid death. Even the Case Fatality Rate (CFR) varies wildly by age group and other factors such as access to hospital care and co-morbidities reflecting variations in demographics. Even among survivors, Long Covid health implications (Chap. 8) may present a grave future public health problem for many who have been infected but survived. Gravity therefore must involve assessments of a range of interacting variables not just one data point.

Covid is almost unique because of the gravity of the problem at the global level, though still far behind the mortality rates of Spanish Flu and the Black Death as yet. The Spanish influenza killed many more (80–100 million) and generally infected younger rather than older people, meaning far more '*life years*' were lost. Not only is there cost in terms of lives from Covid, there are also drastic economic, health and wellbeing consequences of various non-pharmaceutical virus-control measures, including lockdown, quarantine, school closures, travel restrictions, consequences of which will continue for some time into the future as has been discussed in earlier chapters.

It is argued by the anti-mandate proponents that the situation is not grave enough to warrant any vaccine mandate. According to Prof Allan (Weekend Australian 1–2 January 2022), of those who catch Covid and are not vaccinated 99.7% survive. Covid is patently not as lethal as some previous pandemics (noted in the paragraph above) and on that basis, while highly infectious it does not justify huge inroads into the core of liberal democracy. The virus will kill but is selectively dangerous only for those over 80 or have co-morbidities or are immune-compromised, and only these persons need specialist support and treatment. This can be done, and therefore, there is no valid reason ethically to segregate anti-vaxxers and stuff up their lives and careers. Except that data appearing from the Omicron variant are now suggesting that Covid deaths may still head upwards given recent relaxations of vaccination mandates and most other restrictions and will overtake those of the Spanish Flu in some countries. For example, data recently released from the State of Queensland, Australia, reveal that Covid claimed the lives of more citizens in the State of Queensland in the first five months of 2022 than the whole of the Queensland Spanish Flu pandemic, with unvaccinated persons over 10 times more likely to die. During this period, of 4.8 million vaccinated Queenslanders, 223 ($p = 1$ in 0.000048) died from Covid, whereas the unvaccinated cohort on 410,000 lost 235 ($p = 1$ in 0.00057).

Deciding conclusively whether Covid is sufficiently grave perhaps requires both more and better data than we had or even have now (hindsight is a marvellous thing!!) as well as agreement on defining quantitative criteria that would warrant this kind of intervention. ***But given the global scope and impact of the pandemic in not only costing many lives but also destroying economies and societies, most nations have accepted that Covid was and still is a grave public health emergency, with implications that go well beyond health.***

The Vaccines Are Safe and Effective

There are concerns that testing has been rushed and vaccines may not be safe and effective, or some are more effective and safer than others as different countries produce their own. But all have been approved in a few nations and some worldwide. *Safe and effective may not be joint criteria as a vaccine could be effective but not very safe or* vice versa. However, the technology being used in many of these vaccines has been successfully used in other vaccines. On the other hand, no pharmaceutical company or research group has ever produced a safe and effective vaccine so quickly. While there has been apparent pressure to rush the development of various vaccines, they are still subject to stringent tests and evaluation to ensure that licenced Covid vaccines are both effective and safe.

WHO SAGE report (2019) emphasises the inordinate value of vaccines and vaccination. Between 2000 and 2018, an estimated 35 million deaths have been averted through use of vaccines, 96% of them of infants. These efforts have almost halved the number of deaths from vaccine-preventable diseases. Looking forward, the report estimates 122 million deaths are likely to be averted by immunisation over the lifetime of people born between 2000 and 2030. These statistics speak volumes to the extraordinary impact of vaccines. Vaccines are almost uniquely successful interventions, highly effective, extremely safe and mostly free or very affordable.

A wide-ranging analysis in California has given detailed, real-world results highlighting the protection offered by Covid vaccines. The study, with 43,127 Covid cases carried out in Los Angeles County, found unvaccinated people are almost 30 times more likely to be hospitalised once the results are adjusted for age, while 30,801 cases (71.4%of all cases) were found among unvaccinated people (RACGP 2021). While not everyone becomes very sick or dies from Covid, a September 2021 report from the Centers for Disease Control and

Prevention in the United States which has charted the rampant spread in the previous 12 months shows that vaccinated people are 10 times less likely to be admitted to hospital or to die from Covid than those who are unvaccinated. The UK Health Security Agency data weekly vaccine report for the final four weeks of 2021 shows unvaccinated adults are between four and six times more likely to die with Covid for different age groups and between two and six times more likely to require hospitalisation. Similar statistics are appearing from Australian experience with unvaccinated being over 20 times more likely to be in the ICU ward. *Thus, the overall conclusion from experiences worldwide is that Covid vaccines do offer highly significant protection.*

Even so, health authorities are aware that no vaccine has ever been shown to be 100% safe. There will always be side effect risks some of which may take time to show up. This is not to denigrate vaccines or provide support to the anti-vaccination movement. It is only to acknowledge that every vaccine and medical procedure like anaesthesia has risks. The ethical approach is to be honest about the type and extent of those risks and ensure medical authorities and general public understand the limitations of confidence in safety and efficacy relative to the evidence so far discerned.

The ethical dilemma is between introducing a vaccine early and saving more lives from Covid, but risking more side effects or ineffectiveness versus engaging in longer and more rigorous testing and having more confidence in safety and efficacy, but more people dying of the disease in the meantime. Given the original but inaccurate projected modelled figures for infections and deaths with the possibilities of hospitals being overwhelmed and, given the economic and social dislocations of other restrictive measures like lockdown, there was considerable pressure to introduce approved vaccines as early as possible.

The question remains of how safe is safe enough to warrant mandatory vaccination. It is unlikely that there will be absolutely no risk of harm from any biomedical intervention, and the disease itself has dramatically different risk profiles in different groups of the population. In an ideal world, the vaccine would be shown to be 100% safe. But there will likely be some risk remaining and any mandatory vaccination programme would therefore need to make a value judgement about what level of safety and what level of certainty are safe and certain enough. Of course, it would need to be very high, but a 0% risk option is not likely.

Mandatory vaccination is most justifiable when there are benefits to both the individual and close contacts in terms of preventing transmission through the rest of the community. Another justification would be to prevent exhaustion of healthcare services in an emergency (e.g. running out of ventilators or beds), which has been used as a basis of restriction of liberty (it was the main justification for lockdown). It could also be justified in the case of protection of children and others who cannot decide for themselves and the protection of other adults who cannot be vaccinated for medical reasons. But, governments must also demonstrate that alternative policies would be inadequate in responding to such a clear and serious health risk (3rd ethical argument below).

Better than the Alternatives

It is a standard principle of decision theory that the expected utility of a proposed option must be compared with the expected utility of relevant alternatives. In public health ethics, there is a familiar concept of the '*least restrictive alternative*' (Giubilini, 2019). The least restrictive alternative is the option which achieves a given outcome with the least coercion and least restriction of liberty.

Vaccination is the alternative of choice worldwide as it achieves a high level of protection and can be administered easily. Most authorities are unhappy with compulsory vaccination as there is always a small but vocal and well-organised minority who reject any form of vaccination for a variety of reasons and it would involve a high degree of coercion to obtain compliance. The major alternative to compulsory vaccination is obviously voluntary inoculation associated with massive publicity and opinion leader support which is congruent with medical ethics that individuals have the right to reject health advice.

Voluntary vaccination may result in too low a proportion of the population developing immunity as there has been a current slackening of concern to get booster vaccination in 2022 and 2023, a sort of vaccination fatigue, despite it being shown that a booster is highly effective against the current variants spread. The voluntary approach is necessary as some people have allergies, immune problems or other illnesses and cannot be vaccinated. Revaccination is also voluntary but highly encouraged as the elderly are often at more risk as they tend to produce a weak immune response. Even immunity wanes over time, so people previously vaccinated may become vulnerable, may get re-infection, and currently booster shots are being delivered.

Other alternative policies that might obviate the need for mandatory vaccination include strict and long lockdowns, closure of all but essential shops and business and educational establishments, plus abandonment of activities where crowds gather such as sporting activities and church services. All these have been invoked initially in most nations imposing considerable dislocation and stress to individuals, communities and economies and still are invoked in China. The long-term costs and benefits of such policies have never really been evaluated thoroughly and compared with mandatory vaccination. How costs and benefits of alternative restrictive mandates should be evaluated is another ethical question. Are the criteria deaths averted (no matter how old), life years lost, wellbeing changes (how do we measure the latter in a valid and operational way?)? How do we quantify loss of liberty or privacy? It seems that voluntary vaccination supported by massive public health messaging offers a significantly smaller loss of wellbeing or liberty than mandatory vaccination and other complex resource intensive strategies like lockdowns, enforced quarantine with tracking devices, contact tracing and abandoning crowd activities which have imposed considerable economic and social distress.

The alternatives: Failure of Lockdown, Self-isolation and Restrictive Movement

Lockdowns were based on several flawed assumptions, including '*no one is protected until everyone is protected*', '*lockdowns are highly effective to reduce transmission*', '*lockdowns have a favourable cost–benefit balance*' *and* '*lockdowns are the only effective option*'. Most of this ignores the effect on human mental distress and economic devastation (Miles et al., 2022) but without such foresight most countries implemented population-wide lockdowns; hindsight (which obviously no one had) paints a different picture on the human impacts (see earlier chapters).

While in the short-term various forms of quarantine and 'lockdown' policies can be effective initially to manage viral outbreaks in small areas, they are unsustainable when extended over long periods of time across swathes of any nation, because they are socially disruptive and impose obvious threats to economic viability and social life. The relationship between the economy and health has been widely studied. Research in fields as diverse as sociology, economics, psychology, gender and race studies have found that economic downturns are strongly associated with negative health outcomes, including the onset of chronic conditions, long-term disability and early mortality. These effects are unequally distributed and tend to increase health inequities along the lines of class, race, age and gender. *In short, sound public health policy is not one that should cause additional numerous forms of distress across a country.*

The Influence of Early Modelling Estimates

Early modelling made fear-inducing predictions (Lally, 2022). On 16 March 2020, the UK Imperial College COVID19 Response Team published modelling of the impacts of the virus and ways to reduce mortality and healthcare demand in the USA and UK to avoid overwhelming critical care capacity. They argued that imposed non-pharmaceutical suppression measures would be needed for over 2/3 of the next two years without which there would be 510,000 deaths in Great Britain and 2.2 million deaths in the USA by mid-April 2020, surpassing ICU demand by 30 times (Biggs & Littlejohn, 2021. They admitted that neither ethical nor economic implications were included and that effects of the mandated non-pharmaceutical measures would be profound. The Imperial College COVID19 Response Team on 26 March 2020 extended this alarming prediction to an estimated global impact of the pandemic on and reported that without lockdowns 7.0 billion infections and 40 million deaths globally would occur in 2020.

Again their discussion indicated they ignored the wider social and economic costs of suppression, which they admitted would be high and disproportionately so among lower-income groups as well as pharmaceutical interventions. These modelling numbers are only mathematical projections, but the resulting harm is the advocacy and imposition outcomes of human-made policies, not the outcome of a novel virus. There was an excessive overstatement of the likely effects of the virus (Biggs & Littlejohn, 2021). But the harm had been done and the result was a media transmitted contagion of fear and crisis as the dire modelling predictions were reported as headline news without explanation of the basis for the estimates, resulting in conformity and obedience to excessively restrictive mandated policies applied across the world, with popular strong positive support for heads of government, reflecting the '*rally round the flag*' effect. Social media inflamed the panic by focussing on absolute numbers of Covid cases and deaths modelled invalidly in the projections because the modelling had curiously ignored vaccination regime effects, behavioural change and age-dependent variables.

Popular group hysteria, matched with governments' group think, evoked action to reduce risks of infection and deaths from this one particular disease, with an unattainable target of zero Covid initially in some nations to the exclusion of all other health risks or other life concerns. It was a war effort with virtue signalling to the crowd of an unwavering presumption that the cause is morally right, that we will win, that any critics or deniers are essentially traitors, despite the invalidity and unreliability of the modelling estimates as well as the failure to perform adequate cost/benefit analyses, plus banking on low level difficult to monitor non-pharmaceutical methods like masks and social distance (Chap. 1).

It could be argued that the Covid lockdown and other mandates were only wrong in hindsight and unfair to look back blaming nations' leaders. There was no Covid playbook in March–June 2020, and faced with an unknown virus and accepting what turned out to be incorrect modelling providing poorer than '*expert advice*' that millions of people would die without lockdown and isolation, politicians and public health officials believed they were making the correct decision at the time. But by June 2020, it was already known that:

(i) The empirical predictions of the models were wrong.
(ii) The models made a number of questionable assumptions.
(iii) Actual deaths were highly skewed to the elderly.
(iv) The cost implications were large.

By August 2020, there was enough information available to argue that any reasonable cost/benefit analysis would reveal that lockdown was creating more harm than good, and that a review and revision of the policies could have been made in the August/September when the second wave of infections started to hit.

Cost/Benefit Issues

A review of the Covid lockdown cost/benefit literature (Allen 2022; Pak et al., 2021) reveals that the early cases made for lockdown rested on some unrealistic assumptions, viz.:

- The virus continues to spread exponentially until herd immunity is reached.
- Individuals never change behaviour in the light of a viral threat.
- The value of lives lost is independent of age.

However over the course of the last 3 years, research has revealed that:

- The models failed to predict the progression of the virus.
- Individual health protective behaviours to the virus are quite significant and important.
- Old age is a very important factor.

Lockdowns have some effect on cases, transmissions and deaths, but these effects are marginal. Zahariadis et al. (2022) studied the effectiveness of non-pharmaceutical interventions (NPIs) implemented by the national governments of Greece and Cyprus during 2020 to limit the spread of the virus and mitigate the pandemic's economic fallout. He found mask wearing and working from home better managed the pandemic by reducing cases and had less severe economic impacts than lockdowns. The personal, social and economic costs of blanket lockdowns are more far reaching, large and impacting. The conclusion is that lockdowns fail to pass a cost/benefit test.

Pak et al. (2021) present quite a number of critical valid points about the cost/benefits assessments issues:

1. Modelling

The devastating inaccurate original modelling, e.g. the UK Imperial College model noted above, that propelled massive period of quarantine and lockdown did not take into account the obvious changes in behaviour that most individuals would deliberately adopt to keep themselves clear of infection; in the face of danger, people do modify their behaviour to lower or even avoid risk, and ignoring such adjustments would overestimate the benefits of lockdown in terms of the number of cases, hospitalisations and deaths.

2. Mortality

Invoking the number of deaths averted by lockdowns is too simplistic, as clinical evidence was revealing then, and even two years later, that elderly persons, particularly those in aged care/nursing homes had a significant higher risk of death, especially if already carrying some co-morbidities (Levere et al., 2021). There is overwhelming evidence that a significant disproportion of deaths occurs in aged care settings, not simply due to age, but involving a complex of interacting variables such as co-morbidities, inadequate staffing due to staff having the virus or imposed isolation on staff who were close contacts and incomplete vaccination programmes. Thus, the total number of deaths is a less important indicator of benefits when a more appropriate measure would have been residual life expectancy of the average death which can be employed to estimate the number of life years saved due to lockdown.

3. Benefits Analysis

There has been little use of measures to determine the benefit of an intervention. There are two fundamental approaches to this problem: one uses the economic concept of the value of a statistical life (*VSL*) a measure that provides an index to determine the appropriate level of health, safety and environmental regulation in monetary terms, in this case for lockdown and other non-pharmaceutical interventions. This is calculated by assessing individual willingness to pay (say for a PCR test or isolate for a period at home) for a small reduction in mortality risk. The second uses a more popular health approach measure, the value of quality-adjusted life years (*QALYs*) metric that guided public health decisions before 2020 that seemingly was hardly used in any cost–benefit analysis of imposed restrictions to evaluate the cost-effectiveness of medical and mandated interventions and options for Covid suppression. Joffe and Redman (2021) show that in all 11 studies that used *QALY* as a common metric, costs of lockdowns exceeded benefits by between 2.5 times at the lowest to 26 times at the highest end of the cost–benefit ratios. This a rather devastating data on lockdown benefit.

Therefore, the efficacy of lockdowns to reduce transmission, cases and deaths has likely been highly exaggerated. Many studies found that more restrictive lockdowns in different international locations were not associated with any clear effect on '*flattening-the-curve*' of cases or deaths. It is not clear that lockdowns can markedly reduce transmission. Lockdown restrictions in fact create forced congestion in the lockdown location and offers transmission outside and back inside because some people have to continue to carry out their essential activities. For example, young people may have returned to or stayed home (where most transmission occurs) with older parents due to unemployment or university closures, and risk may have simply been shifted from the professional class to the working class, who cannot afford not to work. Personal modification of behaviours like wearing masks, maintaining distance when encountering individuals and limiting large-size gatherings of individuals is likely more important than lockdowns.

Earlier chapters have charted the immense number of harms that emerged from lockdowns over the last couple of years, including economic recession, unemployment, loneliness, poverty and food insecurity, deterioration of mental health with increased suicides and substance use, increased partner violence and child abuse, lost education and future potential in children and delayed/disrupted health care for serious conditions. Unemployment and loneliness are two of the strongest risk factors for shortened lifespan and chronic diseases. Functional coping strategies have been blocked by lockdowns (e.g. eating healthily, seeking social support and exercise). Useful studies of the cost/benefits effects of lockdowns and other measures can be found in the following: Bendavid et al. (2021); Lally (2022); Leffler et al. (2020); Miles et al. 2022; Rangel (2020).

4. Costs Analysis

Finally, to estimate the other side of the equation, that of costs, *GDP* decline has been a favourite of economists as decline represents lost output and foregone services. But this ignores and therefore does not correspond to the true burden of social, economic and psychological costs lockdowns impose. *GDP* thus provides an underestimate of true costs some of which are non-financial but just as devastating in human impact. For example, age demographics are unequally involved in costs as young people lose out on the higher costs of lost occupational and educational opportunities as well as inadequate levels of social contact and increasing risk to mental health compared to older groups (Robinson et al., 2021).

The question is, however, how many lost years of life would have resulted from COVID-19 deaths if there had been no lockdown? The review of the literature suggests that lockdown only had a marginal effect on deaths, then by cost/benefit standards, lockdown has been a public policy disaster (Allen, 2022). This analysis only considers the number of years of lost life. A proper cost/benefit analysis would consider the value of these lost years. As noted above, the value of life is not constant across age. Since the life years lost to Covid deaths were mostly among those older than 60 and since the years of lost life because of lockdown have mostly been among the young, adjusting the above cost/benefit ratios for the value of life will make lockdown an even worse policy.

The conclusion is that lockdowns, implemented in the name of public health, entailed trade-offs that were not adequately considered. Lockdowns may prevent some Covid deaths and lower stress on hospital and healthcare provision, services and staffing. At the same time, lockdowns cause severe adverse effects for many millions of people, disproportionately for those already disadvantaged. The collateral damage included severe losses to current and future wellbeing from unemployment, poverty, food insecurity, interrupted preventive, diagnostic, and therapeutic health care, interrupted education, loneliness and deterioration of mental health and domestic violence. It is time to calibrate the response to the true risks, make rational cost–benefit analyses of the trade-offs, not repeat the lockdown and other mandated groupthink policies and now emphatically encourage a massively dominant role for vaccination plus other simple non-pharmaceutical interventions like masks and social distance as required. National governments have begun this journey with massive lockdowns only evident still in China. As the former UK health minister Steve Brine noted 20,000 Britons died of flu in a bad season, yet it has never been a legal requirement to stay at home if you have flu. Data from the real world contradict, as it has from the beginning, the dire warnings of the doomsday modellers, and indicates we are now in a good place to be able to get through Omicron and other variants with minimal deaths and no more restrictions: just sensible individual precautions based on personal responsibility.

The pandemic is better framed as a public emergency, not a public health emergency. This is because the pandemic is affecting all sectors and activities of society (not just the healthcare system). Governments are no less responsible for children's education, people's livelihoods, mental health and the community emotional wellbeing.

The Swedish Approach—Personal Responsibility

At a practical level, the known potential consequences of alternatives particularly lockdowns informed the 'controversial' Swedish approach (vide Chap. 2) where instead of shock solutions guided by theories of suppression or elimination, public health leadership opted for a sustainability approach, based on personal responsibility. For most of the pandemic, Sweden stood out among European nations for its comparatively hands-off response. The Scandinavian country never went into a lockdown or closed businesses, relying instead on citizens' sense of civic duty to control infections. Authorities have emphasised individual responsibility instead of government health measures (Anderberg, 2022).

The Swedish approach continues to stoke serious discussion for epidemiological and moral debates, but the results show that Sweden may be faring comparably better in terms of excess deaths, i.e. those greater than the usual number of deaths expected in a certain time period. Excess deaths can indicate whether policies intended to combat the pandemic have unintended consequences and are an important measure of the overall efficacy of policy. Sweden recorded 7.9% excess deaths (assumed to be Covid based) in 2021 compared to the years 2016–19, which means that the country had the 23rd lowest annual excess deaths out of 30 European countries; lower than the U.K. (15.1%), France (10.4%) and Spain (18.9%). Sweden also has a lower number of coronavirus deaths per million than those countries at 144.9; other nations have recorded for example UK 206.7, USA 217.5 and Italy 217.8, all of which have gone under strict lockdowns during the pandemic (Our World in Data). Rejecting lockdown policies can lead to sustainable and equitable population outcomes in the middle of this crisis. Even at the beginning of the crisis, some experts recognised that quick solutions are not well-suited for complex public health problems.

However, the rapid expansion of Omicron and a consequent surging death rate as elsewhere jolted Sweden into pursuing a slightly more preventative approach at the beginning of 2022. Sweden's public health authorities advised restaurants, cultural venues and leisure centres, where the risk of spreading of the infection is great, to ask their customers to show digital proof of vaccination. This recommendation from the Swedish Public Health Agency (2022) isn't a legal requirement but voluntary guidance for businesses. In terms of cost–benefit issues, mandated vaccination appears justified as the most effective approach overall.

Coercion Is Proportionate to Risk-Mandated Vaccination

It is important to recognise that coercive vaccination *can* be justified by reference to other coercive interventions that are usually well accepted in the public interest. A few mundane examples include conscription in wartime, seat belts in cars, helmet wearing by cyclists and paying income tax. Taxes benefit individuals because tax revenue allows the preservation of public goods and tends to be levied based on considerations of fairness and utility. Seat belts and helmets are viewed by most as preventing unnecessary deaths. Conscription is acceptable to preserve the sovereignty of a country although some pacifists may disagree. Thus, to impose mandatory vaccination in the context of a grave pandemic situation is difficult to argue against in terms of the four ethical criteria being discussed.

In fact, mandatory vaccination policies for other diseases are already in place in different parts of the world. There are a range of possible penalties or costs which can coerce people. Australia has an existing '*No Jab, No Pay*' scheme which withholds child benefits if the child is not vaccinated with the standard toddler vaccinations and a '*No Jab, No Play*' scheme which withholds kindergarten childcare benefits. Italy introduced fines for unvaccinated children who attend school. In the USA, state regulations mandated that children cannot attend school if they are not vaccinated, and healthcare workers were required to vaccinate.

Coercion to be vaccinated has minimal risk medically speaking. The risks of the mandated vaccination as a condition of employment basically lie in the economic and social areas of life and bring into play concepts of justice, fairness, equality and autonomy. It is considerably harsh producing potential devastating socio-economic consequences likely resulting in closing industries down, grossly interfering with supply chains and flooding hospitals with unvaccinated sick people, who could clog up ICUs preventing those with other issues like road accident victims who need ventilators to be denied them. Who then decides on priorities?

Coercion rarely is effective in a democracy, producing division in society between, in this case, the vaxxed and unvaxxed. None of this compulsion is likely to motivate convinced anti-vaxxers to get vaccinated anyway, and restricting freedoms for the unvaccinated will not further protect the already vaccinated. The unvaccinated have made their choice and are willing to take their chances. Thus, it is not difficult to take the view that vaccination mandates are a dangerous path towards segregation and despotism and can be regarded as ignoring equality before the law. Vaccination mandates may also be in contravention of the UN International Convention on Economic, Social and Cultural Rights (1966) that all people have economic and social rights to choice in health, work and education.

This raises the question of the extent to which an individual's liberty outweighs the collective's drive to contain and protect themselves from diseases, whose spread can be quenched by inoculation. Unfortunately, there is no consensus regarding this predicament. Yet, answers to this ethical dilemma may well provide us with a new social standard reform that can have implications on the employment, health, education and travel sectors; equally, it may impact the perception of vaccinated and unvaccinated individuals in the public eye. On the other hand, the infringement on personal liberty and bodily integrity that is associated with mandatory vaccinations as well as the public scrutiny that may be associated with vaccination refusal may border the transgression of some constitutional and human rights.

A better focus is to use reason not force; explore, listen and understand in open dialogue the issues the unvaccinated have and for many of them it boils down to two factors (a) safety concerns about injecting '*non-natural*' material into their bodies and (b) desire for choice. We actually do not need 100% vaccine uptake, and most nations are well over 90% double dose with many having had additional booster shots. The people we need to focus more support on now are the vulnerable—the aged, pregnant ladies, the immune-compromised and of course the unvaxxed.

Summary of the Implications of the Four Ethical Principles

The evidence and arguments from the above four ethical principles of gravity, safety of procedure, cost/benefit and coercion proportionality to risk appear to be totally in favour of a degree of mandated vaccination, as the prime procedure with only more limited benefits accruing from non-pharmaceutical impositions. The indiscriminate implementation of radical forms of social control, like contact tracing, imposed and self-imposed quarantines and mass-lockdowns possibly had their moment at the onset of the disease, as medical uncertainties on lethality existed and citizens' anxieties were running high. But the accurate and transparent representation of the net harms and net benefits of these policy pathways is paramount for a legitimate argument about the policy choices based on evidence-informed decision making and democratic public deliberation.

Biomedical Ethics: Do No Harm. The Four Principles of Biomedical Ethics

The four Nuffield criteria discussed above can be linked in several ways to four additional principles of biomedical ethics when evaluating the merits and downsides of medical and non-pharmaceutical procedures. To justify a practice to be considered '*ethical*' under the biomedical model, it must also respect the four principles of *justice, beneficence, autonomy and non-maleficence.* (Varkey, 2021).

Beneficence

The principle of beneficence is the obligation of health personnel to act for the benefit of the person and involves a number of moral rules to protect and defend inter alia, the right of others, remove conditions that will cause harm, help persons with disabilities and rescue persons in danger. It is worth emphasising that, in distinction to non-maleficence (below), this principle imposes positive requirements. The principle calls for not just avoiding harm, but also to benefit the public and promote their welfare. Not only encouraging but also mandating vaccination can be for the benefit of the person. Figures from NSW Health show that as of Jan 2, 2022, unvaccinated people are 6 times more likely to be hospitalised for Covid than those who are fully vaccinated. Before the first cases of the Omicron variant were detected in Australia on 27 November 2021, unvaccinated people were 25 times more likely to be hospitalised for Covid, and half the Covid patients in ICU were unvaccinated but account for just 8% of the population, with the unvaccinated 12 times more likely to end up in intensive care (Our World in Data). Thus, beneficence seems to be addressed in the vaccinations debate.

Non-maleficence

Non-maleficence is the obligation of a health professional not to harm the patient. This principle focusses on several moral rules—do not kill, do not cause pain or suffering, do not incapacitate, do not cause offence and do not deprive others of the goods of life. The practical application of non-maleficence is for the health professional to weigh the benefits against negatives of interventions and treatments, dismiss those that are inappropriately burdensome and to choose the best course of action. This is particularly important and pertinent in difficult Covid end-of-life care decisions on withholding and withdrawing life-sustaining treatment, medically administered nutrition and hydration as well as in pain and other symptom control.

In contrast to the positive effects of vaccinations noted worldwide, lockdown restrictions imposed negative effects of malfeasance by causing massive damage to cancer, cardiovascular and diabetes patients; inflicted incalculable harms on hundreds of millions of children worldwide through cancelled schooling and lockdown programmes, reversing decades of progress; loss of job/family income and return to poverty, alcoholism and drug abuse and domestic violence with worsening mental health. It is possibly one of the greatest violations of civil liberties and human rights in the history of Western democracies, with entire populations put under 'house arrest', with states dictating the most intimate aspects of personal relationships and taking charge of essential daily activities as if freedoms are a reward to be handed out at the pleasure of governments rather than inalienable rights held by citizens. Yet it all failed to halt the march of the disease. Lockdowns and movement restrictions should be limited to outbreaks in small zones where serious levels of death may arise such as aged care homes, disadvantaged and remote communities. The principle of non-maleficence does not appear to have been achieved.

Autonomy

The philosophical underpinning for autonomy, as interpreted by philosophers Kant (1724–1804) and J. S. Mill (1806–1873), is that everybody has intrinsic and unconditional worth and, therefore, *should have the power to make rational decisions and moral choices, and to exercise their capacity for self-determination.* Autonomy needs to be weighed against competing moral principles and occasionally may be over-ridden; an obvious example would be if the autonomous action of a person causes harm to another person(s) like your child or work colleague as might occur with refusal to be vaccinated. The principle of autonomy does not extend to infants and children who lack the capacity (competence) to act autonomously or incompetence arising from mental or physical disorder. Healthcare institutions and state governments usually have policies and procedures to assess incompetence.

Even in most advanced Western countries all with heterogeneous cultures, including indigenous as well as immigrant, there are significant minority populations who hold views different from those of the majority population in respect of need for full disclosure, the role of stress and mental health counselling and decisions about life support usually preferring a family-centred approach involving professionals from their own group. However, there is a core of universal human rights that need to be honoured, despite variations in local custom or law which cannot justify abuses of certain fundamental rights, and the right of self-determination on which the doctrine of informed consent is based. Respecting the principle of autonomy obliges the physician to disclose medical information and treatment options that are necessary for the patient to exercise self-determination. In this case, autonomy may mean for an educated person who has well understood the issues the right to reject vaccination on the basis of their reasoned judgement.

Justice

Justice is generally interpreted as fair, equitable and appropriate treatment of persons. Of the several categories of justice, the one that is most pertinent to clinical ethics is distributive justice. Distributive justice refers to the fair, equitable and appropriate distribution of healthcare resources such as vaccines and *RATs*. There are different valid principles of distributive justice, such as distribution to each person by (i) equal share, (ii) according to need, (iii) according to effort, (iv) according to contribution, (v) according to merit and (vi) according to free market exchanges.

Each principle is not exclusive, and can be, and is often combined in application. It is easy to see the difficulty in choosing, balancing and refining these principles to form a coherent and workable solution to distribute medical resources such as vaccines, test kits, ventilators, PPE and levels of nursing care not just in one country but more importantly across the globe. It is obvious from each nation's data that some groups and even whole nations have been considerably disadvantaged in access to some of these resources. For example, government policies in the Western world have in various ways failed the elderly, particularly those in aged care homes. In March 2022, more than one-third of older Australians most vulnerable to serious Covid infections were yet to get boosted, and nearly half of them had been eligible for their third dose for at least a month. Waning immunity is of serious concern for them as the longer the period from completion of two-dose vaccination increases the risk of hospitalisation and mortality clearly, particularly in the older age group. So justice may be absent in some situations and nations.

In summary, whether mandatory vaccination for any disease can be justified will depend on precise facts around the magnitude of the problem, the nature of the disease and vaccination effectiveness, the availability and effectiveness of alternative strategies and the level of coercion. Mandates, by their nature, are discriminatory, contravene the justice, beneficence and autonomy principles. Even if they fulfilled the conditions of being safe, effective and available, it might still be arguable that they impose on people's freedoms in an unfair or discriminatory way. Even the WHO does not support mandatory vaccination of populations.

Ethical Dilemmas in Health Care

Unequal Distribution of Vaccines

WHO called for greater global equity in the distribution of and access to vaccines in 2021. Based on the then current rate of vaccine rollout, 109 countries would miss the WHO's target for 70 per cent of the world's population to be fully vaccinated by July 2022. About 36 nations had not even reached 10 per cent vaccination cover at January 2022. Among severe patients worldwide, 90 per cent were unvaccinated. Wealthy countries including Australia, Canada and the USA struck deals with manufacturers early on to provide their own countries with more than enough doses, leaving lower-income countries unable to immunise but a small proportion of their citizens. China and India have large vaccine industries, which allow them to reserve some of their vaccine supplies for their own populations. WHO Director General Tedros Ghebreyesus have warned that bidding wars over vaccines has led to inequitable distribution and, ultimately, failure to eliminate the risk of new outbreaks, with Covid undoubtedly spreading from less vaccinated countries to the more developed ones with possibly new variants with trade and travel opening up.

It is therefore in every country's interests to adopt humanitarian policies and send vaccines to poorer countries which cannot afford them. Illustrative examples of vaccination rates in poorer countries in 2022 include Chad 0.89%, Nigeria 3.8%, Kenya 14%, Libya 16%, Iraq 17%, Egypt 30%, Pakistan 42% and Bangladesh 47%. However, Dr Fauci in his retirement speech on 22 November 2022 as US Presidential medical advisor regretfully noted that supplies of vaccines and PPE offered freely were declined by some undeveloped nations as they claimed they had no way of distributing and using the vaccines and equipment around their nations leaving unequitable distribution a source of continuing pandemic and mutations which are then still able to travel around the world.

Australia's Stark Health Inequalities—A Moral Policy Failure

Inequitable distribution has also occurred in developed countries involving the aged, indigenous groups and the immunosuppressed. National healthcare services in most countries claim they offer ethically equal, fair and rational care for everyone. But the gap in health outcomes between citizens has been laid bare over the course of the pandemic. This is so in Australia too. Problems of messaging immigrant groups have led in Australia to almost three times as many Covid deaths among people born overseas compared to those who were born in Australia. People born in North Africa and the Middle East were 10 times more likely to die from Covid than those born in Australia, while people who came from Southeast Asia and Southern and Central Asia recorded twice as many Covid deaths. People born in the UK and Ireland had similar death rates to Australian-born Covid cases (ABC, 2022). The language problem was realised too late, and language translations of Covid critical public health information were eventually distributed to multicultural communities' weeks out of date. In some of Sydney's most affected local government areas, more than 60 per cent of people speak a language other than English at home. Lower health literacy is also associated with an increased reluctance to accept vaccines as vaccination messages are ignored.

As a result in NSW, Covid surges have disproportionately impacted Sydney's west and south-west, lower-income areas home to linguistically and culturally diverse communities. Here, people (a) don't have the luxury of being able to work from home, but work in industries like aged and childcare, manufacturing, transport, construction and retail/hospitality jobs that keep the nation running, (b) more likely to live in large, multigenerational overcrowded households, which prevents successful isolation from other household members if they become exposed to the virus. This puts other workers in the same workplace at higher risk of being exposed to infection. A similar situation was seen in Victoria in 2020, when an outbreak forced nine high-density public housing towers in Melbourne with a similarly high concentration of ethnic minority and migrant populations into a hard lockdown.

The pandemic is demonstrating that poverty and social exclusion actually influence health. In Australia, health inequalities are felt most acutely by Indigenous people and those living in socio-economically disadvantaged areas, including in rural and remote Australia. The reasons for health disparities are varied and complex, but can largely be explained by unequal access to resources such as good housing, adequate income, educational opportunities and social support, with those most affected by Covid often facing multiple challenges at once. The clamping down with tough restrictions has a lasting effect to further entrench inequalities in already disadvantaged populations. For example, families with school-aged children, limited resources and space at home can make remote learning an enormous challenge. Holed up in a small flat with limited access to outdoor spaces and not able to get a break from each other offers every opportunity for high levels of mental health impacts.

Covid surged in Australia's impoverished and isolated Aboriginal communities which had limited health facilities resulting in a major crisis for these remote communities where there was already poor underlying health conditions. Again people had not been provided with the necessary resources or public health education to prevent the spread of the virus. As an example of the problems, the Guardian (2022) reported that an elderly Aboriginal woman with Covid was forced to sleep outside and self-isolate under a tree in an effort to avoid infecting her relatives, including a person on dialysis and a young child.

While 95% of the Northern Territories population was fully vaccinated by late 2021, only 67 per cent of the Yuendumu Aboriginal community had received two vaccine doses with more than 140 people out of 800 contracting the virus since the outbreak (ABC News, 2021). According to 2016 census data from the Australian Bureau of Statistics, just 10.8% of Yuendumu residents work full time, and 50% of the population is unemployed. In some remote Aboriginal communities, that figure is as low as 38% vaccinated. The rapid spread of Covid through Aboriginal communities is a stark expression of the class issues at the centre of the pandemic. Decades of neglect have resulted in widespread poverty and third-world health and living conditions.

A similar situation in late 2021 was reported from an aboriginal township Yarrabah south of Cairns in Queensland where 342 homes for 3500 people were penetrated by the virus. One virus-ridden house had 14 people sleeping 4 to a bed with an average in the community of 11 persons per house. Isolation is impossible; vaccination rates are low, and there are limited supplies of masks and PCR tests (The West Australian 2021). It is a third-world situation for many Aboriginal communities in the bush. The government again did not properly engage with remote Aboriginal communities in its public health messaging and failed to anticipate and respond to the risks. Many of these vulnerable communities had fears about vaccination which should have been alleviated by better focussed communication using opinion leaders. The low vaccination rates then left them very vulnerable.

Moral Distress Among Health Staff

At times, decisions can conflict with beliefs, values and the responsibility to provide ethical care. The pandemic has raised many psychosocial, ethical and moral challenges for hospital workers, particularly those in Emergency Departments, Intensive Care and Ambulance paramedics in most Western nations, including Canada, Australia, USA and the UK, significantly impacting their delivery of critical care (Markwell et al., 2020). Emergency and intensive care staff are more vulnerable to experiencing intensified moral distress amid Covid due to issues such as wearing PPE and masks all day, staff shortages as others fall sick or suffer from burnout, increased crowding on wards with fewer staff to deal with more patients, caring for dying patients and feeling unable to prevent death in numerous cases. Emergency nurses and physicians are twice as likely to leave the profession due to moral distress compared with other healthcare professionals (Almutiari et al., 2019).

Nurses have been faced with other issues such as insufficient time to manage competing demands, limited resources such as PPE, the responsibility to implement new no-visitor policies, among many others, and making morally challenging decisions that may result in devaluing patients' wishes and reducing nurse–patient interaction, in crowded emergency wards while observing physical distancing guidelines and having a higher risk of exposure. Decisions about who should be prioritised for intensive and ventilation care take place daily and challenge their moral values and beliefs. Staff must rely on their own professional and moral judgements to make sense of the situation and determine the best course of action to provide competent, responsible and ethical care. These judgements can be influenced by social and cultural norms and values so that both client and/or clinician characteristics, such as age, gender, education and culture will affect moral judgements and decisions according to Graham et al. (2016).

If this is so, can there ever be completely fair and rational decision making within healthcare systems? Because of pressure from increasing number of Covid patients and decreasing staff levels through resignation and required isolation, there has been less time and opportunities for informal discussions when making decisions (Liberati et al., 2021). This creates moral distress in medical staff which is defined as the inability to act according to one's own core values. During the pandemic, moral distress in medical personnel has gained attention, related to pandemic-associated factors, such as the uncertainty of treatment options for the virus, the availability of equipment and the accelerated pace of deaths, as well as the experience of knowing the right thing to do while being in a situation in which it was nigh impossible to do it (Vittone & Sotomayor, 2021; Virani, 2021).

Mental health services in many countries had to rapidly re-organise. Usual practices and decision making via face-to-face consultations, meetings, informal discussions and family/carer involvement were largely dispensed with. For social workers, mental health specialists, clinicians, psychotherapists and psychologists whose work is based on building trusting relationships face to face or by facilitating engagement with the community, practising in the normal professional way which fitted with one's moral values and beliefs about wellbeing became increasingly difficult (Adams, 2021). Ethical decisions about what support could be offered, to which client, where and how, was often uncertain. For example, there were immediate questions about how safe was it to offer clients face-to-face therapy if this was their preference?; what about clients who could not access remote support or use Zoom?; is it fair to restrict a client's leave from hospital in order to reduce the risk of infection?; etc.!

What Next? Moral Progress After COVID-19

Covid may positively impact the future with moral benefits. Over the last three years, unprecedented changes have impacted millions of lives as requirements to obey demanding new rules and accept new risks in a context no one had to face in the last 100 years. The disruption may well raise awareness of and challenge to our ethical thinking, particularly the responsibilities we owe to each other. Both rallies and government policies raise serious debates on such aspects as the ethics of vaccine mandates, restrictions on civil liberties, the limits of government power and the inequitable distribution of health services nationally and globally.

Ethical decision making is rarely something we think about, but the effects of our actions on others are now forefront as governments and health directives had altered the basic rules of life of who we could visit, where we could travel, whether we could work or study, for what purposes could we leave the house, how many vaccinations we would need to relax our personal restrictions, etc. Moral progress into a better society after Covid is feasible. It happened before, after World War II when there was considerable moral progress in many countries involved in the conflicts. Then, a new beginning gradually lowered old class divisions, the welfare states emerged along with more comprehensive health systems providing a new sense of caring, hope and unity.

But new problems loomed as restrictions eased off in stages and at varying rates in different parts of each country, differentially affecting regional areas, demographic and occupational groups, leading to feelings of discrimination, envy and resentment and perhaps local social unrest. Ethical judgements will also be challenged by heightened anxiety caused by the unavoidable consequent infection spread as risk easing occurs, but also by a reduction in perceived social support when we are no longer '*all in it together*' and '*personal responsibility*' becomes more in vogue as most Western governments removed financial subsidisation provided during the first two years. Ethics and economics will need some judicious and acceptable balance. This crisis has emphatically highlighted the value and importance of national and state health services and staff, the similar importance of social care and of our reliance on the legions of poorly paid delivery drivers, hospitality workers, aged care and childcare workers and others in the service sector. This new appreciation could halt the erosion and underfunding of both health and social care and begin to reduce the glaring inequalities in income and housing that leave so many struggling to survive.

References

ABC News. (2021, November 29). Retrieved November, 29 2021 from https://www.abc.net.au/news/2021-11-29/vaccine-uptake-remote-communities-nt/100659052

ABC News. (2022, November, 11). COVID-19 deaths higher among disadvantaged people in Australia. Retrieved November 16, 2022 from https://www.abc.net.au/news/covid-19-deaths-higher-amongst-disadvayaged-people

Acton, L. (1887, April 5). *Power tends to corrupt, and absolute power corrupts*. Letter to Bishop Mandell Creighton. In J. N. Figgis, & R. V. Laurence, (Eds.), *Historical essays and studies*. Macmillan.

Adams, C. (2021). Resilience in the time of pandemic. *The Canadian Journal of Psychiatry., 66*(1), 62–63. https://doi.org/10.1177/0706743720946170

Ahorsu, D. K., Lin, C. Y., Imani, V., et al. (2022). The fear of COVID-19 scale: Development and initial validation. *International Journal of Mental Health and Addiction, 20*(3), 537–1545. https://doi.org/10.1007/s11469-020-00270-8

Allen, W. (2022). Covid-19 lockdown cost/benefits: A critical assessment of the literature. *International Journal of the Economics of Business, 29*(1), 1–32. https://doi.org/10.1080/13571516.2021.1976051

Almutairi, A. F., Salam, M., Adlan, A. A., & Alturki, A. S. (2019). Prevalence of severe moral distress among healthcare providers in Saudi Arabia. *Psychology Research and Behavior Management, 11*(12), 107–115. https://doi.org/10.2147/PRBM.S191037

Anderberg, J. (2022). *The herd: How Sweden chose its own path through the worst pandemic in 100 years*. Scribe Press.

Australian Bureau of Statistics Census Data. (2016). Retrieved March 15, 2022 from https://www.abs.gov.au/websitedbs/censushome.nsf/home/2016

Bendavid, E., Oh, C., & Bhattacharya, J. et al. (2021). Assessing mandatory stay-at-home and business closure effects on the spread of COVID-19. *European Journal of Clinical Investigation, 51*(4). https://doi.org/10.1111/eci.13484,

Bentham, J. (1789). *An introduction to the principles of morals and legislation*. Oxford University Press.

Biggs, A., & Littlejohn, L. (2021). Revisiting the initial COVID-19 pandemic projections. *The Lancet., 2*(3), e91–e92. https://doi.org/10.1016/S2666-5247(21)00029-X

Centers for Disease Control and Prevention. Morbidity and mortality weekly report September 2021: MMWR. https://www.cdc.gov/mmwr/index.html

Coetzee, A. (2021). Reuters News report (28.11.21). Retrieved January 13, 2022 from https://www.reuters.com/world/africa/safrican-doctor-says-patients-with-omicron-variant-have-very-mild-symptoms-2021-11-28/

Economist Intelligence Unit. (2021). Democracy index. Retrieved August 27, 2022 from https://www.eiu.com/n/campaigns/democracy-index-2021/

Giubilini, A. (2019). *The ethics of vaccination*. Palgrave Studies in Ethics and Public Policy Cham (CH). https://doi.org/10.1007/978-3-030-02068-2

Graham, J., Meindl, P., Beall, E., et al. (2016). Cultural differences in moral judgment and behavior, across and within societies. *Current Opinion in Psychology, 8*, 125–130. https://doi.org/10.1016/j.copsyc.2015.09.007

Great Barrington Declaration. (2020). Retrieved October 17, 2021 from https://gbdeclaration.org/

Imperial College London COVIC19 Response Team. Retrieved June 14, 2021 from https://www.imperial.ac.uk/media/imperial-college/medicine/sph/ide/gida-fellowships/Imperial-College-COVID19-Global-Impact-26-03-2020v2.pdf

Independent Scientific Pandemic Insights Group on Behaviours (SPI-B). Retrieved October 26, 2021 from https://www.gov.uk/government/groups/independent-scientific-pandemic-influenza-group-on-behaviours-spi-b

Joffe, A. R., &Redman, D. (2021). The SARS-CoV-2 pandemic in high income countries such as Canada: A better way forward without lockdowns. *Front Public Health, 22*(9). https://doi.org/10.3389/fpubh.2021.715904

Kulldorf, M. (2021, October, 12). Covid, lockdown and the retreat of scientific debate. The Spectator. Retrieved January 04, 2022.

Lally, M. (2022). A cost–benefit analysis of COVID-19 lockdowns in Australia. *Monash Bioethics Review, 40*, 62–93. https://doi.org/10.1007/s40592-021-00148-y

Leffler, C. T., Ing, E., Lykins, J. D., et al. (2020). Association of country-wide coronavirus mortality with demographics, testing, lockdowns, and public wearing of masks. *American Journal of Tropical Medicine and Hygiene, 103*, 2400–2411. https://doi.org/10.4269/ajtmh.20-1015

Levere, M., Rowan, P., & Wysocki, A. (2021). The adverse effects of the COVID-19 pandemic on nursing home resident well-being. *Journal of the American Medical Directors Association, 22*(5), 948–954. https://doi.org/10.1016/j.jamda.2021.03.010

Liberati, E., Richards, N., Willars, J., et al. (2021). A qualitative study of experiences of NHS mental healthcare workers during the Covid-19 pandemic. *BMC Psychiatry, 21*(1), 250. https://doi.org/10.1186/s12888-021-03261-8

Markwell, A., Mitchell, R., Wright, A. L., & Brown, A. F. (2020). Clinical and ethical challenges for emergency departments during communicable disease outbreaks: Can lessons from Ebola Virus Disease be applied to the COVID-19 pandemic? *Emergency Medicine Australasia, 32*(3), 520–524. https://doi.org/10.1111/1742-6723.13514

Miles, A., Andiappan, M., Upenieks, L., & Orfanidis, C. (2022). Using prosocial behavior to safeguard mental health and foster emotional well-being during the COVID-19 pandemic: A registered report of a randomized trial. *PLoS ONE, 17*(7), e0272152. https://doi.org/10.1371/journal.pone.0272152

Mill, J. S. (1859). On Liberty. John W. Parker and Son : London (Original Ed).

Morgan, G. (2021). Covid-19's rebel scientists: Has iSAGE been a success? *BMJ, 375*, n2504. https://doi.org/10.1136/bmj.n2504

Nuffield Council of Bio-Ethics Report. (2007, July 13). Retrieved April 19, 2021 from https://www.nuffieldbioethics.org/publications/public-health

Our World In Data. Updated to 12 Nov 22. https://ourworldindata.org/excess-mortality-covid

Pak, A., Adegboye, O. A., & McBryde, E. S. (2021). Are we better-off? The benefits and costs of Australian COVID-19 lockdown. *Frontiers in Public Health, 2*(9), 798478. https://doi.org/10.3389/fpubh

Royal Australian College of General Practitioners (RACGP). (2021, August 31). Retrieved October 19, 2021 from https://www1.racgp.org.au/newsgp/clinical/new-us-study-shows-profound-impact-of-covid-19-vac

Rangel, J. (2020). A way forward: Considering the sustainability, equity and unintended effects of social control measures as a response to the COVID-19 crisis. *Journal of Evaluation in Clinical Practice, 27*, 3–8. https://doi.org/10.1111/jep.13508

Rayner, G., (2021). Deputy Editor *the Telegraph.* Retrieved May 14, 2021 from https://www.telegraph.co.uk/news/2021/05/14/scientists-admit-totalitarian-use-fear-control-behaviour-covid/Use of fear to control behaviour in Covid crisis was 'totalitarian', admit scientists

Robinson, I., A., Sullivan, R., Shogren, J. (2021). Do the benefits of COVID-19 policies exceed the costs. *Risk Analysis, 41*, 761–770. https://doi.org/10.1111/risa.13561

Rousseau, J. -J. (1762). *The Social Contract.* Swan Sonnenschein & Co.

Savulescu, J. (2021). Good reasons to vaccinate: Mandatory or payment for risk? *Journal of Medical Ethics, 47*(2), 78–85. https://doi.org/10.1136/medethics-2020-106821

Swedish Public Health Agency Recommendations Oct 2022. Retrieved October 31, 2022 from https://abcnews.go.com/Health/wireStory/virus-outlier-sweden-adopts-restrictions-cases-rise-74801875

The West Australian. (2021, December 10). Retrieved December, 11 2021 from https://thewest.com.au/news/coronavirus/concerns-over-low-qld-indigenous-vax-rates-c-4900292

The Guardian (2022, January 14). Retrieved January 15, 2022 from https://www.theguardian.com/australia-news/2022/jan/24/elderly-woman-forced-to-isolate-under-a-tree-in-remote-community-due-to-lack-of-facilities

UK Health Security Agency. Continually updated. Online at https://www.gov.uk/government/publications/covid-19-vaccine-weekly-surveillance-reports

ULCA Survey (2022, June 29). Retrieved July 01, 2022 from https://newsroom.ucla.edu/releases/california-health-interview-survey-covid19-vaccine

Varkey, B. (2021). Principles of clinical ethics and their application to practice. *Medical Principles and Practice, 30*(1), 17–28. https://doi.org/10.1159/000509119

Virani, S. B. (2021). Moral distress amid COVID-19: A frontline emergency nurse's perspective. *Nursing, 51*(12), 39–43. https://doi.org/10.1097/01.NURSE.0000800072.35132.c1

Vittone, S., & Sotomayor, C. R. (2021). Moral distress entangled: Patients and providers in the COVID-19 era. *HEC Forum, 33*, 415–423. https://doi.org/10.1007/s10730-021-09450-y

World Health Organisation. (2019). *Immunization coverage: SAGE report.* World Health Organisation.

Zahariadis, N., Exadaktylos, T., Sparf, J., et al. (2022). Assessing the effectiveness of public health interventions for Covid-19 in Greece and Cyprus. *European Policy Analysis., 8*(3), 345–359. https://doi.org/10.1002/epa2.1153

CHAPTER 11

The Rush to Publish Research on the Pandemic

Abstract Given the vital importance of providing health authorities, governments and organisations with information about the impacts of the disease on the wellbeing of nations, groups and individuals as early as possible, a massive impetus to research was generated. This rush led in numerous cases to sloppy research design, ignoring some of the vital standards of scientific method such as acceptable sample selection and operational definition of variables. This rush also led to the overwhelming of the journal review procedures with the use of preprints many of which were later withdrawn. The logic of enquiry requires valid and reliable evidence and cannot be based on belief, emotion, or misinformation. Three studies are explored as examples of poor research from which unwarranted assumptions were made, viz: Wakefield's Study, hydroxychloroquine and Ivermectin claims. Early statistical modelling made erroneous claims about the severity of the pandemic leading to initial panic by health authorities and governments. The theme of this chapter has been the need to safeguard the integrity of scientific research and evidence which will support maintaining public trust in science and scientific institutions, particularly critical during a pandemic, as we have just experienced globally.

Keyword Scientific method · Research design · Survey research issues · Preprints · Hydroxychloroquine · Ivermectin · Statistical modelling

© The Author(s), under exclusive license to Springer Nature Singapore Pte Ltd. 2023

R. B. Burns, *The Human Impact of the COVID-19 Pandemic*,
https://doi.org/10.1007/978-981-99-1710-5_11

The Scientific Method: Not All Research Is Valid and Reliable

This chapter is a ***caveat emptor*** about the recent plethora of research on Covid particularly from the socio-psychological fields of study. Research, whatever the subject, should involve a rigorous methodology—the scientific method.

Science is not an academic subject; it is a method of investigation that can lead to advancing knowledge and therefore is never settled. The scientific method of investigation in developing knowledge invokes processes such as hypothesis formation and testing, reliable and standardised observation and data gathering, statistical analysis of data, culminating in the objective reporting of results. There is no room for personal beliefs, bias, invalid and unsubstantiated assertions, emotional justifications or conspiracy 'theory'. A scientific approach to an issue discerns what actually is the case rather than offering a patchwork of opinions, likes and dislikes, authoritarian diktats, prejudice, political convenience, woolly armchair theorising or an unthinking willingness to jump on a current bandwagon.

Whether you are from Argentina, Albania or Angola, whether you hold left or right wing views, or whether you are an agnostic or devoted follower of a religion, Delta and Omicron are both variants of the SARS-CoV-2 coronavirus, vaccination is a proven medical method of curtailing epidemics and pandemics of various diseases, and quarantine is a long established method of preventing transmission from an infected person onwards, as science is based on evidence with no room for personal interpretations.

However, scientific research has not and cannot provide all the answers yet about managing the virus or fully understanding all its effects on humans, short and long term, or its implication for life in the 'new normal'. Science has a hard job to compete with most misinformation and conspiracy theory as berating someone with real facts can generally cause a boomerang effect making their mistaken belief more firmly entrenched. A 15 second rant can require a 15 minute boring refutation with rational argument and facts which puts everyone to sleep. Science is also a slow process compared to a constantly evolving virus. Much of science is taken up with obtaining data/information and to get it right can take time, because the science method works by gradually uncovering more valid evidence, thereby refining existing knowledge, offering new explanations and theories, consequently altering knowledge.

The scientific method has one essential characteristic over personal opinion and belief, and that is self-correction, replacing old knowledge with new findings. Therefore, using the scientific method nothing is ever settled for good as it is a logic of enquiry for generating, replenishing and correcting knowledge, constantly advancing knowledge with new research and discovery. This where science differs absolutely from conspiracy theories and misinformation.

The current socio-political environment suffers badly from ideas that are simply the product of ideology and political bias where emotional responses and beliefs are viewed as superior to facts, as in the current anti-vax and

Freedom mob rallies, where activist views are the only acceptable ones, regarded by them as far more important than addressing actual issues. Truth has been trumped by dogma as in the social media myths of the effectiveness of hydroxychloroquine and Ivermectin for the treatment of Covid infection and even of the efficacy of vaccination itself.

Nowadays, research scientists who propose new facts and information from their studies that 'offend' those who myopically focus on their perverse perception of 'truth' are the 'New Age Galileos' to be de-platformed, ridiculed, made lepers and untouchables, enforced with a barrage of anger and hate from the social media (which is far from being social). To seek the truth uncompromisingly, is the keystone of good scientific research. This requires scepticism and 'devil's advocacy' to cut through human bias and vested interests. When others deem it necessary to 'cancel' the truth, and to despise or avoid scepticism, they undermine scientific endeavour, replacing it with a hard line mob 'religion'.

Your evaluation of the validity of research

Whenever you read a research report in any field consider, and where possible investigate, by asking these questions:

- who conducted it; are they qualified in that field?
- do they have any known predetermined views on the research topic?
- was correct methodology used, involving research design, sampling procedure, valid survey questions, and appropriate statistical analysis?
- were only partial results supportive of the known agenda revealed, and
- who funded the research?

In addition, check if you can to determine whether the research meets several essential guidelines below:

- ***Control*** enables the investigator to identify the causes of their observation. Without it the cause of an effect cannot be isolated from the effects of an array of other interacting and uncontrolled variables. This is obviously not a problem in most epidemiological and psychological studies of the virus which is clearly identifiable. However, there are few issues where other interacting variables influence the data, and thus, the implications derived therefrom. For example, deaths of elderly and aged care persons are usually classified as Covid deaths if there is a trace of the virus detected by tests. This may well artificially inflate mortality data as the elderly may well have died **with** but not **from** coronavirus because of serious other illnesses which where the reason for being in aged care in the first place. However, inquests are rarely held to ascertain true cause of death in these aged care deaths.

- ***Operational definitions of variables*** are essential so that there is clear agreement as to what each variable is. This then eliminates confusion in meaning and communication between researchers and in the mass media. Luckily in medical research, variables are well defined. There is no querying for example what the Covid-19 virus is or what a particular medical procedure is.
- ***Replication*** implies that consistent results are found when a study is repeated. If results vary how do we know which one is the correct result? Replication should be a mandatory requirement for all studies where possible.
- ***Hypothesis formulation and testing***. A hypothesis is a focussed, succinct clearly stated proposition or assumption implying relationship between operationally defined variables that is capable of being tested. A hypothesis enables us to focus exactly on what specific questions we are trying to answer. For example, a hypothesis could be, *coronavirus transmission between children below the age of 12 is significantly lower than the transmission rate in adolescents between 13 and 18 years of age*. The results of such a study would have implications for differential managing of the virus between primary and secondary school age children. A hypothesis that cannot be tested does not belong to the realm of science. Additionally, we never say that a hypothesis is proved; this is because proof carries the connotation of finality. We acknowledge a hypothesis is strongly supported when strong statistically significant evidence for it has been produced. The resulting theory/knowledge is then accepted as the best possible answer until further research and evidence suggests that it is not the whole story.
- ***Sampling Methods***. Samples from whom data are sought should be chosen by one of several acceptable random sample selection techniques as this permits generalisation of results from the sample back to the population the sample represents. Choosing anyone available, often called an opportunity sample, means the results cannot be generalised back to any specific group. For example, an attitude survey on mask wearing conducted on a main street will simply pick up those who happen to be around and this of course depends on time of day and location, and results are likely to be significantly different from an opportunity sample of patrons at a night club, or fans at a football match.
- ***Reliable and valid measurements***. Reliable is really the same as replicable in that we need certainty that the measurement instrument usually, psychological surveys and questionnaires, measure consistently. Reliability can be defined as the relative absence of errors of measurement in a measuring instrument. Error and reliability are opposite sides of the same coin. The more error, the less stable, and less accurate is the data. Valid implies that the measuring instrument is measuring what it is supposed to measure, i.e. how accurately a thermometer measures temperature.

It is easy to confuse reliability with validity but understanding their distinction is important. Whilst reliability relates to the accuracy and stability of a measurement, validity relates to the appropriateness of the measure to assess what it purports to measure. A dodgy thermometer may be consistent ***in its inaccuracy*** say measuring 0.5 °C above the person's real temperature on every reading occasion; it is therefore reliable but it is not giving the valid temperature, i.e. it is consistently wrong (invalid) but consistent in its error (reliable).

- ***Correlation or association does not imply cause and effect.*** This is a simple and easy mistake to make when research findings suggest an association between two variables. Yes, in some cases, it does reflect a real cause and effect such as bodily temperature increase with viral infection. However since the correlation coefficient statistic which measures association is simply a mathematical calculation, it means any two measurable variables can be correlated together and produce a mathematical answer no matter how ridiculous the two variables are in terms of a possible relationship such as the monthly rainfall figures for a place correlated with the monthly average price of unleaded fuel.

Methodological Issues Concern

Currently, there are major concerns with existing scientific standards worldwide in most academic areas of investigation. For example, Dr. R. Horton, editor of the medical journal *The Lancet* in a damning assessment of research four years before the pandemic, wrote '*much of the scientific literature perhaps half may be simply untrue. Afflicted by ... flagrant conflict of interests together with obsession for pursuing fashionable trends of dubious importance, science has taken a turn towards darkness*' (*The Lancet*, April 2015). A study (Hunter 2017) in the UK (BBC News) suggested most sciences are facing a reproducibility crisis where more than two-thirds of researchers failed to reproduce another scientist's experiments. These issues are longstanding and have not been eradicated.

The past decade has been a turbulent one for social sciences particularly psychology. Researchers have come to realise that a lot of psychological research rests on rather shaky foundations. The amount of scientific misconduct that occurs in the field is hard to quantify, but one study found that between 0.6% and 2.3% of psychologists admit to falsifying data, and between 9.3% and 18.7% have witnessed another researcher doing so (Stricker & Günther, 2019). Additionally, just under 65% of retractions in the American Psychological Association (APA) Databases *database PsycInfo* were due to misconduct (APA Trends Report 01-01-2022). In another research area, Piller (2022) detailed in the journal Science concerns of possible Alzheimer's research fraud. A well-publicised Alzheimer's trial investigating the experimental drug *simufilam* was based on manipulated images published by scientists years earlier. Pillar reports that Professor Schrag investigated scores of images in scientific papers authored by the head researcher Dr. Sylvain and suggested significant image tampering had consistently occurred. Leading independent image analysts and internationally recognised Alzheimer's researchers have backed Schrag's claims (Piller, 2022). If this is common practice, then volunteer patients to drug trials, including the *simufilam* studies, may be facing unnecessary health risks associated with the experimental treatments, likely with no hope of clinical benefit.

A pivotal study from the Open Science Collaboration (8 August 2015), attempted to replicate the findings of 100 psychology studies published in three influential journals, finding a positive effect for just 36 of the 97 studies that had all originally found a positive outcome. Other replication attempts have cast doubt on well-known findings that appear in many introductory textbooks (BPS Psychologist Jan 2022 Enquiry into reproducible science). Even when reproducibility is demonstrated, results don't necessarily generalise beyond the narrow group from which they were derived, usually participants who are Western and Educated from Industrialised, Rich and Democratic countries (the WEIRD problem). Researchers are more aware than ever of these problems, developing large collaborations to study psychological phenomena with huge numbers of participants across multiple countries. Holmes et al. (2020) suggested the formation of multidisciplinary research teams and outlined priorities for mental health research during the pandemic. Included in these various recommendations, there was a call for work to be conducted at scale with multiple research groups and networks, warning against the waste of time energy and funding on '*the current uncoordinated approach with a plethora of underpowered studies and surveys*' (Holmes et al., 2020).

A systematic review (Jung et al., 2021) looked at the quality of all published research on Covid during 2020 compared to papers from before the pandemic began. When compared with non-Covid articles published in the same journal before the pandemic, Covid papers generally achieved lower quality scores. New studies attempting to understand the pandemic were being rushed out with major flaws; they may have a small number of participants and cannot be generalised across the world. Many were conducted in an artificial environment, usually online, as face to face is impossible under Covid restrictions and are usually of the survey format that may not tap into how people really think or behave in their daily life. As an example, the 'Fear of COVID-19 Scale' (Ahorsu et al., 2020) is a seven-item scale that has already been translated into many languages and asks questions like '*I cannot sleep because I am worried about getting coronavirus-19*'. The surface implication is that higher scores are bad. But detailed analysis suggests that people who scored higher on that item were more likely to practise positive public health behaviours like social distancing. Rather than measuring some pathological 'fear', the scale may actually be tapping into adaptive behaviour that predispose us respond positively to dangerous transmission situations, avoiding disastrous consequences of which we are now well aware.

Dr. Finkel, formerly Australia's Chief Scientist, lamented in the journal Nature 2019 that a significant number of research papers are of such low quality that they should never have made it through to publication. He added that we cannot know how many of the 1.6 million or so papers added every year to the Web of Science database are flawed, and that focus must transfer from quantity to quality to safeguard against shoddy work in research. Unfortunately, financial and career incentives keep researchers on a treadmill, churning out papers.

The incentive to publish and funding

The things that really trump quality for today's scientists are how much grant money they receive, the count of how many studies they publish (never mind the quality feel the width), or how much the topics and results touch emotional nerves in their appeal to the public interest, all of which explain the flood of papers on Covid impacts. Science has become less about quality research and objective findings and more about popularity. The challenge today is maintaining the funding. A vicious cycle commences. To receive grants and funding, scientists need to publish, but to publish work scientists need to have positive results. Scientists therefore choose 'safe' research that is easy to publish or may even publish selectively biased results to appeal to their sponsors, ignoring those which do not fit the agenda, or in several cases, offer faked results.

The major problems include:

(1) incentives to publish (such as promotion and more grant money) lead studies to be shoddily designed, e.g. in terms of sampling and reliable measurement instruments,
(2) replicating results are crucial but there is a lack of funding to do so and also tends to be avoided just in case replication cannot be shown, and it becomes embarrassing for career prospects,
(3) peer reviews are often performed by colleagues or like-minded researchers and therefore can be biased or flawed as mates support each other,
(4) getting access to scientific results is costly leading to cutting corners, e.g. obtaining randomised samples, using specialised equipment,
(5) scientific results are communicated in abstruse and technical ways which denies access to the general public who do not understand whether rigorous scientific methodology has been followed or whether the discussion and implications are valid.

Some issues with Survey Research

Survey research, often the main data source for Covid studies, also carries problems for every realm of scientific investigation. The problem is that the answers people give can be influenced in unintended ways by the wording of the items, the order of the items, the response options provided, the interpretation of the question by the responder and many other factors that can determine or manipulate the answer given. At best, these influences add noise to the data. At worst, they result in systematic biases and misleading results. Clarity of operational definitions is important in deciding what concept the survey is focussed on as respondents will have different attitudes and beliefs about the survey leading them to answer in terms of their personal interpretation.

Survey questions can be written in a way to obtain the answers the researcher would like (and perhaps the funders too). If the question is '*do you believe governments should impose mandated restrictions on the general public to manage infection rates*'? A sizeable majority of respondents will respond '*yes*' since it is obvious to most people that governments need to do this. But if the question is '*do you believe that the answer to controlling infection rates is a six month lockdown*'. Very few would say '*yes*'. Most people agree that action needs to be taken but would prefer other options in the mix too such as mandated vaccination and closed borders rather than one draconian policy. Responses to a single question survey like those thrown out in the mass media may indicate strong feelings about controlling the spread of the virus but be quite misleading about how it should be dealt with.

Mass media surveys are limited in validity and reliability as it is unknown who responded. (It is not unknown for a group of people to respond multiple times!!). The same survey in the Guardian and the Australian will also produce very different responses because their readers are different, and results are often reported in percentages. For any survey, who are the group forming the sample, how large is the sample, and how was the sample selected, are three vital questions to consider when evaluating the results. Who were they; university students, people stopped in a shopping mall, a chosen age group, political allegiance group, etc. The results of a sample can validly only be generalised back to the type of population that they were selected from, i.e. back to university students, those who voted for party X or those belonging to a particular age group. There are a number of valid random sampling methods that will ensure this is feasible but some studies do not apply such rigorous methods leaving biased sampling as a serious criticism. Remember too that people for a variety of reasons can lie deliberately on surveys, or can complete a questionnaire in a slap dash fashion, or really don't know enough about the content of the question to answer validly at all.

In any research, a large percentage from a small sample will be an even smaller number so look for sample size, often the table column labelled '*N*', as well as how the sample was constituted. Percentages should also be quoted so that 100 deaths from 10,000 vaccinated cases are recognised as a far better proportion (1 in 100 or 1%) than 50 deaths from 200 unvaccinated cases (25 in 100 or 25%). Otherwise, it looks as if the vaccinated have a higher mortality rate if only the number of death are recorded.

Savvy questionnaire survey writers can deliver the answers required by choosing the 'right' sample, formulating the question in a particular way and controlling the range of responses available. Therefore, more valid surveys offer some open-ended questions which require the responder to provide a personal response rather than tick fixed response questions where the fixed options are often only a dichotomy between yes and no. The message repeated here again is please conduct a detailed check of methodology, interpretation of results, etc., when reading research reports. A good reference book for those interested in the nitty gritty of survey research is Burns and Burns (2008, Chaps. 9 and 20). It appears that worldwide there is a problem with the quality of scientific research and the biased analyses of results to suit the author's predilections, and this also applies to the plethora of Covid research.

Dodgy Research and Bogus Science in the Covid Pandemic

Current covid research is not immune from these general research methodology problems that can infect most research areas. Several examples of Covid dodgy research are referred to below, viz: The vaccines are unsafe myth; the Ivermectin saga; and the hydroxychloroquine storey. Rigorous research and findings can only be assured by independent peer expert review and greater quality assurance, which will robustly examine all aspects of the research from initial design to final conclusions based on objective interpretation of statistical analyses all involving, where necessary, devil's advocate questioning, scepticism, dissent, access to original data and replication before publication are permitted. This is a very tall order, rarely invoked, and leads to the over-riding rule when reading research findings of '*caveat emptor*' or *buyer beware.*

Some Specific Inaccurate Promotion of Covid Scientific Research

Below are three of the more dodgy representations of science in the context of the Covid pandemic, which carry the tremendous potential to harm people and compromise public trust and public health initiatives.

1. *Vaccines are unsafe; the Wakefield Study*

History shows dodgy research can often fester in the public domain long after being shown false and can be held to blame for continually stoking anti-vaccination movements. They continue to be cited, republished and accepted as fact for decades after debunking. It took 12 years for an erroneous study falsely linking autism to the measles, mumps and rubella vaccines by disgraced scientist Andrew Wakefield to be formally retracted by The Lancet (Eggertson,

2010). His study of just 12 children had been rigged but the damage was done, contributing to vaccine hesitancy around the world leaving children and adults unprotected from serious diseases including Covid. The repercussions are still being felt today, with Dr. Wakefield still being hailed as a hero by Covid vaccine sceptics and considerable erosion of public trust in medical science along with concerns that repeated immunisation protocols may be excessive, redundant or pharmacological profit-making enterprises rather than valid preventive medicine.

2. *The hydroxychloroquine storey*

The hydroxychloroquine controversy stands as a good illustration of both the ways in which things can go wrong and the myriad harmful ramifications. In mid-March, 2020, French researchers published a preprint suggesting that hydroxychloroquine had potential therapeutic benefits in the treatment of Covid. The sample was small ($n = 80$), and almost immediately criticised as being too methodologically flawed to justify publication in a peer-reviewed journal. Indeed, a later academic review of the study suggested it was '*a non-informative manuscript with gross methodological shortcomings*' (Rosendaal, 2020). This study preprint escaped into the mass media and unfortunately was cited close to 2000 times despite the scientific concerns, giving hydroxychloroquine a great deal of disturbing attention and endorsements from prominent individuals including Elon Musk and Donald Trump! Internet searches spiked as a result of these endorsements as well as dangerous increases in off-label prescriptions by doctors.

More and more researchers around the world started investigating the drug, despite the fact that there was (and remains) little evidence to suggest any clinical utility (University of Oxford—News, 4 August 2020). Then, in mid-June 2020, a large study published in the influential *The Lancet* concluded that the drug had the potential to cause significant adverse events, which stopped clinical trials temporarily due to safety concerns (The Guardian, 4 June 2020). More evidence, including both observational and clinical trials of varying methodological strengths has been produced since concluding the drug is unlikely to be beneficial for Covid (Qaseem et al., 2020). Indeed, because of the lack of compelling evidence, and concerns about significant side effects, all key clinical trials have been abandoned, including those sponsored by the National Institutes of Health (Kiley, 2020) and the World Health Organization (WHO Newsroom, 4 July 2020).

3. *The Ivermectin storey*

Around the world, it was originally not opposition to vaccines but a lack of vaccines that led people to Ivermectin. The drug had early on in the pandemic been approved, recommended or prescribed for Covid in India, South Africa, and much of Latin America, as well as in Slovakia. In February 2021, Merck, one of the companies that makes the drug, said there was '*no scientific basis for a potential therapeutic effect against COVID-19*' Health authorities in the

US, UK and EU have found there is insufficient evidence for using the drug against Covid, and key studies that the drug's promoters rely on, contain serious errors. Health authorities in all nations have stopped recommending Ivermectin in treatment guidelines.

A BBC Reality Check investigation (6 Oct 2021) reveals that more than a third of 26 major trials using Ivermectin on Covid had serious errors or signs of potential fraud. None of the rest showed any convincing evidence of Ivermectin's effectiveness. The BBC investigation did not locate a single clinical trial claiming to show that Ivermectin prevented Covid deaths that did not contain '*either obvious signs of fabrication or errors so critical they invalidate the study*'. Out of a total of 26 studies examined, there was evidence in five that the data may have been faked containing virtually impossible numbers or rows of identical patients copied and pasted. In a further five, there were major red flags with numbers not adding up, percentages calculated incorrectly or local health bodies unaware the studies had even occurred.

On top of these flawed trials, there were 14 authors of studies who failed to send their raw data back. Independent scientists have flagged this as a possible indicator of fraud. The Therapeutic Goods Administration in Australia (14 Dec 2021) reported testing a number of imported Ivermectin products and finding a number of them are fake and have smaller doses of active ingredients in them than advertised and some in fact contaminated because of a lack of manufacturing and testing standards.

Calls over suspected Ivermectin poisonings in the US have increased a lot but from a very small base (435 to 1143 in 2021). Patients have had vomiting, diarrhoea, hallucinations, confusion, drowsiness and tremors. But indirect harm can come also from giving people a false sense of security, especially if they choose Ivermectin instead of seeking accepted hospital treatment for Covid, or preferably getting vaccinated in the first place. Some anti-vax media posts still rail about conspiracy theories of Ivermectin coverups, as well as pushing anti-vaccine sentiment or encouraging patients to leave hospital if they aren't getting the drug. These groups have co-ordinated harassment of doctors who fail to prescribe Ivermectin and abuse has been aimed at scientists (Volz, 2021).

There are, of course, other examples of both poor science and poor science communication in the context of Covid-related research. But the hydroxychloroquine controversy, which amplified due to celebrity endorsements of questionable preliminary research, caused numerous disadvantages for science including making it more difficult to recruit participants for well-designed clinical trials, spurring questionable public investment in further research, encouraging unnecessary and potentially harmful prescriptions (Ledford, 2020), and creating unjustified beliefs (e.g. 23% of Canadians, and 30% of Quebecers wrongly believed the drug was effective (Carleton University School of Journalism, 22 May 2020). All the hype and eventually withdrawn papers have increased conspiracy theories and likely decreased public trust of science. A belief in hydroxychloroquine endures for many, despite the load of unsupportive evidence. It is a belief that is part of the baggage of a particular ideological position. As explained in Chap. 4, once internalised a belief becomes a constituent and congruent part of a person's identity, very difficult to alter as the whole identity needs to restructure (Kaplan et al., 2016).

The Danger in Pressure to Undertake Research on an Immediate Problem

As the reality of the coronavirus pandemic set in during March 2020, social scientists and particularly psychologists from a wide range of specialist areas piled in with a plethora of research projects of varying qualities for a rapid attempt to understand how the crisis was affecting individuals, subgroups in society like health and education professionals, single persons, different cultural groups, etc., and even whole nations, covering topics from conspiracy theories to obedience, home working, unemployment, isolation and stress. The sheer speed at which research moved with preprints to swiftly and magically draw tenuous links between their work and Covid to surf the wave to swift publication and impact. Retraction Watch currently lists over 160 Covid papers that have since been withdrawn or retracted from journals mainly in the behavioural science field.

Wanting science to happen quickly during a pandemic is understandable. Covid scientific research is being both undertaken and disseminated at a furious pace. Since the start of 2020, tens of thousands of peer-reviewed academic articles and preprints on Covid issues entered the public domain. Submission rates to prestigious biomedical journals have increased substantially, with some journals receiving triple the usual number of submissions and overwhelming them that sometimes standards of review have dropped, with an astonishing increase in pace of acceptance of around 100 days prepandemic, to some publications progressing through peer review in apparently just one day!!. This has crippled the quality.

The Preprint

The preprint is just what it says where research papers are made public prior to the standard evaluation procedure, the peer review. But this can and has far too often resulted in dodgy research conclusions that can confuse public discourse (the hydroxychloroquine issue started with a preprint) as both news media and Internet media jump in with banner headlines on what they don't realise are results from methodologically unsound studies which seem to promise the earth in new vaccines or New Age medicine. In an effort to overcome delays imposed by peer review, masses of preprints were uploaded to the Internet. And while this increased speed and access to novel findings, it also resulted in unchecked studies being treated as though they were of similar quality to peer-reviewed articles and provide risky citations for scientists and media without realisation of the poor quality and methodological deficiencies raised above which could lead to unreliable results and misleading advice. Of course, methodological problems are not new. The pandemic comes at the end of a decade in which methodological crises in research have really been thrust under the spotlight. While it is inspiring to see the research community responding vigorously to the pandemic crisis, all this Covid research activity has created a churning sea of flotsam and jetsam, conflicting results and exaggerated headlines. This will lower the professional standing of researchers, of what science can offer, and may cause confusion, inappropriate expectations and treatments, and the erosion of public trust.

Fraser et al. (2020) revealed Covid preprints are accessed and distributed at least 15 times more than non-Covid preprints. Not all preprints are later deemed inadequate but many are more like fool's gold reflecting a false glow which dissolves into disaster failing to live up to initial expectations when subjected to the acid test of a sound peer review. So when finding a preprint that looks valuable from its title, search for some reviews of the paper before making any decision on its quality and usability. A recent systematic review on the quality of 66 prediction models for diagnosing Covid reported in 51 manuscripts, 45 of which were non-peer-reviewed preprints, found that the models identified were poorly reported and all had a high risk of bias, with likely overly optimistic performance (Palayew et al., 2020). Locher et al. (2021) warned that the speed of paper acceptance has led to dubious papers which may have been published simply because the authors were not independent from the journals in which they appeared, e.g. they may have already been reviewers for the journal or the editors were colleagues, etc. Locher et al. (op cit.) therefore considered this a new type of publishing entity, '*self-promotion journals*' which could be used to serve the assessment of academic productivity-based metrics, with consequent decisions about academic promotion, tenure and grant funding for those with more publications, a sort of old pals act. One of the fastest ways to create confusion and lose public trust is to publish and publicise weak, careless or worse, fraudulent research (Yarborough, 2014). Unfortunately, this may be happening too often in this era of panicky, pandemic publishing. The desire for quick results should not be allowed to erode scientific standards and give science a bad name when retracted.

Preprints numbers need to be radically reduced with journal editors taking more time, despite external pressures for speed, to ensure peer reviews are adequately undertaken to ensure that what is eventually published is sound, trust worthy and respectable. Those preprints that are offered to the public should emphasise the preliminary nature of the study and conclusions, and that no peer review has been conducted.

Scienceploitation

There must be a halt to tolerating and legitimising health pseudoscience, especially at universities and healthcare institutions. Bogus Covid therapies have infected respected health institutions in the West where, for example, the Cleveland Clinic in Ohio, offers *reiki*, a practice with no science basis to balance the "*vital life force energy that flows through all living things*" using your hands, but not touching the patient who has been told the technique could boost their immune systems and make them less susceptible to the virus. A similar situation occurs in the UK and Canada where, for example, some health providers in the United Kingdom promote homeopathy as a remedy for Covid. Other examples include a range of providers worldwide marketing procedures and products against Covid claiming that spinal adjustment, or intravenous vitamin therapy could fend it off; a total non-sense. Of course there is some evidence that placebo effects from alternative treatments can relieve distress, a common justification used for offering unproven alternative treatments. But it's ethically wrong to deceive people with pseudo magic and damaging for scientists to let such misinformation flourish uncontested.

Those pushing unproven ideas usually make it sound like the language of real science or '*scienceploitation*' to legitimise their products. Homeopathy and energy therapies, proponents argue depending on quantum physics; colonic hydrotherapy is justified using phrases borrowed from microbiome studies; the language of stem-cell research is used to promote a spray claiming to have immune-boosting anti-viral properties. Again none of this makes sense in scientific terms and clear explanations of why this hijacking is incorrect and scientifically dishonest must be strongly pursued by scientists and medical authorities with simple and shareable material in the mass media, stating convincingly that quantum physics doesn't explain homeopathy, and that energy therapies such as reiki nor colonic hydrotherapy will bolster your immune system against Covid. Neither will a supplement spray enhance the functioning of your stem cells. Therefore, science researchers should become active participants in the public fight against misinformation.

There Are Models and Models

While modelling is an important tool to help guide decision making, it cannot be the only tool as the estimates that emerge depend on what variables are believed relevant and the weighting of those variables, and these two issues are subjective. The original apocalyptic modelling projections caused governments worldwide to engage in herd behaviour and lockdown their countries. As islands, this was an easy action for New Zealand and Australia to set up their fortress positions.

Australia has a world class Covid response and this has meant that the estimated numbers modelled previously, particularly early in the pandemic, have not been realised. Early modelling in 2020 at the start of the outbreak suggested that there would be 35,000 ICU beds required within 17 weeks of an uncontrolled outbreak. The modelling predictions were quite wrong in suggesting predictions of tens of thousands of deaths by Xmas 2020 and 600 deaths per day in Melbourne at the peak of the epidemic. In reality, only 909 people died Australia wide in the first year of the pandemic amid 28,000 infection cases. Covid modelling has been inaccurate in Australia, and Australia has consistently defied the predictions. The real figures were far lower than the estimates (news.com.au 10 Sept 2020).

18 months later, modelling, both in Australia and internationally, presented a range of potential scenarios for the developing Omicron variant. As Australia opened up for Xmas 2021, the modelling prediction offered was an astounding 200,000 cases a day based on the following erroneous assumptions that the Omicron variant was as powerful as Delta, a highly limited booster programme, no change to baseline public health measures, an absence of hospital surge capacity and an absence of spontaneous behaviour change in the face of rising case numbers. The Australian Chief Medical Officer described the prediction as most unlikely, as none of the five assumptions above represented the likely state of events, let alone all of them together, therefore presenting a false and highly misleading scenario. The modelling from Warwick University of death in the in the UK in winter 2021/22 contributed negatively to scaring the British general public who did not understand the limitations of the process, and eventually decreasing the level of trust in statistical science when it did not come to pass. It showed average deaths for mid-January 2022 of around 12,500 with maximum range to 20,000 when actual deaths were only around 2500! The London School of Hygiene and Tropical Medicine model for beds occupied winter 2021/22 due to Omicron was also way out with a modelled maximum of 120,000 for mid-January 2022 but the actual turned out to be 18,000 (UK Spectator Newspaper, 16 June 2022).

These are examples that illustrate the divergence of modelling from what actually happened but had formed part of the evidence the UK government used in contemplating what greater or lesser restriction were needed. If these projections had been acted on great harms would have been loaded onto the UK population quite unnecessarily, augmenting existing economic and social damage. Another current situation in Queensland winter 2022 where Omicron variants are running wild impacting large swathes of the population had the Health minister admitting that the modelling done for this particular outbreak was totally incorrect and authorities didn't know where it was all heading!!! Apparently, some of the values or weightings of many variables included in the modelling for the third wave were based on assumptions that were unreliable. (Similar problems arose with some climate modelling on which the UN's IPCC based their predictions of how high temperatures would rise.)

Trust in Scientific Research

The theme of this chapter has been the need to safeguard the integrity of scientific research and evidence which will support maintaining public trust in science and scientific institutions, particularly critical during a pandemic. In France, it was found that regions with high trust decreased their public movements and mingling related to non-necessary activities significantly more than low-trust regions in the early part of the pandemic. (Bargain & Aminjonov, 2020). A similar finding emerged in Australia that demonstrated a relationship between increasing trust levels in government and health authorities with greater adoption of physical distancing and hygiene-related behaviours (Seale et al., 2020). Conversely, distrust of science was strongly correlated with a failure to adopt preventative strategies, like physical distancing, and, not paying attention to public health experts' advice on Covid in a US study (Barry et al., 2020). Behind myths and conspiracy theories, a lack of trust in relevant institutions has also been found (Pickles et al., 2021).

Given the daily diet of medical advice and information on media, the public are not shielded from noting the messy process of building scientific understanding and the obvious later retractions, and the disagreements that appear to deny scientific consensus. This inevitably evokes questions concerning what faith can we place in scientific evidence, especially as the pandemic remorselessly extends its tentacles morphing public concern and fear into frustration and anger as Lwin et al.,(2020) found early in the pandemic. A London School of Economics report (Aksoy et al., 2020) suggested that the Covid crisis "*will reduce confidence in individual scientists, worsen perceptions of their honesty and weaken the belief that their activities benefit the public*" particularly amongst those who have little or no scientific education or understand how scientific knowledge advances. Matthew (2020) found a 10% drop in trust in science, driven mostly by frustration surrounding the two polarising topics: the hydroxychloroquine debacle and policy reversals surrounding the use of masks in France. This provides a fertile seeding ground for anti-vaccine and Freedom 'ralliers' rhetoric. There are also concerns in many countries that scientific research into vaccines is driven more by politics and '*big pharma profits*' than science, with this contention supported by 78% of Americans (Silverman, 2020).

Another way trust is lost in what public health and government officials inform and demand is that without too much experience based on emerging science during a rapidly spreading pandemic, decisions often need to be made quickly using a less than ideal body of evidence. This then leads to frequent revising a position as new evidence and (or) social conditions change but this should not be viewed as a failure of the system. Public health officials must provide strong and unequivocal messaging to modify behaviour as much and as quickly as possible, but it is important to be explicit about the need for future modifications as there is some evidence that being transparent about uncertainties can actually heighten credibility (Drage O'Reilly, 2020). Never forget that scientific research is an iterative and, in general, a slow process.

The developing lack of trust in some science research is unfortunately being paralleled by a developing lack of trust in reputable research publishers too. The leading science journal *Nature Human Behaviour* has recently changed its editorial purpose and becomes politicised where editorial decisions over-ride truth with imposed fictions of ideologies, suppressing any scientific research the editor deems to have the potential to harm the public. This is a very vague criterion but exhibits far reaching disturbing editorial censorship revealing how far science has become weaponised in attempts to shut down debate and argument which does not meet with approval by certain groups. Climate science has already experienced this approach, and it is a dangerous move to invoke such publishing restrictions.

References

Ahorsu, D. K., Lin, C. Y., Imani, V., Saffari, M., et al. (2022). The fear of COVID-19 scale: development and initial validation. *International Journal of Mental Health and Addiction, 20*(3), 1537–1545. https://doi.org/10.1007/s11469-020-00270-8

Aksoy, C., Eichengreen, B., & Saka, O. (2020). Revenge of the experts: will COVID-19 renew or diminish public trust in science? Working Paper No. 243. *European Bank for Reconstruction and Development* [online]: Available from www.ebrd.com/publications/working-papers/revenge-of-the-experts

American Psychological Association Databases. Regularly updated. Online at https://www.apa.org › pubs › database.

American Psychological Association. (2022). Open science is surging. *Trends Report (Helen Santoro), 53*(1). Retrieved 3 March 2022 from https://www.apa.org/monitor/2022/01/special-open-science

Bargain, O., & Aminjonov, U. (2020). Trust and compliance to public health policies in time of COVID-19. *Bordeaux Economics Working Papers* [online]: Available from gretha.u-bordeaux.fr/LAREFI. http://larefi.u-bordeaux.fr/

Barry, C., Han, H., & McGinty, B. (2020). *Trust in science and COVID-19*. Johns Hopkins Bloomberg School of Public Health Expert Insights. Available from www.jhsph.edu/covid-19/articles/trust-in-science-and-covid-19.html

BBC News. Fielden, T. (2017, February 22). *Most scientists 'can't replicate studies by their peers'*. Retrieved 14 May 2021 from https://www.bbc.com › science-environment-39054778

BBC Reality Check. (2021, October 5). Schraer, R., & Goodman, J. *A third of 26 major trials of Ivermectin for use on Covid have serious errors or signs of potential fraud*. Retrieved 6 October 2021 from www.bbc.com/news/health-58170809

British Psychological Society. (2020, July 7). The psychologist. Retrieved 8 August 2020 from tinyurl.com/10replicate

British Psychological Society, Psychologist Jan 2022. Enquiry into reproducible science.

Burns, R. B., & Burns, R. A. (2008). *Business research methods and statistics using SPSS*. Sage.

Carleton University School of Journalism. (2020, May 22). *SJC COVID-19 research series, part 1: conspiracies and misinformation spreading online.* Retrieved 18 September 2020 from https://carleton.ca/sjc/2020/sjc-covid-19-research-series-part-1-conspiracies-and-misinformation-spreading-online/

Davey, M. (2021, December 22) Leaked Doherty COVID modelling shows just the most worrying scenario—not the most likely. *The Guardian.* Retrieved 22 December 2021 from https://www.theguardian.com/world/2021/dec/22/leaked-covid-modelling-shows-just-the-most-worrying-scenario-not-the-most-likely

Drage O'Reilly, E. (2020, June). Retracted coronavirus studies are threatening trust in scientific data. *Axios.* Available from https:\\www.axios.com/coronavirus-scientific-studies-trust-757f38eb-f2dd-40ab-8828-3b8fe43b5044.html

Eggertson, L. (2010). Lancet retracts 12-year-old article linking autism to MMR vaccines. *CMAJ, 182*(4), E199-200. https://doi.org/10.1503/cmaj.109-3179

Finkel, A. (2019, September 19). There is a problem. *Nature Index.* Retrieved 20 February 2020 from https://www.nature.com/nature-index/news-blog/australias-top-scientist-alan-finkel-pushes-to-eradicate-bad-science

Foster, A. (2020, September 10). *Coronavirus Australia: mistake in COVID modelling that informed lockdown.* Retrieved 10 September 2020 from https://www.news.com.au › world › australia › news-story

Fraser, N., et al. (2020). The evolving role of preprints in the dissemination of COVID-19 research and their impact on the science communication landscape. *PLOS Biology.* https://doi.org/10.1371/journal.pbio.3000959

Holmes, E. A., O'Connor, R., & Perry, V. H. (2020). Multidisciplinary research priorities for the COVID-19 pandemic: A call for action for mental health science. *Lancet Psychiatry, 7*(6), 547–560. https://doi.org/10.1016/S2215-0366(20)30168-1

Horton, R. (2015). Offline: What is medicine's 5 sigma? *The Lancet, 385*(9976), 1380. https://doi.org/10.1016/S0140-6736(15)60696-1

Horton, R. (2020, September 26). COVID-19 is not a pandemic. *Lancet, 396*(10255), 874. https://doi.org/10.1016/S0140-6736(20)32000-6

Hunter, P. (2017). The reproducibility 'crisis'. *EMBO Reports. 18*, 1493–1496. https://doi.org/10.15252/embr.201744876

Jung, R. G., Di Santo, P., Clifford, C., et al. (2021). Methodological quality of COVID-19 clinical research. *Nature Communications, 12*(1), 943. https://doi.org/10.1038/s41467-021-21220-5

Kaplan, J., Gimbel, S. I., & Harris, S. (2016). Neural correlates of maintaining one's political beliefs in the face of counterevidence. *Scientific Reports, 6*, 39589. https://doi.org/10.1038/srep3958

Kiley, J. (2020). Effect of hydroxychloroquine on clinical status at 14 days in hospitalized patients with COVID-19. *JAMA, 324*(21), 2165–2176. https://doi.org/10.1001/jama.2020.22240

Ledford, H. (2020). Chloroquine hype is derailing the search for coronavirus treatments. *Nature, 580*(7805), 573. https://doi.org/10.1038/d41586-020-01165-3

Locher, C., Moher, D., Cristea, J., et al. (2021). Publication by association: How the COVID-19 pandemic has shown relationships between authors and editorial board members in the field of infectious diseases. *BMJ Evidence Based Medicine, 27*(3), 133–136. https://doi.org/10.1136/bmjebm-2021-111670

Lwin, M. O., Lu, J., Sheldenkar, A., et al. (2020). Global sentiments surrounding the COVID-19 pandemic on twitter: Analysis of twitter trends. *JMIR Public Health Surveillance, 6*(2), e19447. https://doi.org/10.2196/19447

Mathew, R. (2020). We must not be guided by bad science on covid-19. *British Medical Journal, 369*. https://doi.org/10.1136/bmj.m2241

Merck. (2021, February 4). Retrieved 15 April 2021 from https://www.merck.com/news/merck-statement-on-ivermectin-use-during-the-covid-19-pandemic/

Open Science Collaboration Study. (2015). Estimating the reproducibility of psychological science. *Science, 349*, 6251. https://doi.org/10.1126/science.aac4716

Palayew, A., Norgaard, O., Safreed-Harmon, K., et al. (2020). Pandemic publishing poses a new COVID-19 challenge. *Nature Human Behaviour, 4*, 666–669. https://doi.org/10.1038/s41562-020-0911-0

Pickles, K., Cvejic, E., Nickel, B., et al. (2021). COVID-19 misinformation trends in Australia: Prospective longitudinal national survey. *Journal of Medical Internet Research, 23*. https://doi.org/10.2196/23805

Piller, C. (2022). Research backing experimental Alzheimer's drug was first target of suspicion. *Science, 377*(6604), 363. https://doi.org/10.1126/science.ade0350

Qaseem, A., et al. (2020). Letter update alert 2: Should clinicians use chloroquine or hydroxychloroquine alone or in combination with azithromycin for the prophylaxis or treatment of COVID-19? *Annals of Internal Medicine*. https://doi.org/10.7326/L20-1007

Retractionwatch. Updated regularly. https://retractionwatch.com/the-retraction-watch-leaderboard/

Rosendaal, F. R. (2020). Review of: Hydroxychloroquine and azithromycin as a treatment of COVID-19: Results of an open-label non-randomized clinical trial. *International Journal of Antimicrobial Agents, 56*(1), 106063. https://doi.org/10.1016/j.ijantimicag.2020.106063

Seale, H., Heywood, A. E., Leask, J., et al. (2020). COVID-19 is rapidly changing: examining public perceptions and behaviors in response to this evolving pandemic. *PLoS One, 15*(6). https://doi.org/10.1371/journal.pone.0235112

Silverman, E. (2020, August 31). Most Americans see politics driving Covid-19 vaccine approval process. *STAT*. [online]: Retrieved 24 November 2021 from http://statnews.com/pharmalot/2020/08/31/most-americans-believe-the-covid-19-vaccine-approval-process-is-driven-by-politics-not-science/?utm_source=STAT+Newsletters&utm_campaign

Stricker, J., & Günther, A. (2019). Scientific misconduct in psychology: a systematic review of prevalence estimates and new empirical data. *Zeitschrift für Psychologie , 227*, 53–63. https://doi.org/10.1027/2151-2604/a000356

The Guardian. (2020, June 4). *Unreliable data: How doubt snowballed over Covid-19 drug*. Retrieved 4 June 2020 from https://www.theguardian.com › world › 2020 › jun ›

The Spectator UK. Simmons, M. (2022, January 16). *Sage scenarios versus actual: An update*. Retrieved 20 February 2022 from https://www.google.com.au/search?q=Spectator+newspaper+16.01.22.+UK+covid+modelling

Therapeutic Goods Administration (TGA). Australian Government. (2021, December 14). *Media release. TGA warns about imports of ivermectin*. Retrieved 23 February 2022 from https://www.tga.gov.au/news/media-releases/tga-warns-about-imports-ivermectin

University of Oxford News. (2020, August 24). Retrieved 25 February 2021 from https://www.ox.ac.uk/news/2020-08-24-largest-global-study-hydroxychloroquine-safety-finds-increased-cardiovascular-risk
Volz, M. (2021, December 7). Hospitals refused to give patients Ivermectin. Lockdowns and political pressure followed. *Health.* Retrieved 9 April 2021 from https://www.pbs.org/newshour/health/hospitals-refused-to-give-patients-ivermectin-lockdowns-and-political-pressure-followed
WHO Newsroom News release. (2020, July 4). Retrieved 10 August 2021 from https://www.who.int/news/item/04-07-2020-who-discontinues-hydroxychloroquine-and-lopinavir-ritonavir-treatment-arms-for-covid-19
Yarborough, M. (2014). Openness in science is key to keeping public trust. *Nature, 515*(7527), 313. https://doi.org/10.1038/515313a

Epilogue: The Future

'the pandemic will not be over anywhere until it's over everywhere'.
WHO Director Tedros Gebreyesus.

Facing the 'New Normal'?

The previous chapters have gushed a flood of human distress and despair derived from the effects of the Covid virus augmented by many existing ethical, economic and societal imbalances. It all seems like a dress rehearsal for a tumultuous ride through the twenty-first century for many people and injected a seismic jolt to the presumption of continuing normality for most communities within societies and nations. Human behaviour caused this global pandemic to start and spread. How it ends will depend on current and near future behaviour to determine. Safeguarding human future is the defining challenge of our time as we enter crucial moments in our species history. Technological progress has fuelled our power so considerably that for the first time in human history, we have the capacity to destroy ourselves. Immense success as a species has evolved us into our own worst enemy. The knowledge that behavioural scientists now possess about controlling society is a current temptation to be applied in ways most of us in democracies would baulk at.

The scope and scale of the coronavirus has brought the world to a stuttering and repeated circle of stop and go. Our brains are a whirl of past, present and future scenarios as we long for a return to 'normality', trying to massage future to past and past to future. The rupture is unavoidable and in our distress, provides a chance to rethink how we can live in the future. For many a return to normality would be an unwanted disaster.. With recovery plans uncertain, some governments and organisations are using the crisis to seek out competitive advantage, while others find it immensely challenging to seek any way forward. It is a volatile, uncertain, complex and ambiguous world which will

© The Editor(s) (if applicable) and The Author(s), under exclusive license to Springer Nature Singapore Pte Ltd. 2023

R. B. Burns, *The Human Impact of the COVID-19 Pandemic*,
https://doi.org/10.1007/978-981-99-1710-5

accelerate changes that are already underway in society, community, education, workforce and economics, providing new and innovative ways of living.

Elements in most governments appear to think problems can be solved by modelling equations. But people are not based on some complex underlying equation that, if we can only find it, holds the solution to all our problems. We must acknowledge that the real world is messy, full of uncertainty and impossible to predict, requiring people who understand human society, culture and community, to a greater extent than politicians.

Covid has created not simply a medical and political storm but also a moral one that will rely on community ethos to advance society. We now need an enlightenment that includes moral/ethical purpose as well as an intellectual one creating a less divided and more equitable world. Such an approach must start from the premise that there is no hierarchy of race or culture, only people like ourselves in every nation, who struggle to satisfy their needs and the needs of those they care about in what is becoming an overcrowded, stressed planet. Crisis may facilitate sensible and ethical decisions as seemingly formerly unacceptable ideas suddenly become acceptable that will permit as many people as possible across the world safe, secure and healthy futures.

The steps taken to halt the spread of Covid internationally have exacted a heavy toll on our lives. We now have an option for a new beginning, to the creation of a reconfigured future of a more humane and community focussed on **'we'** rather than **'I'**. We can better evaluate what really matters particularly in where and how work is conducted. With more pathways open to success, living and working in a rural town, starting a business sharing household income and duties, seeking volunteering opportunities become possibilities.

Not only has the pandemic exposed how reliant we all are on each other, but also how events in one nation ripples onto the lives in other nations, how the health of the disadvantaged impacts on the advantaged, how economies are impacted by the health of the people whose work they rely on and how we can only fight some battles united. In taking a lead on this need for cooperation and unity, WHO's new international treaty on pandemic prevention and preparedness is progressing with anticipated delivery of a progress report to the 76th World Health Assembly in 2023, with the aim of ultimate adoption by 2024. The universality of such a document appears necessary because the Covid pandemic has been shown to be a global challenge with single governments or institutions unable to address the threat of future pandemics alone. This international instrument will be legally binding under international law. A sanitised view of such an agreement on pandemic prevention, preparedness and response adopted under the World Health Organization (WHO) mandate would enable countries around the globe to strengthen national, regional and global capacities and resilience to future pandemics appears superficially eminently sensible. But the downside for many countries is that China has a major influence on WHO and it is feared that extreme brutal lockdown response measures like those China has imposed could be included. As a legally binding document such impositions attempted in the next pandemic would evoke serious unrest in democratic countries. The language used is worrying as the proposal for the international instrument on pandemic prevention, preparedness and response is to be guided by '*a spirit of collective solidarity*' perhaps more a Sino than a Western phrase! To be locked down by your own bureaucrats was bad enough for most.